Comprehensive Virology 16

Comprehensive Virology

Edited by Heinz Fraenkel-Conrat
University of California at Berkeley

and Robert R. Wagner
University of Virginia

Volume 1: *Descriptive Catalogue of Viruses* — by Heinz Fraenkel-Conrat

Reproduction

Volume 2: *Small and Intermediate RNA Viruses* — Contributors: J.T. August, L. Eoyang, A. Siegel, V. Hariharasubramanian, L. Levintow, E. R. Pfefferkorn, D. Shapiro, and W. K. Joklik

Volume 3: *DNA Animal Viruses* — Contributors: L. Philipson, U. Lindberg, J.A. Rose, N.P. Salzman, G. Khoury, B. Moss, B. Roizman, and D. Furlong

Volume 4: *Large RNA Viruses* — Contributors: P.W. Choppin, R.W. Compans, R.R. Wagner, and J.P. Bader

Volume 7: *Bacterial DNA Viruses* — Contributors: D.T. Denhardt, D.S. Ray, and C.K. Mathews

Structure and Assembly

Regulation and Genetics

Additional Topics

Virus-Host Interactions

Comprehensive

Edited by
Heinz Fraenkel-Conrat
Department of Molecular Biology and Virus Laboratory
University of California, Berkeley, California

and
Robert R. Wagner
Department of Microbiology
University of Virginia, Charlottesville, Virginia

Virology

16

Virus-Host Interactions
Viral Invasion, Persistence, and Disease

PLENUM PRESS • NEW YORK AND LONDON

Library of Congress Cataloging in Publication Data

Fraenkel-Conrat, Heinz, 1910-
  Virus-host interactions.

  (*Their* Comprehensive virology; 16)
  Includes bibliographical references and index.
    1. Host-virus relationships. I. Wagner, Robert R., 1923-   joint author.
  II. Title. III. Series. [DNLM: 1. Virus diseases. 2. Virus diseases—Immunology.
  3. Viruses—Metabolism.
  QW160 C737 v. 16]
  QR357.F72 vol. 16   [QR482] 576'.64s [576'.64]   80-20780
  ISBN 0-306-40488-5

© 1980 Plenum Press, New York
A Division of Plenum Publishing Corporation
227 West 17th Street, New York, N.Y. 10011

Printed in the United States of America

Foreword

The time seems ripe for a critical compendium of that segment of the biological universe we call viruses. Virology, as a science, having passed only recently through its descriptive phase of naming and numbering, has probably reached that stage at which relatively few new—truly new—viruses will be discovered. Triggered by the intellectual probes and techniques of molecular biology, genetics, biochemical cytology, and high resolution microscopy and spectroscopy, the field has experienced a genuine information explosion.

Few serious attempts have been made to chronicle these events. This comprehensive series, which will comprise some 6000 pages in a total of about 18 volumes, represents a commitment by a large group of active investigators to analyze, digest, and expostulate on the great mass of data relating to viruses, much of which is now amorphous and disjointed, and scattered throughout a wide literature. In this way, we hope to place the entire field in perspective, and to develop an invaluable reference and sourcebook for researchers and students at all levels.

This series is designed as a continuum that can be entered anywhere, but which also provides a logical progression of developing facts and integrated concepts.

Volume 1 contains an alphabetical catalogue of almost all viruses of vertebrates, insects, plants, and protists, describing them in general terms. Volumes 2–4 deal primarily, but not exclusively, with the processes of infection and reproduction of the major groups of viruses in their hosts. Volume 2 deals with the simple RNA viruses of bacteria, plants, and animals; the togaviruses (formerly called arboviruses), which share with these only the feature that the virion's RNA is able to act as messenger RNA in the host cell; and the reoviruses of animals and plants, which all share several structurally singular features, the most important being the double-strandedness of their multiple RNA molecules.

Volume 3 addresses itself to the reproduction of all DNA-containing viruses of vertebrates, encompassing the smallest and the largest viruses known. The reproduction of the larger and more complex RNA viruses is the subject matter of Volume 4. These viruses share the property of being enclosed in lipoprotein membranes, as do the togaviruses included in Volume 2. They share as a group, along with the reoviruses, the presence of polymerase enzymes in their virions to satisfy the need for their RNA to become transcribed before it can serve messenger functions.

Volumes 5 and 6 represent the first in a series that focuses primarily on the structure and assembly of virus particles. Volume 5 is devoted to general structural principles involving the relationship and specificity of interaction of viral capsid proteins and their nucleic acids, or host nucleic acids. It deals primarily with helical and the simpler isometric viruses, as well as with the relationship of nucleic acid to protein shell in the T-even phages. Volume 6 is concerned with the structure of the picornaviruses, and with the reconstitution of plant and bacterial RNA viruses.

Volumes 7 and 8 deal with the DNA bacteriophages. Volume 7 concludes the series of volumes on the reproduction of viruses (Volumes 2–4 and Volume 7) and deals particularly with the single- and double-stranded virulent bacteriophages.

Volume 8, the first of the series on regulation and gentics of viruses, covers the biological properties of the lysogenic and defective phages, the phage-satellite system P 2–P 4, and in-depth discussion of the regulatory principles governing the development of selected lytic phages.

Volume 9 provides a truly comprehensive analysis of the genetics of all animal viruses that have been studied to date. These chapters cover the principles and methodology of mutant selection, complementation analysis, gene mapping with restriction endonucleases, etc. Volume 10 also deals with animal cells, covering transcriptional and translational regulation of viral gene expression, defective virions, and integration of tumor virus genomes into host chromosomes.

Volume 11 covers the considerable advances in the molecular understanding of new aspects of virology which have been revealed in recent years through the study of plant viruses. It covers particularly the mode of replication and translation of the multicomponent viruses and others that carry or utilize subdivided genomes; the use of protoplasts in such studies is authoritatively reviewed, as well as the nature of viroids, the smallest replicatable pathogens. Volume 12 deals with special groups of viruses of protists and invertebrates which show properties that set them apart from the main virus families. These are the lipid-containing phages and the viruses of algae, fungi, and invertebrates.

Volume 13 contains chapters on various topics related to the structure and assembly of viruses, dealing in detail with nucleotide and amino acid sequences, as well as with particle morphology and assembly, and the structure of virus membranes and hybrid viruses. The first complete sequence of a viral RNA is represented as a multicolored foldout.

Volume 14 contains chapters on special and/or newly characterized vertebrate virus groups: bunya-, arena-, corona-, calici-, and orbiviruses, icosahedral cytoplasmic deoxyriboviruses, fish viruses, and hepatitis viruses.

Subsequent volumes deal primarily with virus–host interactions and one (Volume 17) with biophysical, biochemical, and serological methods used in virus research. Volume 15 is concerned with immunological reactions to viruses and to virus-infected cells.

The current volume is concerned with viral invasion of cells, factors controlling persistence of viruses in cell cultures and animals, and responses to viral infection of animal and plant cells, as well as certain diseases caused by viruses. At least one additional volume will be devoted to other aspects of cell responses to viral infection, including cell death.

Contents

Chapter 4

Persistence and Transmission of Cytomegalovirus

Fred Rapp

Chapter 7

Host Plant Responses to Virus Infection

R. E. F. Matthews

Viral Invasion: Morphological, Biochemical, and Biophysical Aspects

C. Howe, J. E. Coward, and T. W. Fenger

Department of Microbiology and Immunology
Louisiana State University Medical Center
New Orleans, Louisiana 70112

1. INTRODUCTION

The first encounter of an infectious viral particle with the surface of a susceptible cell initiates a complex series of events, the outcome of which determines whether or not penetration and subsequent takeover of cellular machinery for viral replication ensue. Recognition of factors which govern these interactions derives from knowledge of the molecular structure of virus and target cell, as well as from the effects of the environment in which the interactions occur. This chapter will deal with animal viruses and will be limited to a consideration of the interactions at the cellular membrane which in sequence govern attachment and penetration of the virion up to the point at which the viral genome is uncoated. Early events in the viral replicative cycle have been the subject of several excellent reviews (Dales, 1973; Lonberg-Holm and Philipson, 1974, 1978).

With few exceptions, the most sensitive criterion of "intactness" of a viral particle is its infectivity, or its capacity to initiate self-replication in a susceptible cell. In order to be infectious, the viral nucleic acid must be associated with the requisite capsid proteins, enzymes, and, in

TABLE 1

Summary[a]

Naked viruses	Viral component(s)	Cell receptor	Viral attachment/ penetration	Associated changes
Adenovirus	Penton fiber (Arg)	3 proteins (KB cells) ?lp; receptor "families"	VP Direct entry	Partial loss of penton fiber; uncoating at NP
Papovavirus (SV40, polyoma)		Ec lp (SV40) Ec gp (polyoma)	VP: Monopino- cytotic envelop- ment, Nu inter- membrane fusion (SV40, polyoma)	Increased mem- brane fluidity (polyoma)
Parvovirus MVM	"Light" particles activated by cell factor(s)		VP (Pinocytosis)	
Reovirus	Nonglycosylated capsid protein = HA (σ^1) (RE03)	?gp	VP	
Picornavirus (enterovirus rhinovirus)	Four capsid proteins	Receptor families ?glp Under genetic con- trol; correlated with suscepti- bility; N-ase insensitive	VP Direct entry	D → A particles Receptor- mediated uncoating; early loss of Vp4; increased membrane fluidity

Abbreviations: Ag, antigen; Arg, arginine; ASA, attachment site activity; ASLV, avian sarcoma leukemia viruses; CEF, chick embryo fibroblasts; Cv, C virus; Ec, erythrocyte; F_0,F_1,F_2, fusion protein complex; Fu, fusion; gl, glycolipids; glp, glycolipoprotein; gp, glycoprotein; HA, H, hemagglutinin; Hc, histocompatibility; HL, hemolysis; HSV-1, Herpes simplex virus type 1; k, kilodalton; lc, lymphocyte; LIS, lithium diiodosalicylate; MLV, murine leukemia virus; MMTV,

Enveloped viruses	Viral envelope component(s)	Cell receptor	Viral		Associated changes
			Attachment	Penetration	
Orthomyxovirus (Influenza A)	HA, (gp) → HA₂ (N)	Essential NANA Ec glycophorin cilia	HA	VP (HA cleavage)	Increased membrane fluidity; ?lipid exchange
Paramyxovirus (NDV, Sendai)	HN gp F₀ → F₁, F₂ (?phosphatase tase) (?host agent)	2 → 3 NANA Ec glycophorin	HN Surface ion rearrangement	Fu, VP (Ec: Fu/HL)	?Membrane dephosphorylation (?Ec band 3); lipid exchange; Ag dispersal
Morbillivirus (measles)	H gp F → F₁, F₂ No N	No NANA required; Rh monkey Ec PAS-2, 4 T lc	H	Fu (Ec: Fu/HL)	Ag dispersal
Pneumovirus (RS)	Spikes No HA, N (1 glycosylated protein)	?		Fu	Ag dispersal
Rhabdovirus (VSV)	G protein Component II (spikes)	?Protein No NANA; ?lipid		VP (Fu)	Viral lipid depletion
Togavirus (Sindbis, SFV)	1 gp, 50 k spikes "Loose" vs. "tight" particles	pl, (gl) CEF:ASA HC ag	Envel. essential	VP pH, ionic strength dependent	Increased membrane fluidity
RNA TV (MLV, MSV, avian TV, MMTV)	Spikes gp71 (MLV)	Transforming strain-specific ASA, LIS-soluble; Cv budding sites; β2-microglobulin	ASLV:CEF gap junctions	VP Direct (? Fu)	
Poxvirus	Vaccinia, lipoprotein envelope DNV (Amsacta)	Relatively unspecific	Electrostatic, relatively unspecific	VP, Fu Fu, VP	Ag dispersal
Herpesvirus	HSV-1 Envelope gp (B2, C2) EBV	? EBV:C3, Fc	?Envelope glycoprotein(s); under genetic control	VP, Fu	Regulatory balance (gpB2, C2)

mouse mammary tumor virus; MSV, murine sarcoma virus; MVM, minute virus of mice; N or N-ase, neuraminidase; NANA, N-acetylneuraminic acid; NDV, Newcastle disease virus; NP, nuclear pore(s); Nu, nuclear; PAS, periodic acid Schiff; pl, phospholipid(s); Rh, rhesus; RS, respiratory syncytial; SFV, Semliki Forest virus; SV40, simian virus 40; TV, tumor virus(es); VP, viropexis; Vp, viral protein; VSV, vesicular stomatitis virus.

the case of enveloped viruses, lipids, to ensure relatively efficient transport of the viral genome across the host cell membrane. The viral subunits involved in these infectious processes are now quite clearly recognized in a number of major taxonomic groups. The naked nucleic acid of certain positive-stranded RNA viruses (e.g., poliovirus, encephalomyocarditis virus) and a few DNA viruses (e.g., herpesviruses, SV40) can transfect cells not normally susceptible to the corresponding whole virus. Infection initiated in this manner bypasses the receptor components of the cell membrane with which virions must interact in order to penetrate into the cytoplasm. While readily demonstrable experimentally, this mode of genomic entry is not known to have a role in naturally occurring infection and so will not be discussed in detail.

The term "viropexis" was coined to describe the penetration of intact viral particles through the cell membrane by energy-dependent processes assumed to be equivalent to normal phagocytosis (Fazekas de St. Groth, 1948). In the light of accumulated knowledge of endocytotic mechanisms, the present concept of viropexis may now be broadened to include mechanisms of entry by viruses into cells not normally phagocytic. In these instances specialized phagocytic reactions are triggered by the irreversible attachment of viral particles and the "recruiting" of receptor molecules to the attachment site. These specialized processes include receptor-mediated alteration of virions, as with adenoviruses and picornaviruses, or the envelopment of virions by plasma membrane prior to transcytoplasmic migration, as with papovaviruses. Intramembranal events, even though still incompletely understood, are as important as the specificity of surface receptors in governing viropexis and the outcome of initial viral contact. In addition it is apparent that, while most if not all viruses can penetrate by some form of viropexis, only those possessing a lipid-containing envelope can enter the cell by fusion with the plasma membrane.

In considering the susceptible cell, particular attention has been focused on the concept of viral "receptors." This term denotes chemical groupings on the cellular surface, the presence of which determines to a large extent whether viral attachment and penetration can take place. The chemical specificity of receptors underlies the long-recognized "tissue tropisms" of different viruses. It is increasingly clear, however, that receptor specificity alone does not account for the spectrum of susceptibility to viruses, genetic and other biological factors being of equal importance. The reader is referred to recent reviews of these questions (Smith, 1977; Lonberg-Holm and Philipson, 1978). The term "receptor" should be reserved for the attachment function associated with the cell membrane and should not be used to designate reactive sites on viral surfaces or even viral antigens which may appear at the cell surface during viral maturation. Surprisingly little is known about the biochemical composition of receptors for animal viruses, with the exception of those for orthomyxoviruses and paramyxoviruses. Investigation of cell receptors has broadened to include interrelationships between histocompatibility antigens and susceptibility to viruses, as well as the complex problem of persistent viral infection (e.g., paramyxoviruses, measles virus, and herpesviruses). Problems in the identification of receptors and approaches to their solution have been summarized recently (Gallaher and Howe, 1976; Lonberg-Holm and Philipson, 1978).

Viruses representative of almost every taxonomic group have now been analyzed with respect to the morphology of attachment and penetration. In spite of extensive data available, variation in the strains within a single species, as well as different experimental conditions make it impossible to generalize or even to repeat individual experimental observations, some of which must therefore stand alone. However, interpretations of electron micrographs have in many instances been fortified by other kinds of evidence. We have therefore included results of pertinent biochemical and biophysical analyses, as outlined in Table 1. Only those viruses which have been examined by electron microscopy during early stages of infection are represented in this tabular summary.

2. METHODS

Some of the morphological and biochemical–biophysical approaches toward the elucidation of virus–receptor interactions are listed below, followed by a brief discussion of salient features in each category:

I. Approaches to morphology
    A. Transmission electron microscopy (TEM)—ultrathin sectioning, negative staining techniques
    B. Scanning electron microscopy (SEM)
    C. Freeze-fracture, freeze-etching, immunofreeze-etching
    D. High-resolution autoradiography
II. Biochemical and biophysical approaches
    A. Surface and intracellular components analyzed by fluorescence microscopy, fluorescence probes

B.   Alteration of viral and/or cell surfaces to affect susceptibility to infection, hemolysis, fusion, attachment–elution of viruses, membrane stability: enzymes, lectins, antibody to cellular and viral constituents, superinfection, interference

C.   Uptake and fate of radiolabeled virus
   1.   Quantitative measurement of attachment
   2.   Quantitative measurement of inoculum deficit
   3.   Cytochemical localization and autoradiography

D.   Competitive inhibition of viral binding: infection; viral subunits: envelopes, capsomeres

E.   Liposomes
   1.   Artificial membranes and vesicles
   2.   Incorporation of proteins, glycoproteins, lipids to mimic "receptor" or "viral" activity

F.   Viral hemagglutination/fusion/hemolysis; equivalent to the first step in infection: adsorption, attachment, penetration (restricted)

G.   Identification of "receptor" activity in solubilized isolated membrane components, receptor analogs
   1.   Inhibition of infection, hemagglutination
   2.   Adsorption to purified virus
   3.   Controlled modification of inhibitors to abolish or enhance reactivity

Interpretation of the morphology of viral entry is subject to numerous limitations which are imposed by the techniques used and are inherent in the systems examined. Transmission electron microscopy (TEM) affords the degree of resolution which most nearly approaches events at the subcellular level. These events, however, must occur with sufficient frequency in a given system to be detectable in ultrathin sections, which by their nature severely restrict the sample. Within this framework, the effect of fixation and embedding, and the artifacts introduced by planes, angles, and thickness of sections, must be taken into account. Many aspects of the primary and secondary structure of viruses have been elucidated by application of negative staining or negative contrast techniques, in which salts of heavy metals, e.g., uranyl acetate, phosphotungstate, outline ultrastructural details which may not be revealed in ultrathin fixed and embedded specimens. Immunoelectron microscopy is applied to the detection of structures by reaction with antibody or other ligands which have been coupled with electron-dense molecules (ferritin) or with horseradish peroxidase. In the first instance direct visualization of ferritin granules signals the locus of the specific reaction, whereas in the second system the enzyme label mediates the deposition of electron-dense reaction product (e.g., benzidine). The latter system has the advantage that the same label provides permanent samples which can be visualized by light microscopy. Both methods are applicable by either direct or indirect techniques. In order to be of maximum utility in ultrastructural analysis, both methods require that the specificity and class of immunoglobulins involved be known with great precision.

Scanning electron microscopy (SEM), while sacrificing resolution, provides a "three-dimensional" effect which has given important information on structural interrelationships in many systems. However, SEM has relatively limited utility in analyzing cellular interactions with viruses or viral subunits which are beyond the resolution of this system. In freeze-fracture, freeze-etching, or immunofreeze-etching techniques, ultrastructural relationships are preserved in a more natural and undisturbed state than with chemical fixation. Since cleavage planes follow the hydrophobic interior of lipid bilayers, freeze-fracture electron microscopy has yielded important information on the internal structure of biomembranes, including viruses and their interaction with cells. In describing the complexities of membranes and fracture plane relationships, a uniform nomenclature should be used (Branton *et al.*, 1975).

In trying to define the morphology of viral penetration, a gray area is encountered in which interpretation of images becomes increasingly subjective. Moreover, the number of systems which have been critically examined by different observers is quite small. These considerations added to profound variations in both viral strains and cell types preclude any generalizations regarding mechanisms of entry within even a single taxonomic group. Ancillary biological data are therefore of utmost importance in lending credence to observed ultrastructural changes.

In examining the dynamics of viral reactions with cell membranes in relation to morphological observations, a number of correlative experimental approaches have been applied. Fluorescence microscopy with singly or doubly labeled antibody or other ligands provides a useful guide to defining the areas of greatest potential ultrastructural interest. With unfixed cells, immune reactions are generally confined to the surface of membranes, whereas fixation, usually with acetone or alcohol to disrupt the lipid barrier, allows penetration of macromolecules to intracellular sites. Here again, as with immunoelectron microscopy, the specificity, potency, and class of antibody, in both direct and indirect techniques, influence the validity of interpretations.

In the search for receptor specificity, viral and/or cell surfaces can be chemically altered in order to enhance or abolish a given biological reaction and thereby provide indirect evidence for the nature of chemical groupings involved. Identification of receptor activity in soluble form is usually accomplished through the demonstration of interference with attachment of virus or viral subunits. Modifying reagents include proteases, saccharases, lectins with specific binding sites, and antibody to cellular or viral components. In certain instances specificity of receptors has been demonstrated by the resistance of persistently infected cells to superinfection with homologous virus, implying blockade, elimination, or internalization of the receptors involved (e.g., persistent measles virus infection). Conversely, cells transformed by a given RNA tumor virus may retain receptors specific only for the transforming virus (e.g., murine leukemia viruses).

Quantitative analysis of viral binding can be achieved by measuring directly the uptake of radiolabeled virus or, alternatively, by determining a deficit of inoculum after adsorption to cells. Radiolabeled virus has also been used to trace the distribution, among cell fractions or by autoradiography, of virions, viral proteins, and genomic subunits following adsorption and penetration. Based on the same quantitative techniques, specificity of interactions with cells has been analyzed in various systems by competitive inhibition by highly purified viral subunits, as in the adenovirus system in which fiber antigen has been identified as the organelle of attachment. Receptor activity likewise can be detected by inhibition of viral attachment with purified membrane constituents or receptor analogues obtained from noncellular sources. Controlled, enzymatic, or chemical degradation of such soluble inhibitors has provided additional insight into the specifically reactive groupings on the cell surface.

Information regarding receptor groupings has also been obtained through the use of artificial membranes and vesicles into which putative "receptor" macromolecules can be introduced and which can then be shown to react more or less specifically with virus. While not functionally simulating the natural membrane, liposomes and related constructions are useful in examining surface interactions which do not require energy. Analogous approaches have been used in attempts to recombine isolated viral subunits into functional entities corresponding to whole virions (e.g., paramyxoviral envelope subunits combined with defined lipids).

The capacity to adhere to the surface of erythrocytes and cause their agglutination was first described in connection with influenza viruses. Hemagglutination (HA) has since been found to be characteristic of a number of otherwise unrelated groups of viruses (see reviews of Howe and Lee, 1972; Bächi et al., 1977a). This characteristic offers a means other than infectivity for quantitating viral particles and, by specific hemagglutination inhibition (HI), for detecting antibodies directed to viral surface components. While the same general visible effect is seen with all hemagglutinating viruses, the molecular basis underlying this restricted interaction may vary for each major group. As with initiation of infection, these differences have to do not only with the viral capsid or envelope subunits involved but also with the nature of specific interactions with receptors on the erythrocytes of different species. A brief summary of current concepts of erythrocyte membrane structure has been included subsequently in connection with the discussion of orthomyxoviruses and paramyxoviruses, the prototypic hemagglutinating viruses.

3. INVASION OF CELLS BY NAKED VIRUSES

3.1. Adenoviruses

In the adenovirus system the penton fiber complex has been well defined as the mediator of viral attachment. Purified adenovirus type 2 or 5 fiber protein completely inhibited attachment of ^{32}P-labeled adenovirus of either type to HeLa cells but not the attachment of poliovirus (Philipson et al., 1968).

Adenoviral receptors have been shown to be distinct from those for picornaviruses as demonstrated by cross-saturation experiments with representative picorna- and adenoviruses. Attachment of radioactive viruses was generally inhibited only by homologous viruses or viral subunits. However, there was some communality of receptors between adenovirus type 2 and Coxsackie B3 virus (Lonberg-Holm et al., 1976a). In buoyant density gradient centrifugation analyses, virus–receptor complexes banded at a density of 1.2 g/cm^3 and were sensitive to ionic detergent. These findings, and the binding of virus to plasma membrane fragments, indicated that receptor activity was associated with a membrane fraction.

A clue as to the chemical nature of receptors for adenoviruses has been derived from analyses of proteins solubilized from KB cell membranes with SDS or Triton X-100 (Hennache and Boulanger,

1977). A polypeptide of 78,000 molecular weight, probably the main constituent of tonofilaments, was thought to be the component to which primary binding by penton fibers might occur. A 42,000 molecular weight protein may also be part of this primary binding site. The smaller polypeptide may correspond to actin and thereby implicate microfilaments in this receptor activity and possibly also in transport of adenoviruses through the cytoplasm. This also implies that, as suggested in electron micrographic studies, virions which penetrate the membrane, whether directly or by viropexis, may appear to be intact during their transcytoplasmic migration (see below). Receptor activity for adenovirus has been found in a protein fraction of erythrocyte ghosts solubilized with SDS (Philipson *et al.*, 1976) but not otherwise characterized.

Based on results of extensive biochemical and biophysical investigations, a model has been proposed for the early adenovirus–receptor interaction (Lonberg-Holm and Philipson, 1969; Philipson *et al.*, 1976). The first step is attachment of virions by penton fibers to receptors and is temperature independent. This is followed by recruitment of additional receptor units to the receptor site, resulting in the formation of a multivalent virus–receptor complex which causes invagination of the cell membrane and may trigger pinocytosis. The translational movement of receptor proteins is dependent on the fluidity of the membrane lipid matrix and is therefore temperature dependent. As a result of complexing with receptors at the plasma membrane, virions are irreversibly altered. Only a small portion of such altered particles (B particles) elute, the majority entering the cytoplasm where the DNA in the partially uncoated virions (C particles) is found to be sensitive to nucleases (Lonberg-Holm and Philipson, 1978). The virus ultimately reaches the nucleus where uncoating is completed. This sequence is consistent with the apparently "direct" penetration of adenoviruses observed by TEM, as described subsequently.

In electron microscopic analyses of infection by adenovirus type 7 (Dales, 1962), phagocytosed viral particles were found in cytoplasmic vacuoles from which they appeared to pass into the nucleus. In extensive subsequent studies (Chardonnet and Dales, 1970*a,b*) attachment of virions was synchronized by adsorption at 4°C. With subsequent warming to 37°C virions were rapidly transferred to the region of the nucleus. Gradient analyses showed that type 7 virions penetrated less efficiently than type 5 virions and became preferentially concentrated in lysosomes, in which they were not uncoated. Type 5 particles on the other hand reached the nuclear membrane within 10 min, where they were converted to empty capsids, the DNA cores reaching the confines of the nucleus.

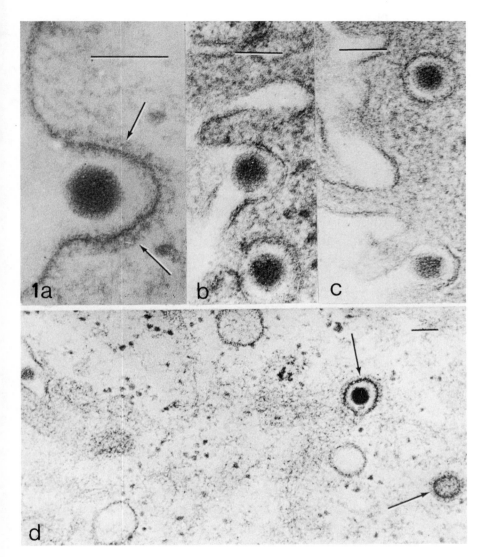

Fig. 1.   Stages in viropexis of adenovirus type 5 in HeLa cells. Invaginated segment of
plasma membrane (a) has acquired dense inner coating (arrows) which is still evident
around cytoplasmic vacuoles, each of which contains a viral particle (b,c,d). From
Chardonnet and Dales (1970a), by permission of the publisher. Bar = 100 nm.

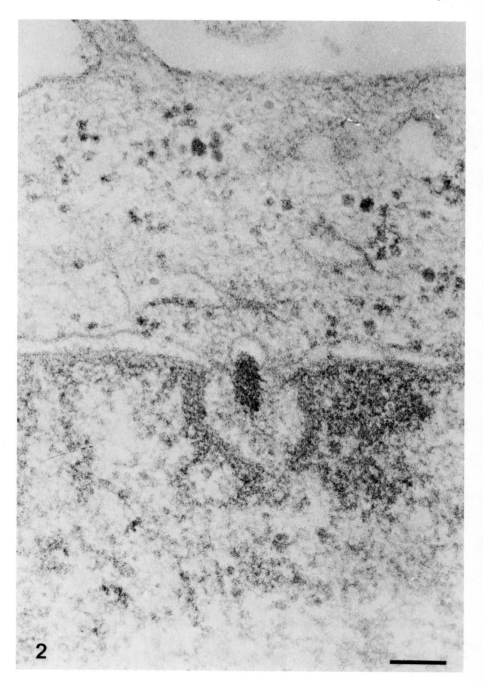

Fig. 2. Adenoviral nucleoprotein passing into the nucleus from a capsid remnant in the cytoplasm. From Morgan *et al.* (1969). Reprinted by permission of the publisher. Bar = 100 nm.

The difference in behavior noted between types 1 and 5 on the one hand and types 7 and 12 on the other could not be ascribed to differences in fiber length, since types 1, 5, and 12 all possess relatively long fibers in comparison to those of type 7. In analyses of type 5 adenoviral penetration, morphological evidence was presented to show that transfer of inoculum virions with dense cores into HeLa cell nuclei occurred via the nuclear pore complexes along with the accumulation of empty capsids at the site later in the process (Fig. 1). An altered adenoviral particle observed in passage from cytoplasm to nucleus via a nuclear pore is depicted in Fig. 2.

Recent evidence has shown that, after adsorption and viropexis, encapsidated virions are released into the cytoplasm and, after binding specifically to microtubules, move vectorially toward the nuclear pores. Intracytoplasmic virus retained most of the identifiable radiolabeled polypeptides present in purified extracellular virus. However, PAGE analyses showed that there was a small deficit in the penton fiber polypeptide in cytoplasmic virus when compared to inoculum virus. This deficit may represent a portion of the penton fiber complex broken away during passage of virus through the phagolysosomal barrier into the cytoplasm (Lyon *et al.*, 1978).

Evidence in support of apparently "direct" penetration by adenovirus 2 has come from analyses of freeze-etched preparations (Brown and Burlingham, 1973) in which virions were found to be embedded in the plasma membrane 10 min after infection. Moreover, there were configurational changes from hexagonal to round forms in the transition from extracellular to intracellular loci. This change in shape, previously observed by TEM (Morgan *et al.*, 1969), may signal selective loss of capsid protein from the vertices. However, the PAGE analyses alluded to above would tend to argue against this interpretation. One possible explanation of this discrepancy may relate to the proportion of plaque-forming units (PFU) to particles. The higher this ratio, the less likely the particles are to end up in vacuoles. By contrast, the larger the proportion of noninfectious particles, the more likely these are to be phagocytized and remain surrounded by vacuolar membrane. The truth may lie somewhere in between and may emerge when a precise account can be given of the role of individual capsid proteins in the progression of events from viral entry to emergence of viral progeny.

3.2. Papovaviruses

The early events in papovavirus invasion were analyzed in permissive cells (Barbanti-Brodano *et al.*, 1970) on which radioactive virus combined irreversibly with cell receptors. The latter were thought to be lipoprotein in nature. SV40-transformed permissive cells, however, were resistant to superinfection with SV40, but the isolated viral DNA could still be introduced into the cell, suggesting that homologous receptors on transformed cells were blocked or no longer present. Entry of SV40 was rapid and took place by pinocytosis at altered membrane sites. Fifty percent of input virus was adsorbed within 2 hr, some penetrating within 30 min to the nucleus where uncoating took place. In the process of internalization virions became enveloped and thus increased in size (Fig. 3) (Hummeler *et al.*, 1970).

In an extensive analysis of SV40 infection in permissive and nonpermissive cells, entry of virions into different cellular compartments was seen to occur by a process which entailed sequential envelopment of viral particles by membrane which then fused to other membranes (Maul *et al.*, 1978). The sequence most consistently observed depicts initial envelopment of virions at the plasma membrane, passage in pinocytotic vesicles through the cytoplasm, fusion with the nuclear membrane, and the release of naked virions into the intracisternal space of the nuclear envelope. Virions then attain their final goal first by inducing the inner nuclear membrane to invaginate, thus gaining entrance into the nucleoplasm. The presence of specific receptors on the nuclear membrane, as in the plasma membrane, may underly the penetration of virions from cytoplasm to nucleus. Removal of the acquired (?pinocytotic vesicle) membrane was not recognizable by electron microscopy but must be assumed to occur as a necessary prelude to uncoating and transcription.

A somewhat similar mechanism appears to govern the invasion of either permissive or nonpermissive cells by polyoma virus (Mackay and Consigli, 1976). Under saturation conditions of infection, virus was identified intracellularly by radiolabeled DNA or capsid proteins. Pseudovirions were identified by prelabel with horseradish peroxidase. Virions were also identified immunologically with horseradish-labeled Fab′ fragments of antibody to virus. Intact virions with nuclease-resistant DNA were detected in the nucleus at 15 min after infection, indicating that uncoating occurred after the virion reached the nucleus. The main steps detected morphologically were (1) attachment of virions and pseudovirions to receptor sites at which, at 37°C, invagination occurred with engulfment of complete virions into monopinocytotic vesicles; (2) passage of virions in this form through the cytoplasm to the outer nuclear membrane; and (3) direct penetration of the nuclear membrane. Uncoating was not observed electron microscopically. The presence of a "nuclear transport recognition factor" (NTRF) was pos-

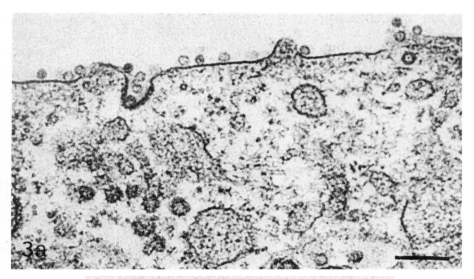

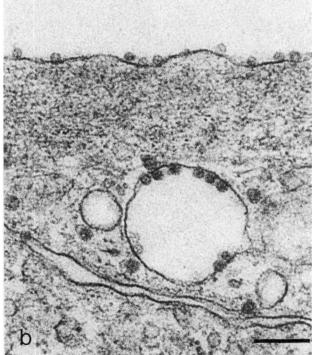

Fig. 3. Penetration of African green monkey cells by simian virus 40. (a) Pinocytosis of viral particle (left) and completed uptake of single virion (right). Particles increase in diameter by acquisition of a second coat derived from the cell membrane. (b) Pinocytotic vesicle containing particles 10 min after infection. From Hummeler *et al.* (1970), by permission of the publisher. Bar = 200 nm.

tulated to explain the observation that only virions and pseudovirions reached the nucleus and that capsids, without DNA, were taken up into phagocytic vesicles and disposed of without ever reaching the nucleus. NTRF (?cellular histone) in the virion may also mediate the attachment of virus to receptors through which the signal for internalization is given. The direct penetration of papovaviruses (SV40 and polyoma) to the nucleus appears to occur by a mechanism distinctly different from that observed with adenoviruses, which undergo irreversible immunological and structural alterations at the cell membrane. The mechanism whereby polyoma virus in monopinocytotic vesicles is transported to the nucleus is obscure but appears to be independent of microfilaments and microtubules.

As a result of the adsorption of polyoma virus to BHK and mouse 3T3 cells, a rapid increase in the degree of fluidity (decrease in microviscosity) of membrane lipids was detectable by a decrease in fluorescence polarization (Levanon *et al.*, 1977). The increase in fluidity was proportional to the number of virions adsorbed and required effective union of virus and receptors. The effect of these nonfusing viruses was the opposite of that following the action of certain syncytiogenic viruses (e.g., Newcastle disease virus, NDV) which effected a decrease in fluidity (increase in microviscosity) (Levanon and Kohn, 1978). Papovaviruses contain no lipid. Consequently, the changes noted could not have been the result of lipid intermixing since, as will be noted with enveloped togaviruses, the change was opposite to what might be expected from a mixture of viral lipids with membrane lipids. The same effect was noted with three entirely different agents (West Nile, encephalomyocarditis, and polyoma viruses) and therefore must involve activation of membranal enzymes triggered by the pinocytotic process.

3.3. Parvoviruses

Among the parvoviruses, the genome of which is single-stranded DNA, only minute virus of mice (MVM) has been examined in the early stages of infection (Linser *et al.*, 1977; Linser and Armentrout, 1978). A9 cells, a line of murine cells derived from L929 fibroblasts, were exposed in subsaturating amounts to labeled MVM at high multiplicity for 2 hr at 4°C. Virus was seen by electron microscopy to be bound to receptor sites on the cell surface which were randomly distributed and were morphologically distinct from intervening normal areas of the cell. Virions, singly and in clusters, attached to filopodial surfaces as well as to apparently undifferentiated areas of the membrane. Segments of membrane to which particles were attached appeared to be thickened, possibly signaling the initiation of phagocytosis. The presence of saturable binding sites was correlated with susceptibility to infection. Wtihin 30 min of incubation at 37°C, most adsorbed virus had become internalized in vacuoles and by 2 hr had reached the nucleus. Virus bound to filopodia was also internalized by pinocytosis triggered by viral crosslinking of separate cell membrane surfaces or by internalization of filopodial bases to form channels which pinched off into smooth vesicles in the cytoplasm (Fig. 4).

A major structural protein (B) of 72,000 occurs in MVM. This protein is apparently cleaved to yield a smaller (69,000), activated protein which adsorbs more rapidly than its precursor. This cleavage-activation process, also effected by cell-conditioned medium, is presumably a membrane-associated function which might influence susceptibility to infection with MVM (Clinton and Hayashi, 1976).

3.4. Reoviruses

Within the three serotypes of reoviruses further differentiation may be made on the basis of hemagglutinating activity with erythrocytes of different species. Human erythrocytes are agglutinated by all three serotypes, whereas type 3 also reacts with bovine erythrocytes to somewhat higher titer. In addition, human erythrocytes bearing determinants of blood group A are more reactive with all three serotypes than are cells of groups O or B. This and other indirect evidence suggests that the receptors for reoviruses may be glycosylated. Beyond this, relatively little is known about the nature of receptors on either erythrocytes or on nucleated cells (see review by Howe and Lee, 1972). Through use of recombinants of reovirus types 1 and 3, the outer reovirus 3 capsid protein (σ1) has recently been identified as HA and hence as probably the principal mediator of attachment to susceptible cells (Weiner *et al.*, 1978).

Penetration of reovirus 3 into L-strain mouse fibroblasts occurs by viropexis. After absorption of type 3 reovirus at 4°C, phagocytosis of virions occurred rapidly once the cells had been warmed to 37°C. During the first 30 min, there was rapid decrease in extracellular virus and increase in undegraded viral particles in lysosomes, in which uncoating presumably occurs. Virus was also found in phagocytic vacuoles in smaller numbers (Fig. 5) (Silverstein and Dales, 1968).

Rotaviruses are biologically akin to reoviruses because of their double-stranded RNA core; they have a particular tropism for intes-

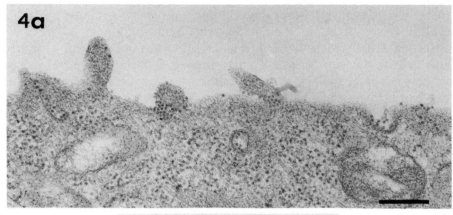

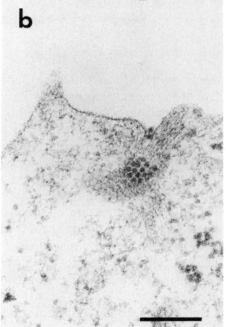

Fig. 4.   Murine A9 cells infected with minute virus of mice. (a) Stages in viral uptake into coated vesicles by invagination (right and left) and formation of "autonomous" coated vesicles (center). Clusters of virions are seen between the plasma membrane surface and the edge of the filopodium. (b) A filopodium bearing a patch of virions is folded into the cytoplasm forming a channel which contains two viral particles. Courtesy P. Linser and R. W. Armentrout. Bar = 200 nm.

tinal epithelial cells. It has been proposed that lactase, the concentrations of which are higher in young animals than in adult animals, might serve a dual function as both receptor and uncoating enzyme for rotaviruses, the major capsid protein of which (protein 7) is glycosylated. In contrast to reoviruses which can be reduced to cores by intracellular proteases, rotaviruses are resistant to proteases but can be uncoated *in vitro* by lactase (Holmes *et al.*, 1976). Electron microscopic observations have been limited to infected intestinal columnar epithelium in intact animals and to limited extent in organ culture. Precise determination of the mode of entry into cells must await a satisfactory cell culture system in which the virus will replicate.

3.5. Picornaviruses

The complexities of early molecular interactions between picornaviruses and cells are beyond the scope of this chapter and are dealt with elsewhere in this volume (see also reviews by Lonberg-Holm and Philipson, 1974, 1978). However, certain relationships can be singled out as probably having an important bearing on the mode of penetration. While there are demonstrable differences in behavior between the relatively stable enteroviruses and the acid-labile rhinoviruses, the biochemical events surrounding attachment and penetration are doubtless essentially similar for all members of the picornavirus group.

All four proteins in the capsid probably participate in the attachment process. Viral interaction with specific cell receptors is temperature dependent and can be variously inhibited by metabolic poisons, indicating that transmembranal migration is an energy-dependent process. Once the virion becomes firmly attached, irreversible alterations occur which are catalyzed in the membrane and which place the virus thus eclipsed (A particles) beyond the reach of antibody. Loss of capsid proteins, notably VP4, is accompanied by corresponding alterations in antigenic structure. These membrane-associated changes constitute the first steps in uncoating and release of the viral genome into the cytoplasm. A certain proportion of A particles may elute but are found to be noninfectious because they lack VP4.

Interference studies have clearly demonstrated sharp differences in specificity among several of the picornaviral subgroups (Lonberg-Holm *et al.*, 1976a). Little information is available, however, as to the biochemical nature of the receptors involved. A lead on this problem may have been provided by the demonstration that poliovirus can be uncoated by plasma membranes isolated from calf kidney or BHK21

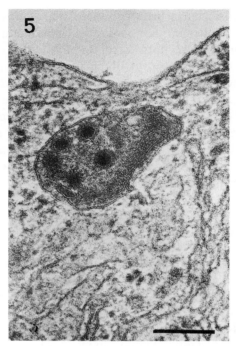

Fig. 5.   Portion of cytoplasm of an L cell 2 hr after penetration of reovirus type 3.
Several inoculum particles are enclosed in a lysosome. From Silverstein and Dales
(1968), by permission of the publisher. Bar = 200 nm.

cells. Glycoproteins solubilized from plasma membranes by extraction
with butanol had a similar action (Chan and Black, 1970). However,
there is no evidence to indicate which portions of the glycoproteins
contain activity.

  Isolated plasma membranes of HeLa cells were separated into two
fractions, one of which was shown to elute previously attached Coxsackie B3 virus or to uncoat it. The second membrane fraction from
which virus could also elute did not show any uncoating activity, but
was inhibitory for uncoating by either whole membrane homogenates
or the other membrane fraction derived from them. These findings were
interpreted to suggest that elution and uncoating might be two separate
and distinct activities of the membrane receptors (Roesing *et al.*, 1975).
Details of the foregoing series of events which accompany and follow
the binding of picornaviruses to cells and which effect internalization of
functional viral mRNA are beyond the reach of morphological observation by electron microscopy. Their end result, however, is viropexis.

Accordingly, polioviral particles were found inside of phagocytic vacuoles within 10 min of inoculation of HeLa cells at high MOI (Dales, 1973) (Fig. 6). The sequence of subsequent steps in the dismantling of the virions remains to be elucidated.

Poliovirus neutralized by 7 S antibody may retain its capacity to adsorb to susceptible cells (Mandel, 1967a) but does not elute as readily as unneutralized virus. Following adsorption, neutralized virus may undergo penetration by some form of viropexis in the same manner as naked virus (Fig. 6), and uncoating may also occur but with divergent results. Following penetration of neutralized virus, viral RNA is found in degraded form, and replication therefore does not ensue as it does with normal virus, uncoating of which releases intact viral messenger RNA into the cytoplasm (Mandel, 1967b). These findings suggested an alternative mechanism for antibody inhibition of viral synthesis. Antibody may prevent initial adsorption, but, once internalized, complexed to virus, it may also suppress a reaction necessary for release of intact RNA and/or stimulate a speedy degradative attack on any RNA that is released. The extent to which loss of VP4 and other capsid proteins may be prevented or minimized and uncoating thus interfered with is not clear. It is possible that by its very presence antibody complexed to virus may effect rearrangements of retained capsid protein and thereby expose the RNA to degradative processes to which intact RNA released from internalized infectious virus is not as susceptible. What appears to be direct penetration of virions into the cytoplasm has also been observed by electron microscopy. In KB, FL, or Vero cells, viral particles were found free in the peripheral cytoplasm 2–5 min after inoculation, the virus having apparently passed directly through the plasma membrane without observable pinocytotic changes (Dunnebacke et al., 1969). A possible basis on which to explain direct penetration by picornaviruses and perhaps other unenveloped viruses was provided by the demonstration of the lipophilic nature of picornaviral A particles. For this purpose, A particles were obtained from purified poliovirus type 2 by incubation in dilute buffer at 37°C and from rhinovirus type 2 by treatment with acid. The A particles but not the intact virions could be adsorbed to liposomes containing phosphatidylcholine and other lipids. This observation led to the suggestion that after primary interaction with intact cell receptors A particles might intercalate into the lipid bilayer of the membrane and then be transferred to the cytoplasm (Lonberg-Holm et al., 1976a). A similar mechanism was suggested by the demonstration that purified poliovirus could be engulfed by phospholipid liposomes and in this form be

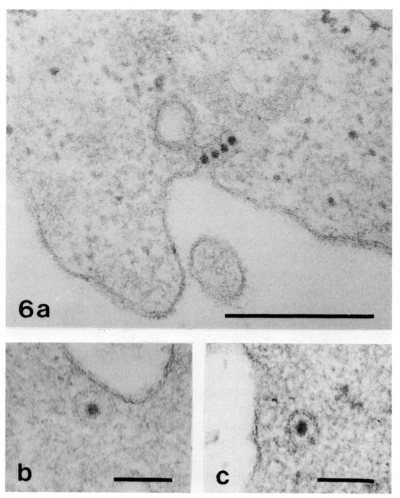

Fig. 6. (a) Viropexis of poliovirus type 1 by HeLa cells 10 min after initiation of penetration. Bar = 500 nm. (b,c) Individual poliovirions within phagocytic vacuoles close to the cellular surface. From Dales (1973), by permission of the publisher. Bar = 100 nm.

introduced by membranal fusion into cells normally resistant to infection by naked virus (Wilson *et al.*, 1977).

4. ERYTHROCYTE MEMBRANE STRUCTURE IN RELATION TO VIRAL HEMAGGLUTINATION

More perhaps is known about the erythrocyte membrane than about any other type of cell membrane with respect to functional surface groupings reactive with viruses, immunoglobulins, lectins, and other ligands. This is true in part for the obvious reason that mammalian erythrocyte membranes free of cytoplasmic constituents can be obtained in large quantity, and the individual components, retaining biological activities representative of the cell surface, can be subjected to quantitative biochemical and biophysical analysis. While the receptor for a hemagglutinating virus may be the same type of macromolecule on both erythrocyte and susceptible nucleated cell, these two types of cell differ with respect to the conformation of their plasma membranes and hence in the distribution and exposure of receptors. The erythrocyte membrane is relatively rigid and unpliable in comparison to nucleated cells, which are characteristically studded with microvilli and are to a varying degree capable of phagocytosis. Some receptors on erythrocytes are found at the distal end of macromolecules such as glycolipids, and glycoproteins which traverse the membrane. The carboxy-terminal end of the latter interacts with peripheral proteins, particularly the spectrin complex (Shotton *et al.*, 1978), which may be related to the actin–myosin (?kinase) complex in nucleated cells. Through this protein–protein interaction, events at the cell surface such as viral attachment and membrane fusion affect cytoskeletal mechanisms which, in nucleated cells, apparently trigger the phagocytic process. Reactions which occur at the surface of the erythrocyte and which exert transmembranal and intramembranal effects thus provide a model for analysis of entry mechanisms in the initiation of infection by hemolytic viruses (Bächi *et al.*, 1977*a*). Erythrocytes do not support viral replication so that their interaction with hemagglutinating viruses is clearly restricted to attachment and, in certain instances, elution, with or without alteration of virions and cell membranes at receptor site(s).

The membrane of mammalian erythrocytes comprises a lipid bilayer in which integral proteins move with relative freedom, subject only to restrictions imposed by interaction with peripheral proteins on the cytoplasmic side. The major glycoprotein (glycophorin A) of human erythrocytes is asymmetrical and accounts for many of the carbohydrate groupings at the cell surface, including all the NANA. Glycophorin A contains the receptor for influenza viral HA (Howe and Lee, 1972; Jackson *et al.*, 1973; Tomita and Marchesi, 1975; Marchesi *et al.*, 1976), Sendai virus, and perhaps other unrelated hemagglutinating viruses (Enegren and Burness, 1977), as well as determinants for the M and N blood groups.

The relationship of glycophorin to structural subunits in the membrane has been the subject of investigation by a number of laboratories. By freeze-fracture electron microscopy, intramembranal particles (IMP) of average diameter 8.5 nm are seen more or less evenly distributed in the plasmatic (P) face of erythrocyte membranes. Evidence based on alteration of IMP distribution patterns by surface reaction with influenza virus, lectins, and alloantibodies suggested that the IMP might be connected to the integral proteins, chiefly glycophorin and a second glycoprotein constituting polypeptide band III (molecular weight approximately 100,000) in the PAGE profiles of hemoglobin-free membranes. Recent analyses, however, have shown that some or all of the glycophorin A may be independent of IMP and hence probably not contributory to their formation. The number of individual receptor sites for convanavalin A (Con A) (Bächi and Schnebli, 1975; Schnebli and Bächi, 1975) or for antibody to glycophorin (Howe and Bächi, 1973) was significantly less than the number of IMP on the P fracture face of erythrocytes. The results of studies with limulin, a lectin specific for sialoglycoproteins (Bächi, 1978), have also indicated a lack of association between glycophorin and the IMP. Additional evidence against such a structural association has come from freeze-etching analysis of erythrocytes of the rare genotype En (a^-). These cells lack glycophorin but appear to have a normal complement of IMP (Bächi et al., 1977b). Vesicles rich in glycophorin and endogenous lipids but lacking IMP were prepared by exposing membranes to low ionic strength and pH to remove spectrin, and then extracting them with Triton X-100, a nonionic detergent. This procedure solubilized glycophorin, separating it from protein band III, which remained in the membranes (Lutz et al., 1978, 1979). These several findings argue for the lack of structural association between glycophorin A and IMP without, however, providing any evidence as to the composition of IMP other than to implicate band III. Insight into the nature of receptors for hemagglutinating enveloped RNA viruses has come mainly from extensive biochemical and ultrastructural analyses of erythrocyte membranes and soluble fractions derived from them in which receptor activity can be detected by inhibition of HA or infectivity.

5. INVASION OF CELLS BY ENVELOPED VIRUS

5.1. Orthomyxoviruses

Influenza virus has now been extensively dissected at the molecular level, and precise information on the structure and function of its envelope constituents is at hand.

The two principal constituents are the HA (molecular weight 75,000–80,000) and neuraminidase (molecular weight 50,000–60,000), both glycoproteins, each coded for by separate segments of the viral genome. Normally maturing virus does not contain NANA, which is cleaved from the viral particle during morphogenesis at the cell surface (Palese *et al.*, 1974; Palese and Compans, 1976). Temperature-sensitive mutants lacking neuraminidase activity have been shown to retain cellular NANA and, when they bud from the cell surface, to undergo aggregation through mutual interaction of viral NANA with hemagglutinin. Maturation of wild-type orthomyxoviruses and some paramyxoviruses is inhibited when neuraminidase activity is blocked with 2-deoxy-2,3-dehydro-N-trifluoroacetylneuraminic acid (FANA), an analogue of NANA. These findings underscore the importance of neuraminidase in the release of these enveloped viruses. Neuraminidase also mediates orthomyxoviral elution from erythrocytes, with concomitant enzymatic cleavage of NANA from receptors.

The HA glycoprotein is the principal mediator of viral attachment to sialoglycoprotein receptors of erythrocytes or susceptible nucleated cells. The functional grouping on the HA glycoprotein, however, has not been absolutely defined. Treatment of influenza virus with bacterial glycosidases cleaved up to 25% of the carbohydrate (galactose and N-glucosamine) from the virion, mostly from HA_1, without altering hemagglutination or infectivity. Similar treatment of purified HA resulted in loss of 50% of carbohydrates, including oligosaccharides, but little or no loss of HA activity. These findings suggest that carbohydrate accessible to enzyme may not be essential for attachment (Collins and Knight, 1978). Following *in vitro* sialylation of influenza viral HA_1, HA activity was destroyed without affecting neuraminidase activity; binding of virus to cells was unaffected and infectivity was enhanced. Apparent enhancement of plaque formation by sialylated virus was ascribed to the infectious units resulting from aggregation of defective and complete virions. NANA residues on viral envelope glycoproteins, possibly by conformational rearrangement of HA, may affect the initial reaction of virions with membranes and viral penetration (Lakshmi and Schulze, 1978). Infectivity of influenza virus was increased following proteolytic digestion of virus and the cleavage of peptides from HA_1, leaving phenylalanine as the terminal amino acid. This finding is consonant with the possibility that some sort of intramembranal proteolytic cleavage of HA occurs during viral morphogenesis in certain host cells (Scheid, 1978). This type of cleavage may be necessary for or, at the least, may enhance the infectivity of viral progeny.

The morphology of penetration by orthomyxoviruses has been variously described. Phagocytosis of influenza virus by leukocytes was reported as early as 1957, and it was noted that the process was enhanced by antibody and was more pronounced with leukocytes from immune animals. It is of interest that these early observations were made in the days before cell-mediated immune mechanisms were clearly identified (Boand et al., 1957).

An alternative mechanism of entry was proposed as a result of morphological analysis of influenza viral penetration into cells of the chicken chorioallantoic membrane (Morgan and Rose, 1968). Viral attachment to cells occurred within the first 5 min of incubation at 37°C, followed in rapid succession by apparent dissolution of the "viral coat," change and loss of definition of the segment of membrane in close proximity to the virion, disappearance of most of the intact particles, rupture of the viral core, and apparently direct introduction of ribonucleoprotein into the cytoplasm. This was followed by "repair" of overlying membranes. The precise mechanism of rapid uncoating of virions at the cell membrane remained unexplained but was thought on the basis of the electron microscopic evidence to involve a process of membrane fusion. Throughout the period of observation, however, intact viral particles were seen in phagocytic vacuoles. This latter finding was in accord with observations by other workers who examined the penetration of influenza A2 virus into chicken CAM cells. Virions were rapidly internalized by viropexis into clear cytoplasmic vacuoles which did not contain lysosomal enzymes, and thence into the cytoplasm by dissolution of viral envelope and vacuolar membrane. No evidence of fusion of viral envelope to plasma membrane was found (Dourmashkin and Tyrrell, 1974). Entry by phagocytosis was demonstrated in a study of Ehrlich ascites tumor (EAT) cells which were subjected to synchronized infection at high multiplicity (Bächi, 1970). Massive internalization of viral particles into phagocytic vacuoles was noted. By 10 min after infection virus had been transported by these means to the perinuclear spaces (Fig. 7). Disintegration of virions soon followed, and virtually all cells became hemadsorbing and produced infectious viral progeny. Despite the multiplicity of infection used, no morphological evidence of fusion was encountered.

In order to minimize the probability of direct contact between infected virus and cell membrane and hence lessen the opportunity for virus–cell fusion, small numbers of active virions were incorporated, along with large numbers of ultraviolet-light-inactivated particles, into aggregates by reaction with histone, a polycationic substance. Such aggregates were as infectious as similarly formed clumps of infectious

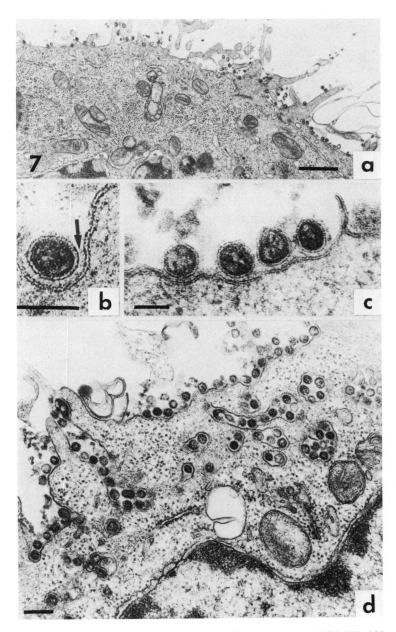

Fig. 7. Ehrlich ascites tumor cells exposed to influenza virus at MOI 200–300 at 4°C, showing (a) massive adsorption of particles and at high magnification (b,c) showing the envelope spikes interposed between virion and invaginated (?prephagocytic) segments of membrane. (d) After 10 min at 36°C, many virions, still apparently intact, are in various stages of engulfment and enclosure into cytoplasmic vacuoles. Courtesy, T. Bächi. Reprinted by permission of the publisher. Bar = 100 nm.

virus alone, or active monodisperse virus without histone. Electron microscopic analyses clearly demonstrated that aggregates of whole viral particles were internalized by phagocytosis, without evidence of interaction between virions and cell membranes other than initial attachment through envelope spikes (Dales and Pons, 1976). Moreover, virus rendered noninfectious by prior complexing with antibody, when similarly incorporated into histone aggregates with inactivated virus, regained infectivity after internalization by viropexis.

Influenza virus adsorbs rather specifically to cilia and to surfaces of respiratory epithelial cells in culture, in which viral replication occurs (Gould et al., 1972). However, morphological analyses of interactions of influenza virus with ciliated epithelial cells have yielded discrepant results. In one study influenza virus appeared to attach to cilia and then to enter apparently by fusion with ciliated as well as with unciliated epithelial cells, no phagocytosis being observed (Blaskovic et al., 1972). In contrast, with guinea pig tracheal epithelial cells, influenza virus was seen to adhere to cilia but not to undergo fusion with them, whereas parainfluenza type 1 (Sendai) virus in the same system penetrated by envelope-membrane fusion (Dourmashkin and Tyrrell, 1970).

The weight of evidence then points to viropexis as the mode of entry by orthomyxoviruses in which discernible fusion of viral envelope with cell membrane appears not to be involved. However, host-specific enzymatic cleavage activation of HA glycoprotein (to yield HA_2) accompanies penetration and is required for initiation of infection. Here there is a functional analogy with fusing paramyxoviruses (e.g., Sendai, NDV) in which intramembranal cleavage of F glycoprotein (to yield F_1) is prerequisite to infectivity. Accordingly, there is also striking homology between HA_2 and F_1 in N-terminal amino acid sequences, the region which in each of these molecules is apparently involved in viral penetration infection (Choppin and Scheid, 1980). Studies with electron spin resonance have indicated that there is an increase in the fluidity of the bilayer of chicken erythrocytes on primary reaction of influenza h surface glycoprotein receptors (Lyles and Landsberger, 1976). anges were not observed with human erythrocytes or with a membranes, neither of which retain the microtubular chicken erythrocytes. A similar signal may trigger viro-tible cells.

agglutinin and neuraminidase activity (HN, molecular weight 65,000). In systems embodying the requisite proteolytic enzymes, the second viral glycoprotein (F_0, molecular weight 65,000) cleaved to yield a smaller polypeptide (F_1, molecular weight 53,000–56,000). The latter is recognized as the "fusion factor" (Scheid and Choppin, 1974; Scheid, 1978) which appears to mediate the entry of paramyxoviruses into susceptible cells. HN and F glycoproteins of Sendai virus are immunologically distinct from one another (Örvell and Norrby, 1977). The F glycoprotein represents one form of envelope spike lacking H and N activity, the HN glycoprotein representing the other (Shimizu *et al.*, 1974); the two kinds of spikes are separable from one another by sucrose density isoelectrofocusing of Tween-20-disrupted virions.

As with orthomyxoviruses, interaction with erythrocytes has revealed some of the essential features which may also govern viral penetration into susceptible nucleated cells. Fusion of erythrocytes by Sendai virus requires initial fusion of virions to the cell via sialoglycoprotein receptors. For some strains at least, receptor activity requires the presence of NANA in 2→3 linkages (Fidgen, 1975). The specificity of Sendai virions for NANA is underscored by the failure of virus to bind or to agglutinate horse erythrocytes (Yamamoto *et al.*, 1974) in which the sialic acid is exclusively N-glycolylneuraminic acid. Virus could be attached to equine erythrocytes which had been pretreated with concanavalin A (con A), a lectin which also reacts with the surface of Sendai virions. Under these circumstances hemolysis occurred due to the direct action of the virions attached to the cells through the bifunctional lectin. Influenza virus, which does not agglutinate equine erythrocytes, likewise attached to con A treated cells but did not show any signs of lysis. Treatment of cells (fibroblasts, calf kidney, and BHK cells) in culture to a critical degree with *V. cholerae* neuraminidase enhanced attachment of Newcastle disease virus (NDV). It was surmised that partial hydrolysis of NANA residues effected reduction and rearrangement of negatively charged surface groupings, thereby increasing viral binding efficiency (Wassilewa, 1977). A more acceptable explanation is found in prior observations (Bratt and Gallaher, 1972) indicating that strains of NDV differ in their requirements for neuraminidase-sensitive receptors. This requirement was less for those strains which were capable of rapid exofusion and which presumably attached to portions of the receptor molecule lacking exposed NANA residues, as proposed for the erythrocyte model (Poste and Waterson, 1975).

Erythrocyte receptors for parainfluenza viruses, along with those for orthomyxoviruses, are contained in the glycophorin molecule which spans the membrane. Sequencing studies have elucidated the composition of glycophorin and its relation to the membrane (Jackson *et al.*, 1973; Marchesi *et al.*, 1976). All of the carbohydrate residues, including NANA, are found at the amino-terminal end at the cell surface. The central portion of the polypeptide is made up of hydrophobic amino acids which interact with the lipid bilayer. On the cytoplasmic face, the carboxy-terminal end interacts with peripheral proteins, including the spectrin complex and possibly also catalase (Deas *et al.*, 1978). An important interaction between spectrin and intramembranal particles (IMP) was brought to light by examining the effects of Sendai virus on human erythrocyte ghosts, which by themselves cannot be fused by virus. However, ghosts which had been loaded with bovine serum albumin (BSA) were susceptible to fusion by virus. Fusion of BSA ghosts was accompanied by release of BSA, presumably through sites at which viral envelope had fused with the membrane. When antibody to spectrin was introduced into the ghosts along with BSA, leakage of BSA still occurred but fusion of membranes to one another was inhibited (Sekiguchi and Asano, 1978). These findings suggested that cross-linking of spectrin by antispectrin acted late in the fusion process to prevent clearing of IMP from portions of the membrane, a change shown to be a prerequisite for fusion at these virus-free sites (Bächi *et al.*, 1973).

The liberation of hemoglobin which may accompany virus–cell fusion occurs probably as a result of several concurrent events. There is evidence which suggests that particles with damaged envelopes fused with the cell membrane offered the chief avenue of escape for hemoglobin. Particles not permeable to uranyl acetate ("early harvest" virus) were nonhemolytic; those permeable to the stain because of damaged envelopes were hemolytic (Homma *et al.*, 1976; Shimizu *et al.*, 1976). This interpretation does not correspond with the observation that fusion was seen to occur at intramembranal junctions where no viral remnants, morphological or antigenic, could be detected (Bächi *et al.*, 1973). Recent studies with "early harvest" egg-grown Sendai virus, which fuses cells without escape of hemoglobin, have shown that in addition to the virus–cell fusion events, which perturb the normal membrane structure, there is an increase in passive permeability of the membrane to ions. This in turn results in the development of transmembranal ionic equilibrium and osmotic swelling. All of these changes, the exact sequence of which is still not clear, disrupt the normal interaction of spectrin with integral proteins which are themselves displaced. As already noted,this is a necessary prelude to cell–cell fusion (Knutton and Bächi, 1980).

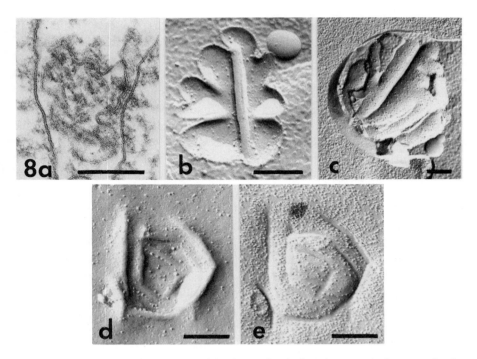

Fig. 8. Type 1 parainfluenza (Sendai) virus adsorbed to human erythrocytes in the cold and incubated at 37°C. (a) Viral remnant between the membrane of two cells showing spikeless convolutions of viral envelope and fragments of nucleocapsid. On the E face (b) and the P face (c) of freeze-fracture replicas at sites of virus–membrane fusion, smooth linear ridges free of intramembranal particles correspond to the convolutions seen in a. (d) E face and (e) P face of complementary replicas of a fusion site. From Knutton (1977), by permission of the publisher. Bar = 200 nm.

Changes in viral envelope structure which accompany fusion to erythrocyte membranes is less well understood. Electron microscopic studies (Knutton, 1977), using freeze-fracture and thin sectioning techniques, have shown that distinctive changes occur in the conformation of the paramyxoviral envelope during the process of fusion to erythrocyte membranes (Fig. 8). "Ridges" free of IMP were seen to develop along with the incorporation of viral membranes into the cell surface. The ridges may represent aggregates of long filaments or rods composed of viral M protein which, with the rearrangement of the interior of the viral envelope, becomes integrated into the plasma membrane at a stage in the fusion process which is not Ca^{2+} dependent (Volsky and Loyter, 1978). While the IMP were temporarily displaced during the initial stages of union with viral envelope, they soon regained their random distribution as the viral envelop ridges dispersed and viral antigen was disseminated through the membrane. The simultaneous removal of cellular NANA residues by the action of viral neuraminidase probably reduced the electrostatic repulsion and enhanced the molecular contact of initially apposed viral envelope and cell membrane. As previously demonstrated, diffusible NANA is released from erythrocyte membranes through the action of neuraminidase during the course of viral hemolysis (Howe and Morgan, 1969). Cell-to-cell fusion is apparently initiated through the intermediary action of viral particles already incorporated into the membrane of one or more cells in the aggregate. Polyerythrocytes are thus formed which contain cytoplasmic bridges between partially fused cells in which viral remnants are no longer visualized. This is consistent with the possibility, although it does not prove, that direct cell-to-cell fusion occurs at virus-free sites probably at relatively late stages in the process, in which the polyerythrocyte has become stabilized. The net result of the clearing of IMP from areas of the membrane is the transient exposure of membrane phospholipid at these sites, resulting in fusion of the two apposed membranes at protein-free areas. A correlation was demonstrated between dephosphorylation of membrane polypeptides, exposure of membrane phospholipids, and clustering of IMP. Dephosphorylation of membranes by virus was dependent on the initial union of virus with sialoprotein receptors and probably the subsequent incorporation of viral proteins into the cell membrane. It may be of significance in this connection that phosphatase activity was found in association with Sendai viral particles and was specifically inhibited by antiviral antibody (Milner et al., 1978). A possible target of the virus-associated phosphatase is erythrocyte band 3, the principal phosphoprotein which may be implicated in the formation of IMP. This virus-associated dephosphorylation, along with the increase in passive permeability noted earlier, promotes dissociation of spectrin from its interaction with transmembranal proteins, thereby abrogating its stabilizing function. This allows the lateral movement of IMP noted on freeze-fracture analysis.

One additional feature which has been observed to accompany fusion of erythrocytes by Sendai virus is the discharge of viral core material (ribonucleoprotein) into the internal confines of the erythrocyte which has been partially or wholly depleted of hemoglobin as a result of virus-induced permeability changes (Howe and Morgan, 1969; Bächi et al., 1973). This ejection of RNP has a parallel in the morphology of paramyxoviral invasion of susceptible cells (see below).

The fusion of Sendai virus to chicken erythrocyte membranes and consequent release of hemoglobin was found to be independent of Ca^{2+}, whereas the cell-to-cell fusion which is a consequence of viral action was entirely calcium dependent (Volsky and Loyter, 1978), as with viral dephosphorylation of human erythrocyte membranes (Loyter *et al.*, 1977). Moreover, along with the virus–cell fusion, Ca^{2+} was accumulated intracellularly when hemolysis was minimal. This transfer inward of Ca^{2+} and perhaps other ions accounts for the swelling of the cells which, as with mammalian erythrocytes, would tend to promote cell-to-cell fusion. In addition, the density of IMP decreased on the P and E fracture faces within the first 2 min at 37°C. This thermotropic separation of IMP was reversible initially, but the IMP were resistant to separation in fused cells. The Ca^{2+} requirement for subsequent steps in cell-to-cell fusion relates to the microtubule system and to spectrin, which are present in nucleated cells, including chicken erythrocytes. As already noted, only spectrin is present in mammalian erythrocytes. The clustering of IMP noted above may be related in both species of erythrocytes to virus-induced dissociation of spectrin from its restrictive interaction with the transmembranal integral proteins.

The process of erythrocyte fusion by Sendai virus may be summarized as follows. Attachment of virus to sialoprotein receptors and cross-linking of cells by virions takes place at 4°C as well as at 37°C, and is Ca^{2+} independent. Folding of the viral envelope follows as a prelude to its incorporation into the cell membrane. This change is accompanied by "ridge" formation seen on the E face of freeze-etched cells. Lateral, radial intramembranal diffusion of viral envelope antigens occurs, along with dephosphorylation, by viral enzyme (phosphatase), of band 3 and perhaps other integral proteins. Spectrin becomes dissociated from its peripheral interaction with the cytoplasmic end of integral proteins and hence no longer exerts control over cell shape. Transient increase in passive permeability to ions and hypotonic swelling ensue. Close apposition of membranes to one another is enhanced through desialylation of receptors on one membrane by viral neuraminidase in the other, with release of diffusible NANA. IMP then become clustered, allowing fusion by interaction of lipids in the intervening protein-free portions of apposed membranes. Ultimately, there is reversal of ATP depletion, rephosphorylation, and reconstitution (repair) of fused membranes and redistribution of IMP, with stabilization of polyerythrocytes. All the steps in this sequence except initial attachment require that a state of fluidity exist in the membrane and hence are temperature dependent.

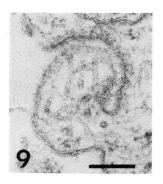

Fig. 9. Sendai virus was adsorbed to isolated chorioallantoic membrane fragments at 4°C for 45 min. After 4 min at 37°C, fusion of viral envelope to cell membrane has occurred. Formation of a phagocytic vesicle may be beginning above the attached virion. From Morgan and Howe (1968), by permission of the publisher. Bar = 100 nm.

The foregoing steps in Sendai viral hemolysis/fusion probably parallel those which occur following the attachment of paramyxoviruses to susceptible nucleated cells, although the sequence is not as readily analyzed as it is with erythrocytes. Transient damage to the permeability barrier noted with EAT cells following early stages of reaction with Sendai virus are probably explained on this or a similar basis (Okada *et al.*, 1975).

Morphological analyses by electron microscopy suggested that the genome of Sendai virus is introduced into susceptible cells through fusion of viral envelope with the membrane, thereby establishing continuity between the interior of the virion and the cytoplasm (Morgan and Howe, 1968). Virus was adsorbed to replicate isolated chorioallantoic membrane fragments or to mouse L929 cells in the cold. With shift of temperature to 37°C, fusion of viral envelope to cell membrane was observed (Fig. 9). Additional observations with other paramyxoviruses indicate that phagocytosis of viral inocula may also have a role in the initiation of infection. In a comparative analysis of SV5 in primary monkey kidney and in BHK21 cells (Compans *et al.*, 1964), virus was adsorbed to monolayers for 1–2 hr at 37°C and then examined after 10–30 min. Viral particles were seen in prephagocytic membrane invaginations and in cytoplasmic vacuoles in which there was morphological evidence of viral dismantlement. Neither fusion of virus with cellular membranes nor disintegration of virus at the cell surface were seen (Fig. 10).

These apparently divergent mechanisms of entry were reconciled in part by the results of another study in which SV5 was examined in

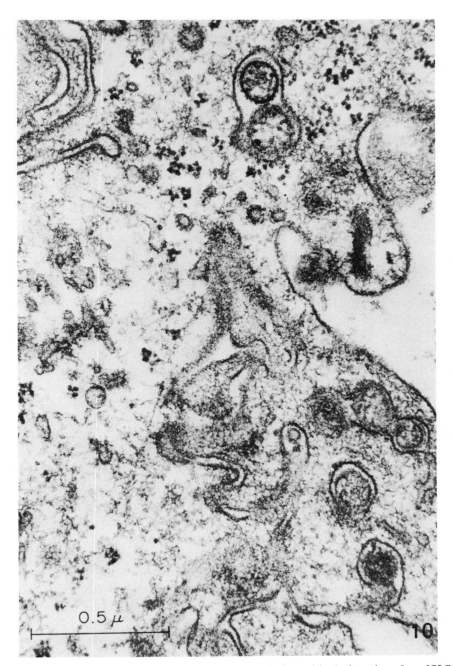

Fig. 10. Monkey kidney cell 20 min after inoculation with simian virus 5 at 37°C. Viral particles with intact envelopes are seen in deep invaginations of membrane or within vacuoles. Courtesy R. W. Compans. Bar = 500 nm.

HEp2 cells in suspension (Dermott and Samuels, 1973). Virus at a multiplicity of 50 was adsorbed in the cold for 1 hr; cells were then washed free of unadsorbed virus and incubated for various times at 37°C. Within 15 min, virions, singly or in clusters, were seen to enter cells directly by apparent fusion of viral envelope with cell membranes, with liberation of viral RNP into the cytoplasm. From 5 to 60 min after adsorption, however, single or clustered virions were also seen to undergo phagocytosis. Disintegration of viral envelopes took place simultaneously with release of RNP from the vacuoles into the cytoplasm. In contrast to the direct penetration by fusion, internalization by phagocytosis continued further into the period of incubation. The possibility was suggested that virus in critical amount which had fused with membrane at an early stage might in itself inhibit the direct entry of more particles by fusion and thus shift the trend toward viropexis in this particular system. From what is now known, particularly about the diffusion of viral envelope constiuents through the membrane from primary sites of viral attachment, this enforced "shift" to fusion resistance is not an unreasonable supposition. Besides the difference in effect between high and low MOI, variations in susceptibility among host cell types and virus strains must be considered, particularly with respect to fusion. Strains of NDV which showed little or no fusing activity were as infective as strongly fusing strains (Bratt and Gallaher, 1972; Poste and Waterson, 1975).

Sendai virus was found to interact specifically with model membranes (liposomes) composed of phosphatidylcholine, cholesterol, and gangliosides, the latter containing sialylated groupings necessary for interaction with viral HA (Haywood, 1975). The reaction of "receptor"-containing liposomes with virus could be directed toward either "fusion" or "engulfment" depending on the presence of auxiliary lipids. This suggested that the lipid composition in the area of primary viral adsorption might in the intact cell influence the mechanism of internalization toward either fusion or viropexis. Other studies related to viral fusion and involving the use of artificial membranes have been reviewed (Gallaher et al., 1979). Gangliosides in lipid bilayer model membranes have also been shown to bind influenza virus (Sharom et al., 1976), which, in contradistinction to Sendai virus, did not show a tendency to "fuse."

The initial interaction of HeLa and chicken embryo fibroblast cells with syncytiogenic strains of NDV and Sendai virus results in an increase in microviscosity (decreased fluidity) (Levanon and Kohn, 1978) measured as an increase in fluorescence polarization. These findings strengthened the view that during the process of direct penetration a mixture of viral envelope and cell membrane lipids occurred. As already pointed out, the change in microviscosity which accompanied influenza viral attachment was in the opposite direction, i.e., decrease in microviscosity, hence increased fluidity. This further lessened the probability that viral envelope–cell fusion actually occurs during direct penetration of orthomyxoviruses.

5.3. Morbilliviruses

Of the morbilliviruses, measles virus has received the most attention, directed primarily to late stages of morphogenesis (*cf.* Fraser and Martin, 1978). There is still some uncertainty regarding the number and function of the envelope proteins which mediate attachment, adsorption, and possibly penetration. This is due largely to the fact that the virus itself is difficult to purify to the complete exclusion of cellular material. A number of studies using PAGE analysis of maximally purified virus have established the presence in the virion of at least five polypeptides, three of which represent, respectively, nucleoprotein, P (?transcriptase-associated) protein, and membrane or matrix (M) protein. Of the remaining two, the largest is glycosylated (H, molecular weight 76,000–80,000) and appears to be the functional hemagglutinin of the virus. A second protein (F_1, molecular weight 42,000) is the reduction product of a large precursor glycoprotein (F, molecular weight 62,000) along with a smaller glycoprotein (F_2, molecular weight 15,000–20,000). F presumably mediates fusion and is therefore analogous to the F_1 protein of Sendai virus (Graves *et al.*, 1978; Hardwick and Bussell, 1978; Tyrrell and Norrby, 1978). The same two envelope components have been identified by immunoprecipitation with viral antibody on the membranes of cells lytically or persistently infected with measles virus (Fenger *et al.*, 1978). Measles virus H glycoprotein has no neuraminidase activity.

Measles virus agglutinates and lyses only erythrocytes of certain primate species, including rhesus monkeys and baboons (Periés and Chany, 1962). The same host restrictions apply to hemadsorption. In addition to the H component, which constitutes the normally functional hemagglutinin, disrupted virions or cells infected with certain strains of measles virus produce a smaller particle which agglutinates monkey erythrocytes in high salt concentrations only (e.g., 0.8 M ammonium sulfate) (Schluederberg and Nakamura, 1967) and not in isotonic saline. Hemadsorption to cells infected with these strains likewise is salt dependent. This salt-dependent agglutinin (SDA) appears to be a stable property of the infectious virion and to have the same erythrocyte receptor specificity as the normal hemagglutinin. An association has been reported between SDA and distinctive plaque morphology among SSPE isolates. These observations prompted the suggestion that SDA, with or without normal HA, might be a mutational characteristic of early isolates from which, on repeated passage in culture, normally hemagglutinating variants are selected (Shirodaria et al., 1976; Gould et al., 1976). The genetic basis for expression of the SDA property was further substantiated by controlled nitrosoguanidine mutagenesis of conventional strains of virus. One strain was encountered which, while fully as infectious as the parental strains, showed only the SDA. In comparison to the wild-type virus, the nonhemagglutinating mutant strain adsorbed as well to susceptible cells, was equally neurovirulent for neonatal hamsters, and gave identical protein PAGE profiles. The mutation reflected in the exclusively SDA was surmised to be due to minor alterations(s) in the main H glycoprotein (Breschkin et al., 1977).

As with Sendai virus, measles virus reacts with receptors which are contained in a glycoprotein. Unlike Sendai virus, however, the presence in the receptors of NANA is not required for primary interaction with the virus. In fact, desialylation of erythrocytes enhanced viral HA activity as well as adsorption to susceptible cells and subsequent penetration. Preinfection of cells with a paramyxovirus (mumps virus) did not block superinfection with measles virus. Conversely, primary infection of cells with measles virus did not interfere with the attachment and cell-fusing properties of Sendai virus (Wainberg and Howe, 1973). The receptors for measles virus are thus distinct from those for Sendai virus, a conclusion which has been supported by analyses of erythrocytes susceptible to agglutination by measles virus.

Glycoproteins with receptor activity have been isolated from rhesus monkey erythrocytes by treatment of hemoglobin-free membranes with lithium diiodosalicylate-phenol (LIS-ph) (Fenger and Howe, 1979). Five components were found which stained in PAGE with the periodic acid Schiff (PAS) reaction and were also positive for NANA by the resorcinal procedure. Of these, two (PAS2 and PAS4) were found to bind preferentially to measles virus. The receptor for measles virus on nucleated cells has not been identified, although indirect evidence indicates that NANA is not an essential part of the receptor.

The majority of human T lymphocytes have been found to possess binding sites for measles virus demonstrated by "rosetting" to persistently infected cells. The rosetting was specifically inhibited by antibody to virus. On the other hand, neither neuraminidase treatment of lymphocytes nor fetuin, a soluble receptor analogue, inhibited the binding of lymphocytes to infected cells, further suggesting that NANA was not involved in receptor activity. The "receptor" on T lymphocytes was unrelated to the donors' state of immunity, implying that specific sensitization to virus was not the mechanism for the observed rosetting (Valdimarsson *et al.*, 1975). Measles virus replication in lymphoblastoid B- and T-cell lines has been demonstrated by infectious center assays on African green monkey kidney cells. Since only a small proportion of either type of lymphocyte absorbed virus at any one time as revealed by subsequent viral replication, it was concluded that the necessary receptors were expressed only during certain phases of the cell cycle, possibly the S phase (Gallagher and Flanagan, 1976).

The ability of measles virus to cause giant cell formation in culture was one of the chief characteristics noted in the original report of the isolation of measles virus (Enders and Peebles, 1954). Along with rapid exofusion of nucleated cells by inactivated virus (Toyoshima *et al.*, 1960) and hemolysis, these effects of measles virus can now be ascribed to the same enveloped glycoproteins, namely, the H glycoprotein by which the virus attaches to cells and the separate "fusion factor" (Cascardo and Karzon, 1965) now recognized as a second envelope polypeptide, F.

Analysis of measles virus HA and hemolysis–fusion has provided a model for the probable mode of entry into nucleated cells capable of supporting viral replication (Bächi *et al.*, unpublished). Virus adsorbed to rhesus monkey erythrocyte poly-L-lysine monolayers (Bächi *et al.*, 1980) in the cold caused lysis of cells and resulted in fusion of contiguous erythrocytes with each other on warming to 37°C. This reaction was inhibited by antibody to virus but was enhanced by prior treatment of the monolayers with neuraminidase. Parallel monolayers of human erythrocytes pretreated with neuraminidase were resistant to hemolysis–fusion with Sendai virus, again emphasizing the requirement for NANA in receptors for some of the paramyxoviruses.

Electron microscopic examination showed a sequence of events very similar to those which occur with Sendai virus on human cells. Measles virions were seen to be attached by close apposition to invaginated segments of the erythrocyte membrane. With incubation at 37°C, viral envelope and cell membrane fused, viral antigen was dispersed along the membrane, and individual cells became fused with one another to form polyerythrocytes (Fig. 11). The loss of hemoglobin occurring during the fusion process varied in extent from cell to cell. Once formed, the polyerythrocytes appeared to be stable.

Measles virus was shown to react with Vero cells by a similar mechanism (Dubois-Dalcq and Barbosa, 1973). The penetration of an SSPE strain (McClellan) of measles virus was examined using peroxidase-labeled antibody. Virus was adsorbed to Vero cells for 1 hr at 37°C at a multiplicity greater than 10. One hour later attached virus was seen to have fused with cell membranes as with paramyxoviruses, continuity between virus and cytoplasm being thereby established. At this early stage the viral envelope and adjacent cell membrane with which it was continuous were specifically reactive with peroxidase-labeled antibody, indicating radial spread of viral antigen within the membrane (Fig. 12).

5.4. Pneumoviruses

Respiratory syncytial virus does not agglutinate or lyse any species of erythrocyte. Little is known regarding the specific nature of the cor-

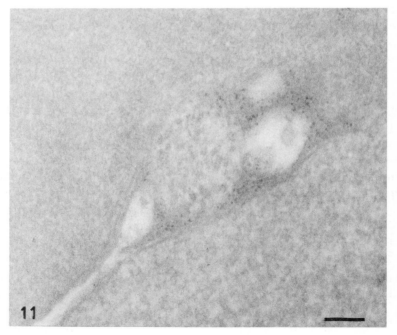

Fig. 11.   Early stage in the fusion of rhesus monkey erythrocytes by measles virus. Ferritin-labeled antibody identifies viral envelope antigens. Bar = 100 nm.

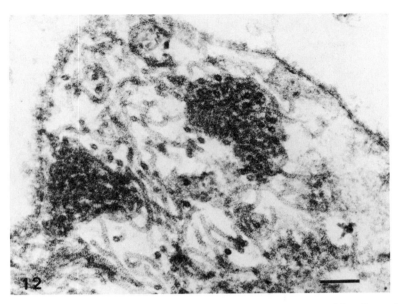

Fig. 12.   Internalization of measles virus by fusion of viral envelope with cell membrane 1 hr at 37°C after inoculation. No morphological remnants of viral envelope remain. However, viral surface antigen is identified by direct reaction with peroxidase-labeled human (SSPE) antibody to measles virus. From Dubois-Dalcq and Barbosa (1973), by permission of the publisher. Bar = 100 nm.

responding cell receptors. As with paramyxoviruses, however, RS virus appears to be capable of fusing with the cell membrane and thus introducing its genome into the cytoplasm (Fig. 13). Also, as with paramyxoviruses, viral antigen is disseminated into the membrane bilayer from sites of initial viral attachment (Howe *et al.*, 1974). Along with the characteristic endofusion which occurs during active infection (Bächi and Howe, 1973), these findings constitute suggestive evidence for the presence in the viral envelope of a "fusion factor" analogous to the F_1 protein of Sendai and the F protein of measles virus, respectively.

5.5.   Rhabdoviruses

The surface spikes of vesicular stomatitis virus (VSV) correspond with component II (Cohen *et al.*, 1970; Cohen and Summers, 1974) or the G envelope protein (Schloemer and Wagner, 1975) of molecular weight 69,000 (Morrison and McQuain, 1978) which contains NANA.

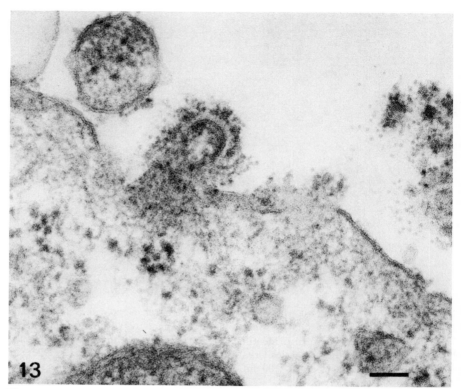

Fig. 13. Vero cell newly infected with RS virus. A viral particle heavily tagged with ferritin is seen attached to the membrane but incompletely fused with it. Internal structure is still visible within the virion, courtesy T. Bächi. Reprinted by permission of the publisher. Bar = 100 nm.

The G glycoprotein of VSV produced in mutant Chinese hamster ovary (CHO) cells reflected defects in glycosylation which formed the basis for resistance of the cells to lectins. Accordingly, virus produced by these lectin-resistant mutant CHO cells lacked NANA and other oligosaccharide structures, but was as infectious as fully glycosylated virus produced in HeLa cells. These findings indicate that the carbohydrate moieties of mature viral capsid glycoprotein probably do not have a critical role in viral adsorption (Robertson *et al.*, 1978).

In contrast to the orthomyxoviruses and paramyxoviruses, NANA is not an essential part of the cell receptor for VSV, virus being able to attach after desialylation by treatment of cells with either neuraminidase or trypsin (Schloemer and Wagner, 1975). The precise groupings which constitute the receptor are not known, except for their capacity specifically to recognize viral capsid protein. However, the wide host range of VSV among various cell lines suggests that the receptor is a common constituent of cell membranes, possibly involving lipid and/or lipoprotein, which in the human erythrocyte may contain receptors for VSV hemagglutination (Cohen and Summers, 1974).

The entry of VSV into L cells was shown to occur by engulfment or phagocytosis (Simpson *et al.*, 1969). At a MOI of 500, VSV adsorbed to L cells for 90 min at 4°C, attachment occurring usually by the rounded tip of the virion to invaginated sites in the cell membrane (Fig. 14). The latter appeared to be coated, signalling the initiation of active phagocytosis. Following elevation of temperature to 37°C, engulfment proceeded and was completed in a time period corresponding to that required for eclipse of the infectious inoculum. It was concluded that viropexis was an obligatory step for the initiation of infection.

An alternate mode of entry by VSV has been recognized in the same cell system (Heine and Schnaitman, 1969, 1971). VSV particles were adsorbed at 4°C for 15 min and then incubated at 37°C for 15 min. At this point viral particles were seen to fuse completely by their square ends to the plasma membrane, with which the viral envelope became continuous (Fig. 15). The fusion process was temperature dependent. Viral antigen could be detected over the membrane of infected cells by specific reactivity with hybrid antiviral-antiferritin antibody. The specifically stained areas of cell membrane were otherwise morphologically identical to adjacent nonreactive segments of membrane and there were no morphological remnants of viral envelope. These results are consistent with the fluid model of the cell membrane in which viral antigens are transported along the plane of the bilayer to areas remote from the sites of initial viral attachment. It might be noted here that, in contrast to paramyxoviruses and HSV, VSV does not induce cell-to-cell fusion exogenously and is not known to elaborate a "fusion factor," the G protein being the only mechanism of viral attachment to cell. Since temperature-dependent fusion of viral envelope and cell membrane is a necessary prelude to penetration of the viral genome, some mixture of lipids in viral and cellular bilayers probably occurs. The effect on the virion, once attached and fused, may relate to such an exchange, a possibility strengthened by studies on the interaction of VSV with unilamellar vesicles composed of phosphatidylcholine (Moore *et al.*, 1978). As a result of contact with these vesicles, viral particles lost infectivity and membranes were depleted of cholesterol. The implications of these findings with artificial vesicles are not yet clear, particularly as they may relate to the mechanism of viral penetration through a natural membrane barrier. However, lipid exchange between apposed membranes may occur during initial union of virus and cell.

Quantitative studies on VSV penetration have shown that viropexis is the principal mode of entry. Following synchronized adsorption of virus to L929 cells at MOI of 10–100, fusion was a rarely observed event, even with centrifugation and in the absence of serum (Dahlberg, 1974).

5.6. Togaviruses

Sindbis virus, an alphavirus which has been widely used in analyzing the molecular biology of togaviruses, interacts with erythrocytes to

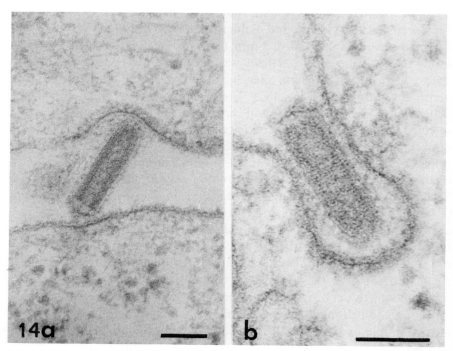

Fig. 14. Viropexis of vesicular stomatitis virus after adsorption to L cells in suspension. (a) Attachment of VS virions by round end to L cell at site showing submembranal thickening (upper) not evident in lower membrane. From Simpson *et al.* (1969). Reprinted by permission of the publisher. (b) An intact particle almost completely internalized by viropexis. Note the thickening of the cell membrane which marks, at an earlier stage, the site of interaction of the virus with cell. (c) A viral particle in a nearly completed vacuole, the wall of which is thickened as in (b). Courtesy S. Dales. Bars = 100 nm.

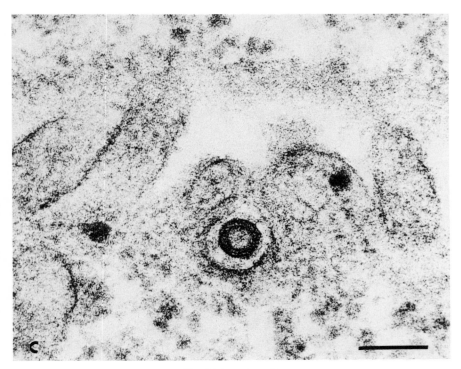

Fig. 14 (*continued*)

cause agglutination within a relative narrow range of pH (6–7). The character of the corresponding erythrocyte receptors, however, remains obscure. Evidently, neither proteins nor glycoproteins are directly involved because Sindbis HA can be inhibited by lipids extractable from human serum. Radiolabeled Sindbis virus could bind to protein-free liposomes containing sheep erythrocyte phospholipids and cholesterol. The interaction displayed the same pH dependence as that governing agglutination of sheep erythrocytes by virus. Phosphatidylethanolamine and cholesterol were the most active lipids in the system, whereas erythrocyte glycoproteins and gangliosides were not required (Mooney *et al.*, 1975). The question remains unresolved as to the identity of the putative phospholipid "receptor," either on liposomes or erythrocytes, with receptors on susceptible nucleated cells. A hint that protein may form part of the receptor on chick embryo fibroblasts is afforded by the finding that tryptic digests, which contained the attachment site activity (ASA) for Rous sarcoma virus, also blocked the attachment of Sindbis virus to the cells (Moldow *et al.*, 1977*b*).

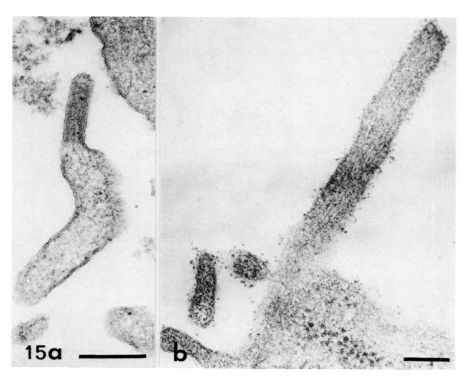

Fig. 15.   Vesicular stomatitis virus adsorbed to L cells at 4°C for 15 min and then incubated at 37°C for 15 min. (a) Envelope of one virion is fused by its square end to the tip of a microvillus. From Heine and Schnaitman (1969). (b) Pseudopodium from an infected cell stained with hybrid antiviral-antiferritin antibody. Viral antigen is widely distributed over the cell membrane which contains no morphological viral residue. From Heine and Schnaitman (1971), by permission of the publisher. Bar = 200 nm.

Evidence has recently been presented to indicate that receptors for Semliki Forest virus (SFV) may be closely associated or even identical with histocompatibility antigens coded for in human cells by the *HLA-A* and *HLA-B* loci, and in mouse L cells by the *H-2K* or *H-2D* loci. Spike glycopeptides isolated from intact virions as 29 S complexes blocked complement-dependent cytolytic antibody to murine antigens; HLA-A and -B antigens incorporated into liposomes competitively inhibited viral binding to human cells by forming complexes with virus which were specifically precipitable by antibody to virus (Helenius *et al.*, 1978).

From studies of SFV, it appears that envelope glycoproteins constituting the viral spikes mediate attachment to erythrocytes and to susceptible cells. Other than providing a hydrophilic environment for the viral particle, viral NANA residues are not involved in viral attachment or antigenicity, which is probably mediated by the envelope polypeptide(s) (Kennedy, 1974). Accordingly, removal of the spikes and hence all of the polypeptide portion of the viral envelope reduced infectivity, hemagglutination, and reactivity with antiviral antibody, and left viral cores intact. By subjecting purified SFV to disruption with NP40, it was possible to show the separate antigenic identities of envelope and core proteins (Appleyard *et al.*, 1970). Hemagglutinin and neutralizing antibody-blocking activity were found to be associated with the principal protein antigen on the viral envelope, which in both Sindbis and SFV has a molecular weight of 50,000–60,000. This corresponds with the earlier finding that envelopes of Sindbis virus contain but one glycoprotein which is in this size range and which does not penetrate through the lipid layer (Compans, 1971). The intact viral envelope is therefore required for internalization of attached virus (Bose and Sagik, 1970), which apparently occurs principally by viropexis. The importance of the ionic environment to the interaction of alphaviruses with cell surfaces is underlined by the results of studies on the binding of Sindbis virus to chicken embryo fibroblasts (Pierce *et al.*, 1974). Under graded conditions of ionic strength, maximal binding of ^{14}C-labeled virus occurred at ionic strength 0.15 at 37°C, at which 80% of the virus became resistant to elution with buffer of 0.25 ionic strength. These findings were consistent with the possibility that eclipse and penetration had perhaps occurred as a result of irreversible fusion of viral envelope with the cell membrane, although there was no direct morphological evidence for this interpretation. There appears to be a significant effect of ionic strength of the medium in sorting out "loose" and "tight" particles, the former eluting, the latter being destined to penetrate. This ionic effect may have some relationship, as yet undefined, to the observed effect of low ionic strength in inhibiting the early stages of viral maturation. Budding of progeny virus at the cell surface is greatly retarded in medium of low ionic strength (Waite *et al.*, 1972). In these latter studies, freeze-etching electron microscopy was the basis for distinguishing emerging virions from those which had already been completed but were still adherent to the intact cell surface. It was surmised that low ionic strength partially inhibited the primary interaction of nucleocapsid with the inner aspect of the membrane, a necessary prelude to maturation. The latter change took place in patches distributed over the cell surface. Concordantly, membrane-associated particles were displaced as morphogenesis proceeded to completion, and the cell membrane was reformed by fusion behind freshly formed virions (Brown *et al.*, 1972). Adsorption of West Nile virus (an alphavirus) caused a marked increase in the fluidity of the cell membrane as shown by fluorescent polarization analysis (Levanon *et al.*, 1977). The observed changes were temperature dependent and required effective union of virus with receptors. Similar changes accompanied adsorption of naked viruses (EMC and polyoma), indicating that the effect was more than simple intermixing of viral and cellular lipids. Activation of intramembranal enzymes and concomitant changes in membrane structure and permeability may pave the way for entry by viropexis. That viropexis is the principal mode of penetration is further substantiated by results of quantitative analysis of virus-specific immune lysis of cells early in infection (Fan and Sefton, 1978). Cells to which either Sindbis virus or VSV had been adsorbed, even at very high MOI, were significantly less susceptible to lysis by antibody to homologous virus and complement than cells newly infected with Sendai virus. As already noted, Sendai virus penetration is preceded by incorporation of viral envelope antigens into the host cell membrane. This occurs to only minimal extent with the other two enveloped viruses, even though fusion has occasionally been observed electron microscopically.

5.7. RNA Tumor Viruses

The RNA tumor viruses, especially those in the avian and feline groups, have been classified according to the cell types which they infect. This classification is based on the specificity of viral receptors expressed on the surface of susceptible cells. Accordingly, avian RNA tumor viruses can be divided into five subgroups, each with different receptor specificities.

Receptors for virus subgroups B and D, however, display some functional cross-relationships. For example, patterns of interference show that infection with a given virus confers resistance to superinfection by others of the same subgroup. The classification of RNA tumor viruses into subgroups is also based on antigenicity of viral envelope proteins (reviewed by Tooze, 1973).

Studies of the specific interactions of Rauscher murine leukemia virus (MuVL) with cell surface receptors have provided evidence that the 71k envelope glycoprotein (gp71) is the principal mediator of attachment (Delarco and Todaro, 1976). Purified ^{125}I-labeled gp71 binding was used to measure the specific interaction. Receptors were· found on all murine cells tested in culture but not on human, rhesus monkey, or hamster cells. The host range in cultured cells corresponds to the restricted range of susceptibility to infection among different animal species. Cells already infected with mouse-tropic viruses failed to bind gp71. It was suggested that, as a result of primary infection with murine virus, receptors on the surface of cells prior to infection become involved in the process of viral maturation and as a result can no longer bind superinfecting virus or exogenous viral components.

Seemingly contradictory results have been obtained with thymotropic murine leukemia virus (Baird *et al.*, 1977). T-lymphoma cells transformed by the Maloney strain of MuLV retained receptor activity for the homologous virus but not for Gross MuLV. A hypothesis derived from these data suggested that a small number of target cells with M-MuLV receptors were transformed to yield a clone of T-lymphoma cells exhibiting receptors for the transforming virus. In contrast to the gp71-binding studies cited above (Delarco and Todaro, 1976) in which receptors for infecting virus became cryptic, the receptors on the lymphoid cell lines remained functional. The selection hypothesis has gained support from fluorescence-activated cell sorter (FACS) analysis of the binding of fluoresceinated and rhodaminated murine retroviruses to lymphoid cells (McGrath *et al.*, 1978). It was shown by blockade experiments that cells of thymic lymphomas induced by radiation leukemia virus (RadLV) bore receptors highly specific for RadLV, but none for nonleukemogenic retroviruses. The recognition of receptors by oncogenic retroviruses may therefore be central to the process of leukemogenic transformation and/or the selection of malignant clones during leukemogenesis *in vivo*. In addition, the presence of receptors as well as their number may be a function of the state of differentiation and the type of cell which in the intact host serves as the target of viral invasion. Along with later steps in penetration, the distribution of receptors may be under genetic control. Virus attached to genetically resistant as well as to susceptible cells but, in the former, penetration was blocked (Piraino, 1967; Moldow *et al.*, 1976). In both types of cells the reaction with virus occurred at "attachment sites" signaled by the presence of dense reticular material. At these sites (?gap junctions), Rous-associated virus (RAV2) was shown to attach and then to become internalized by viropexis (Fig. 16) (Dales and Hanafusa, 1972). Attachment sites for avian tumor viruses have been solubilized by treatment of chicken embryo fibroblasts with lithium diiodosalicylate (LIS) (Moldow *et al.*, 1977*a*). Using the Bryan strain of Rous sarcoma virus and Rous-associated viruses 1 and 2 labeled with [³H]uridine, inhibition of viral binding to CEF by the soluble material was measured quantitatively. Similarly, LIS extracts of human erythrocyte ghosts, comprising

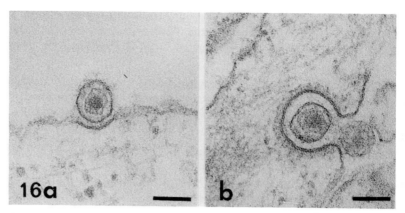

Fig. 16.   Secondary culture of chicken embryo fibroblasts exposed to avian sarcoma virus (Rous-associated virus 2) for 60 min at low temperature and then for 20 min at 37°C. Single virion (a) and one of another pair of virions (b) contained in a membrane invagination which possesses an internal coating perhaps representing receptor sites. From Dales and Hanafusa (1972), by permission of the publisher. Bar = 100 nm.

mostly glycophorin, were examined and found not to bind directly to RSV, although there was some interference with attachment of avian tumor virus. Tryptic digests of chicken embryo fibroblasts containing attachment site activity competitively interfered with viral infectivity. Receptor sites for other viruses are included in these protease-derived surface components, as already pointed out in connection with Sindbis virus (Moldow *et al.*, 1977*b*).

In attempting to analyse initial events of attachment and penetration of tumor viruses into susceptible cells, one of the hazards has been the occurrence of indigenous viral particles in primary mouse cell cultures. The availability of Swiss mice reportedly free of latent viruses has now made it possible to examine the penetration of murine leukemia virus. Primary cultures of Swiss (NIH) mouse embryo cells were exposed at 37°C to DEAE dextran in order to promote subsequent attachment of Rauscher leukemia virus at 4°C. Cultures were warmed to 37°C and examined at short intervals up to 3 hr (Fig. 17). Simultaneous dissolution of viral and cell membranes occurred at the site of viral attachment. By 30 min after adsorption, unenveloped nucleoids from mature inoculated particles were seen in the peripheral cytoplasm beneath the "openings" in the membrane. Alternatively, enveloped particles were also seen to penetrate intact to the cytoplasm through breaches in the cell membrane. Under the same conditions, phagocytosis of viral particles occurred even after 5 min at 37°C. The

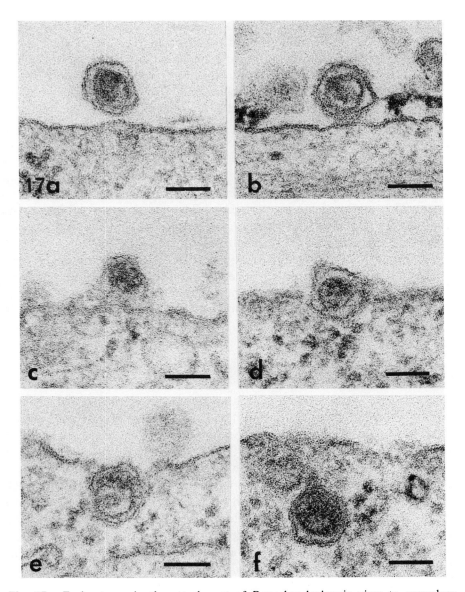

Fig. 17. Early stages in the attachment of Rauscher leukemia virus to secondary mouse (NIH Swiss) embryo fibroblasts free of indigenous type C virus. Virus was adsorbed at 4°C for 1 hr and then warmed to 37°C. Samples were taken from 2 to 180 min. (a) Mature virion in close proximity to cell membrane after 10 min at 37°C. (b) Beginning of dissolution of viral envelope after 30 min at 37°C. (c) Advanced dissolution of viral envelope at 60 min. (d,e) Dissolution of attachment site after 45 min at 37°C (f) Internalization of virion and apparent repair of cell membrane after 30 min at 37°C. From Miyamoto and Gilden (1971), by permission of the publisher. Bar = 100 nm.

activation of an unidentified enzyme was invoked to explain what appeared to be dissolution of viral envelope and release of viral cores. In the studies cited no fusion of viral envelope and cell membrane was unequivocally demonstrated. While the mode of entry was apparently by "direct penetration," phagocytosis could not be ruled out as an additional mechanism (Miyamoto and Gilden, 1971). It should be noted that even though no fusion was visualized, leucoviruses have been shown to be capable of exofusion of XC rat cells in culture (Johnson *et al.*, 1971). This cell line was derived from a tumor induced in rats by Rous sarcoma virus. The results of the studies cited suggested that formation of syncytia by mutual fusion of membranes was due to the action of MuLV-specific component(s). The additional possibility exists that simple attachment of leucoviruses to susceptible cells constitutes a transmembranal signal for internalization.

Among the oncornaviruses, mouse mammary tumor virus (MMTV) has been shown to penetrate by viropexis. B particles were seen at the surface of mouse embryo cells; these underwent phagocytosis over a 4-day period of incubation at 37°C and disintegrated in phagocytic vacuoles (Sarkar *et al.*, 1970).

5.8. Poxviruses

Vaccinia virus, being the largest animal virus and having characteristic morphology, was one of the first to be analyzed by electron microscopy in early stages of infection. In studies of penetration of virus into mouse L cells (Dales and Siminovitch, 1961; Dales and Kajioka, 1964), it was shown that entry was dependent on active phagocytosis by the cell, was energy dependent, and occurred with both infective virus and virus which had been heated or neutralized by antibody. Mutual dissolution of envelope and host cell membrane at the site of attachment also occurred. Radiolabeled virus was uncoated within the phagocytic vesicle, allowing the viral core to penetrate into the cytoplasm where viral replication was initiated.

Further insight into the initial interactions of vaccinia virus with cells has been gained by comparing the behavior of intracellular naked virus (INV) with that of extracellular enveloped virus (EEV). It was found that INV particles, with half the infectivity of EEV, penetrated only under conditions of unimpaired membrane function, as shown by reduced rate and failure to enter the cells at lower temperature or in the presence of inhibitors of endocytosis. In contrast, EEV penetrated by normal, uninhibited endocytosis and also under conditions which inhibited normal endocytosis (e.g., reduced temperature) and therefore also inhibited penetration of INV particles. It was implied that the major factor accounting for this behavioral difference between INV and EEV particles was the initial interaction with cell receptors, which was required for penetration even at reduced temperature. This interaction was specific only for EEV particles, since INV particles presumably lacked the necessary viral envelope component(s) for attachment to receptors. INV particles were therefore regarded as being only passive objects of normal endocytosis (Payne and Norrby, 1978).

In contrast to the foregoing concepts of entry by poxviruses, an alternative mechanism has been demonstrated in which the lipid-containing external viral envelope fuses with the cell membrane to allow the viral core to pass directly to the cytoplasm where uncoating takes place. This sequence is demonstrated in studies of *Amsacta moorei* insect poxvirus (Granados, 1973). Virus was administered *per os* to larvae of *Estigmene acraea* and the larval intestines were then sequentially examined by electron microscopy over a 2-hr period (Fig. 18). Intact viral particles were most frequently found fused to the apices

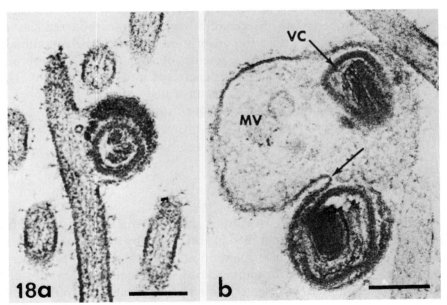

Fig. 18.   Penetration of pox virus (*Amsacta moorei*) into intestinal epithelial cells of the larva of *Estigmene acraea*, inoculated *per os* with 5×10^7 viral inclusion bodies. (a) Virus attached to the tip of a villus. (b) Core internalized after fusion of cell membrane with viral envelope (arrow). MV, microvilli, VC, viral core. From Granados (1973), by permission of the publisher. Bar = 200 nm.

of microvilli. At the time of penetration the viral envelope was lost, the cores, frequently several at a time, progressing to the bases of the microvilli and the lateral bodies disappearing in transit. In contrast to vaccinia virus, viropexis was a rarely observed event under the experimental conditions used. A similar process of entry has been shown with a baculovirus, *H. zea* nuclear polyhedrosis virus (Granados, 1978) and other insect poxviruses (Kawanishi *et al.*, 1972).

Further morphological evidence for viral fusion with cell membrane was offered by Armstrong *et al.* (1973). Fusion of vaccinia virus to cell membranes was shown to occur almost immediately at the end of the adsorption period, allowing viral cores to establish contact directly with the peripheral cytoplasm. In the published micrograph, there was unequivocal continuity between the triple layering of the two joined membranes. Little or no phagocytosis of viral particles was observed initially, but this was seen with increasing frequency as incubation progressed. These observations have been extended to an examination of vaccinia virus interacting with L and HeLa cells (Chang and Metz, 1976). In both systems entry occurred by fusion of virus to cell, followed by dispersal of viral antigens into small patches on the surface of the cell as revealed by reactivity with ferritin-labeled antibody. These foci of viral antigen were discernible in platinum–carbon replicas of cells fixed immediately after viral adsorption. Ferritin-labeled antibody was specifically reactive with segments of infected cell membrane overlying viral cores which had just penetrated into the cytoplasm. The entry of vaccinia virus was first demonstrated to occur by viropexis. More recent evidence supports the conclusion that membrane fusion mechanisms are also important modes of penetration by vaccinia virus. Both are illustrated in Fig. 19.

5.9. Herpesviruses

The mechanism whereby Herpes simplex virus (HSV) penetrates into susceptible cells was examined in HeLa cells by initial adsorption at 2–4°C for 1 hr followed by incubation at 37°C (Dales and Silverberg, 1969). It was found that disappearance of inoculum from the cell surface, as estimated by electron microscopic enumeration of cell-associated virions, was most rapid during the initial period of 30 min at 37°C. Apparently enveloped virions as well as naked particles were handled in the same manner by the cell. The rupture of the viral envelope did not interfere with attachment or envelopment of the parti-

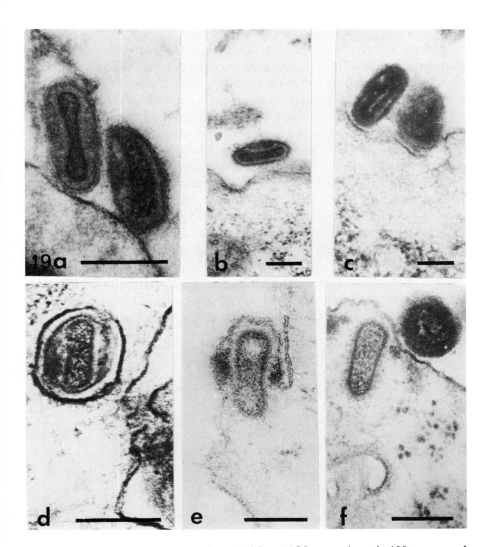

Fig. 19. Vaccinia virus adsorbed 1hr at 37°C at MOI approximately 100 to mouse L cells in suspension. (a,b) Attachment of virions to cell surface. (c) Early stage of engulfment of virus indicated by slight invagination of cell membrane at site of contact. a,b,c: Dales and Siminovitch (1961). (d) Viral particle in a cytoplasmic vacuole. From Dales (1963). (e) Viral envelope has fused with cell membrane 20 min after infection. Lateral bodies identify the segment of membrane to which they remain attached. (f) Viral core has reached the cytoplasm. Remnants of lateral bodies can be seen in close proximity to the plasma membrane. An enveloped virion remains outside the cell. (e,f) From Dales et al. (1976). All (a–f) by permission of the publisher. Bar = 200 nm.

cles by the plasma membrane and their ultimate rapid dismantlement in phagocytic vacuoles (Fig. 20).

In an autoradiographic analysis seeking to trace the path of inoculum radiolabeled DNA from adsorption to nucleus, the results tended to support viropexis as the main mode of entry. Evidence was presented to suggest that after passage through the cytoplasm, in which parental labeled DNA was found without attendant morphological viral remnants, some capsids were seen still in vesicles in which the viral envelopes appeared to be fused to the vesicular wall (Fig. 21). Ultimately, direct continuity appeared to be established between vesicular and nuclear membranes (Fig. 21). Parental DNA had reached the nucleus within 30 min after infection, the major portion of the viral inoculum having been engulfed by the cell within 15 min. The number of particles fused with the plasma membrane was relatively low, suggesting that pinocytosis was the predominant mode of entry (Hummeler *et al.*, 1969).

Further support for viropexis as the principal mode of entry for herpesviruses has come from analysis of the early stages of infection by equine abortion virus (EAV) (Abodeely *et al.*, 1970). Enveloped EAV,

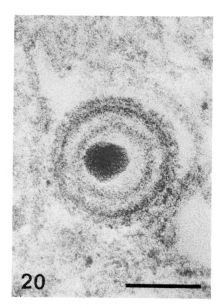

Fig. 20.   Herpes simplex virus at MOI of 20 adsorbed to HeLa cells 1 hr at 4°C. A completely enveloped virion is found in a phagocytic vacuole after 2 min of incubation at 37°C. From Dales and Silverberg (1969), by permission of the publisher. Bar = 100 nm.

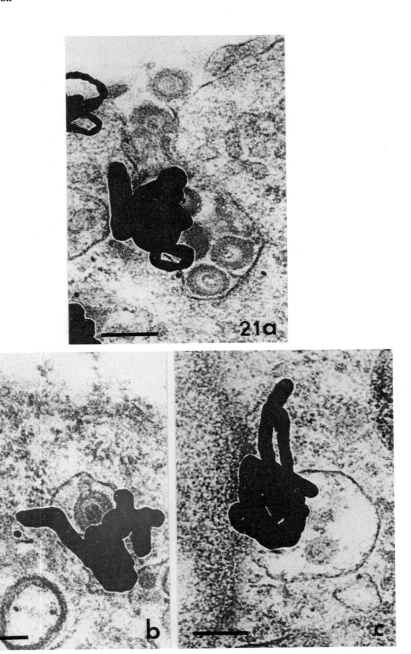

Fig. 21. [³H]Thymidine-labeled herpes simplex virus adsorbed to BHK21 cells. (a) Labeled viral particles internalized by pinocytosis within 15 min. (b) A few naked capsids in the cytoplasm. (c) Enveloped capsid being digested in vacuoles. Final transfer of labeled parental DNA took place through fusion of vesicular and nuclear membranes. From Hummeler *et al.* (1969), by permission of the publisher. Bar = 200 nm.

as well as EAV stripped of envelopes by treatment with NP-40 and sonication, were found to penetrate rapidly by viropexis into mouse L-M cells (Fig. 22). No evidence for fusion of viral envelope with cell membrane was found at any stage. Although the de-enveloped particles penetrated as well by viropexis as the enveloped virions, much lower levels of infectivity resulted than following penetration of normal virus. However, the fact that de-enveloped virions penetrated at all seemed to minimize the importance of the envelope to the process of entry since fusion would not be expected to occur in the absence of the viral lipid. In this latter study no morphological evidence was presented to suggest how the viral genome, once internalized, might progress to the site of transcription. HSV has been reported to enter the cell by fusion of viral envelope with cell membrane (Morgan *et al.*, 1968). The appearance of this process suggested that simultaneous dissolution of cell membrane and viral envelope was occurring at the sites of viral contact during the first 2 hr after infection.

In a subsequent analysis (Miyamoto and Morgan, 1971), two morphologically distinct types of HSV capsids were seen in the inoculum in approximately equal numbers. The more electron-dense type of capsid

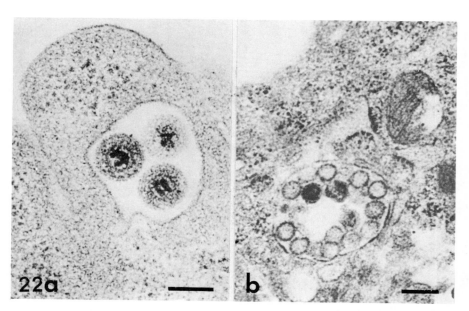

Fig. 22. Enveloped and unenveloped equine abortion viral particles in cytoplasmic (phagocytic) vacuoles. (a) 5 min and (b) 15 min postinfection. From Abodeely *et al.* (1970), by permission of the publisher. Bar = 200 nm.

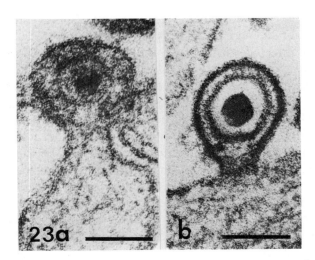

Fig. 23. Herpes simplex virus adsorbed at high multiplicity to HeLa cells at 4°C for 1 hr, then incubated at 37°C. (a) 5 min, (b) 2 min. Viral envelope apparently fused to cell membrane. From Miyamoto and Morgan (1971), by permission of the publisher. Bar = 100 nm.

was thought to undergo disruption in the cytoplasm immediately underlying the plasma membrane. Actual sites of fusion were difficult to find. In cells to which virus had been adsorbed at 4°C, penetration was seen to occur rapidly with elevation of the temperature to 37°C. Nevertheless, morphological evidence of fusion of viral envelope with plasma envelope was presented, including what were thought to be remnants of viral envelope seen as aggregates of dense material inserted into the plasma membrane immediately overlying the internalized virions (Fig. 23). Possession of an envelope seemed to be essential for the viral particle to employ this mechanism of viral penetration by fusion with the plasma membrane. Accordingly, it was inferred that any viral particles, whether dense or light, infectious or noninfectious, as long as they were enveloped, entered the cell. Some evidence was presented to suggest that a substantial number of virions might begin to undergo dissolution before actually penetrating into the cell. The significance of the different types of capsids, as seen before their dissolution, remains obscure. In the same preparations a small but significant number of virions were found in pinocytotic vesicles. From the available morphological evidence, then, it appears that HSV penetrates into the susceptible cell mainly by viropexis, fusion to cells perhaps being an auxiliary mechanism. This is consistent with the fact that HSV in sufficient concentration can cause exofusion. Certain other enveloped viruses, e.g., VSV and Sindbis virus, which do not cause exofusion, appear to enter cells predominantly by viropexis.

In cells infected with HSV the promotion and suppression of cell fusion, or syncytiogenesis (endofusion) late in viral infection have been shown to be the expression of two different viral glycoproteins. These deductions were based on studies with temperature-sensitive HSV1 mutants (Manservigi *et al.*, 1977). Both glycoproteins in question (C2 and B2) are constituents of the viral envelope and are also found in infected cell membranes. While most attention has been focused on late events in viral replication, it is not unreasonable to suppose that B2 may also play an essential role in the initiation of infection by promoting fusion of envelope to cell membrane (Sarmiento *et al.*, 1979). The B2 glycoprotein may also have a regulatory function in the later stages of viral infection characterized by endofusion. The role of the C2 glycoprotein is not clear.

The cytochalasins have a primary effect on membrane-mediated functions, particularly phagocytosis. They affect viral uptake in surprisingly varied manner, and also modify later stages of viral replication (see review by Koch and Koch, 1978). Indirect evidence for the role of envelope glycoproteins in attachment has come from analysis of the effect of cytochalasins on late events in the synthesis of herpes simplex viral proteins (Dix and Courtney, 1976). Cytochalasin B, by blocking membrane hexose transport, inhibited glycosylation of viral protein(s), with substantial reduction in the total yield of virus. Viral progeny also lacked infectivity. As shown also with poliovirus, cytochalasins enhanced the competence of cells for infection by isolated herpes viral DNA. Also, in analogy to polioviral infection, cytochalasin may be able to substitute for the function of viral protein(s) in suppressing cellular protein synthesis during infection of cells with the isolated viral DNA (see review by Koch and Koch, 1978). However, the effect of cytochalasin in enhancing infectivity was not due to increased adsorption or uptake of either poliovirus or herpesvirus nucleic acids (Farber and Eberle, 1977).

There is limited information regarding the nature of specific receptors for herpes simplex viruses. With Epstein-Barr virus (EBV), however, evidence for an apparently close association or relationship between receptors for complement component C3 and those for the virus on B lymphoblastoid cell lines has been adduced (Yefenof *et al.*, 1976, 1977). Receptors for C3 undergo "capping" by antibody to either attached C3 or attached EBV particles. EBV receptors may therefore be included in the same macromolecular complex within the membrane and be distinct from receptors for Fc or IgM, and from β2-micro-

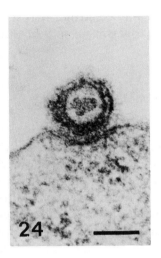

Fig. 24. EB virus interacting with lymphoblastoid T cell (MOLT 4), 90 min after infection. There is a suggestion of fusion between viral envelope and cellular membrane, which is thickened at the site of interaction. No penetration followed despite incubation up to 7 hr at 37°C. From Menezes *et al.* (1977), by permission of the publisher. Bar = 100 nm.

globulin. This was also consistent with the observation that only B lymphocytes can be infected and transformed into permanent lines by EBV.

In an extension of these studies it has been shown that EBV can be introduced into epithelial cells by fusion with B lymphocytes containing the viral genome (Glaser *et al.*, 1976). Cell hybrids made between Burkitt lymphoma cells and EBV-positive lymphocytes contained receptors for EBV which could then be induced. These findings provide a possible explanation not only for the penetration of epithelial cells by EB virus which may be shed into the oropharynx, but perhaps also for the initiation of tumors. The close association of C3 with EBV receptors was further suggested by results of studies of a unique T-cell line (MOLT 4) which, while lacking evidence for the viral genome, could be shown both to possess C receptors and to adsorb EBV. However, viral penetration did not occur. These findings indicate that additional factors besides cell receptors govern susceptibility to viral invasion. Figure 24 shows the adsorption of an EBV particle to the surface of a MOLT 4 cell exposed to a high MOI. There is a thickening of the membrane at the site of adsorption, presumably the start of viropexis, and even a suggestion of fusion of envelope to plasma membrane. However, no penetration occurred as evidenced by the total lack of subsequent new viral protein synthesis or any electron microscopic evidence of entry of viral particles into the cytoplasm up to 7 hr after infection (Menezes *et al.*, 1977).

6. SUMMARY AND CONCLUSION

In this chapter, we have attempted to bring together the morphological, biochemical, and biophysical concepts of viral attachment and penetration. Since the earliest electron microscopic observations, it has become increasingly evident that other technological approaches would be necessary in order to answer some of the questions inherent in this problem. For this reason we have also attempted to review briefly those biological, biochemical, and biophysical data which bear on the electron microscopic observations. From today's vantage point, it appears that no single modality governs the penetration of a given virus. Indeed, viral penetration is profoundly affected by the genetically controlled components of cell surfaces in relation to specific receptors, the nature of the viral surface, by uncontrolled variations among cell strains, and by the milieu in which the initial reactions between virus and cell take place. Virtually all of the observations on viral penetration have been made on cells in culture. Consequently, almost nothing is known about how the analogous phenomenon takes place in the living host. One nonetheless assumes that the mechanisms described have some bearing on the initiation of natural infection despite the necessity for high multiplicity input in order to enhance the statistical probability of finding, by TEM, virions undergoing penetration. Moreover, the onslaught on the single cell by many viral particles probably subjects the membrane to abnormal stresses which may not occur in the course of natural infection *in situ*.

All viruses, to greater or lesser extent, appear to be capable of entering cells by phagocytic mechanisms, which in this context have been subsumed by the term viropexis. Viropexis must now be understood to include the apparently direct penetration observed with certain of the naked viruses which are themselves irreversibly altered through initial reactions with receptors in the host cell membrane. Of the enveloped viruses, only paramyxoviruses (Sendai and NDV), measles, respiratory syncytial and vaccinia viruses have been shown unequivocally to penetrate into the host cell through fusion of viral envelope with cell membrane. Despite earlier claims, there is no valid biological evidence that orthomyxoviruses have this capability. We have attempted to illustrate variations of each of these mechanisms as they apply to the major viral groups and to relate the morphological aspects to salient biological features of the dynamic process of penetration. Newer techniques of electron microscopy, particularly freeze-etching and immunofreeze-etching, as well as antibody labeled with ferritin or peroxidase, have greatly extended the horizon of electron microscopy and have led the way to pertinent biological observations. This combined approach should continue to be productive in the future.

ACKNOWLEDGMENTS

Work by the authors cited in this review was supported by grants from the National Institutes of Health (AI 10945; AI 05744) and the Edward G. Schlieder Educational Foundation. The excellent clerical assistance of Sharon Delaney is gratefully acknowledged.

7. REFERENCES

Abodeely, R. A., Lawson, L. A., and Randall, C. C., 1970, Morphology and entry of enveloped and deenveloped equine abortion (Herpes) virus, *J. Virol.* **5**:513.

Appleyard, G., Oram, J. D., and Stanley, J. L., 1970, Dissociation of Semliki Forest virus into biologically active components, *J. Gen. Virol.* **9**:179.

Armstrong, J. A., Metz, D. H., and Young, R., 1973, The mode of entry of vaccinia virus into L cells, *J. Gen. Virol.* **21**:533.

Bächi, T., 1970, Elektronen mikroscopische Untersuchungen über den Infektionszyklus von Influenza A-viren in Ehrlich Aszites Tumor Zellen, *Pathol. Microbiol.* **36**:81.

Bächi, T., 1980, Morphological characterization of the erythrocyte membrane related to myxovirus receptors, *Acta Histochem. Suppl.* **XXII**:291–297.

Bächi, T., and Howe, C., 1973, Morphogenesis and ultrastructure of respiratory syncytial virus, *J. Virol.* **12**:1173.

Bächi, T., and Schnebli, H. P., 1975, Reactions of lectins with erythroyctes. II. Mapping of Con-A receptors by freeze-etching electron microscopy, *Exp. Cell Res.* **91**:285.

Bächi, T., Aguet, M., and Howe, C., 1973, Fusion of erythrocytes by Sendai virus studied by immuno-freeze etching, *J. Virol.* **11**:1004.

Bächi, T., Deas, J. E., and Howe, C., 1977a, Virus–erythrocyte interactions, in: *Virus Infection and the Cell Surface* (G. Poste and G. L. Nicolson, eds.), pp. 83–127, North-Holland, Amsterdam.

Bächi, T., Whiting, K., Tanner, M. J. A., Metaxas, M. N., and Anstee, D. J., 1977b, Freeze-fracture electron microscopy of human erythrocytes lacking the major membrane sialoglycoprotein, *Biochim. Biophys. Acta* **464**:635.

Bächi, T., Eichenberger, G., and Hauri, H. P., 1978, Sendai virus hemolysis: Influence of lectins and analysis by immune fluorescence, *Virology* **85**:518.

Baird, S., Raschke, W., and Weissman, I. L., 1977, Evidence that MuLV-induced thymic lymphoma cells possess specific cell membrane binding sites for MuLV, *Int. J. Cancer* **19**:403.

Barbanti-Brodano, G., Swetly, P., and Koprowski, H., 1970, Early events in the infection of permissive cells with simian virus 40: Adsorption, penetration and uncoating, *J. Virol.* **6**:78.

Blaskovic, P., Rhodes, A. J., Doane, F. W., and Labzeffsky, N. A., 1972, Infection of chick embryo tracheal organ cultures with influenza A₂ (Hong Kong) virus, *Arch. Gesamte Virusforsch.* **38**:250.

Boand, A. V., Jr., Kempf, J. E., and Hanson, R. J., 1957, Phagocytosis of influenza virus. I. *In vitro* observations, *J. Immunol.* **79**:416.

Bose, H. R., and Sagik, B. P., 1970, The virus envelope in cell attachment, *J. Gen. Virol.* **9**:159.

Branton, D., Bullivant, S., Gilula, N. B., Karnofsky, M. J., Moor, H., Mühlethaler, K., Northcote, D. H., Packer, L., Satir, B., Satir, P., Speth, V., and Staehlin, L. A., 1975, Freeze-etching nomenclature, *Science* **190**:54.

Bratt, M. A., and Gallaher, W. R., 1972, Biological parameters of fusion from without and fusion from within, in: *Membrane Research* (C. F. Fox, ed.), pp. 383–406. Academic Press, New York.

Breschkin, A. M., Walmer, B., and Rapp, F., 1977, Hemagglutination variant of measles virus, *Virology* **80**:441.

Brown, D. T., and Burlingham, B. T., 1973, Penetration of host cell membranes by adenovirus 2, *J. Virol.* **12**:386.

Brown, D. T., Waite, M. R. F., and Pfefferkorn, E. R., 1972, Morphology and morphogenesis of Sindbis virus as seen with freeze-etching techniques, *J. Virol.* **10**:524.

Cascardo, M., and Karzon, D. T., 1965, Measles virus giant cell inducing factor (fusion factor), *Virology* **26**:311.

Chan, V. F., and Black, F. L., 1970, Uncoating of poliovirus by isolated plasma membranes, *J. Virol.* **5**:309.

Chang, A., and Metz, D. H., 1976, Further investigations on the mode of entry of vaccinia virus into cells, *J. Gen. Virol.* **32**:275.

Chardonnet, Y., and Dales, S., 1970a, Early events in the interaction of adenovirus with HeLa cells. I. Penetration of type 5 and intracellular release of the DNA genome, *Virology* **40**:462.

Chardonnet, Y., and Dales, S., 1970b, Early events in the interaction of adenovirus with HeLa cells. II. Comparative observation on the penetration of types 1, 5, 7, 12, *Virology* **40**:478.

Chardonnet, Y., and Dales, S., 1972, Early events in the interaction of adenoviruses with HeLa cells. III. Relationship between an ATPase activity in nuclear envelopes and transfer of core materials: A hypothesis, *Virology* **48**:342.

Choppin, P. W., and Scheid, A., 1980, The role of viral glycoproteins in adsorption, penetration, and pathogenicity of viruses, *Rev. Infect. Dis.* **2**:40–61.

Clinton, G. M., and Hayashi, M., 1976, The parvovirus MVM: A comparison of heavy and light particle infectivity and their density conversion *in vitro*, *Virology* **74**:57.

Cohen, G. H., and Summers, D. F., 1974, *In vitro* association of vesicular stomatitis virus proteins with purified HeLa and erythrocyte plasma membranes, *Virology* **57**:566.

Cohen, G. H., Atkinson, P. H., and Summers, D. F., 1970, Interactions of vesicular stomatitis virus structural proteins with HeLa plasma membranes, *Nature (London) New Biol.* **231**:121.

Collins, J. K., and Knight, C. A., 1978, Removal of carbohydrate from influenza A virus and its hemagglutinin and the effect on biological activities, *J. Virol.* **27**:164.

Compans, R. W., 1971, Location of the glycoprotein in the membrane of Sindbis virus, *Nature (London) New Biol.* **229**:114.

Compans, R. W., Holmes, K. V., Dales, S., and Choppin, P. W., 1964, An electron microscopic study of moderate and virulent virus-cell interactions of the parainfluenza virus SV5, *Virology* **30**:411.

Dahlberg, J. E., 1974, Quantitative electron microscopic analysis of the penetration of VSV into L cells, *Virology* **58**:250.

Dales, S., 1962, An electron microscopic study of the early association between two mammalian viruses and their hosts, *J. Cell Biol.* **13**:303.

Dales, S., 1963, The uptake and development of vaccinia virus in strain L cells followed with labeled viral deoxyribonucleic acid, *J. Cell Biol.* **18**:51.

Dales, S., 1973, Early events in cell-animal virus interactions, *Bacteriol. Rev.* **37**:103.

Dales, S., and Hanafusa, H., 1972, Penetration and intracellular release of the genomes of avian RNA tumor viruses, *Virology* **50**:440.

Dales, S., and Kajioka, R., 1964, The cycle of multiplication of vaccinia virus in Earle's strain L cells. I. Uptake and penetration, *Virology* **24**:278.

Dales, S., and Pons, M., 1976, Penetration of influenza examined by means of virus aggregates, *Virology* **69**:278.

Dales, S., and Silverberg, H., 1969, Viropexis of *Herpes simplex* virus by HeLa cells, *Virology* **37**:475.

Dales, S., and Siminovitch, L., 1961, The development of vaccinia virus in Earle's L strain cells as examined by electron microscopy, *J. Biophys. Biochem. Cytol.* **19**:475.

Dales, S., Stern, W., Weintraub, S. B., and Huima, T., 1976, Genetically controlled surface modifications by poxviruses influencing cell-cell and cell-virus interactions, in: *Cell Membrane Receptors for Viruses, Antigens and Antibodies, Polypeptide Hormones and Small Molecules* (R. F. Beers, Jr. and E. G. Bassett, eds.), pp. 253–270, Raven Press, New York.

Deas, J. E., Lee, L. T., Howe, C., 1978, Peripheral proteins of human erythrocytes, *Biochem. Biophys. Res. Commun.* **82**:296.

Delarco, J., and Todaro, G. J., 1976, Membrane receptors for murine leukemia viruses: Characterization using the purified viral envelope glycoprotein, gp71, *Cell* **8**:365.

Dermott, E., and Samuels, J., 1973, Electron microscopic observations on the mechanisms of entry of simian foamy virus in HEp-2 cells, *J. Gen. Virol.* **19**:135.

Dix, R. D., and Courtney, R. J., 1976, Effects of cytochalasin B on Herpes simplex virus type 1 replication, *Virology* **70**:127.

Dourmashkin, R. R., and Tyrrell, D. A. J., 1970, Attachment of two myxoviruses to ciliated epithelial cells, *J. Gen. Virol.* **9**:77.

Dourmashkin, R. R., and Tyrrell, D. A. J., 1974, Electron microscopic observations on the entry of influenza virus into susceptible cells, *J. Gen. Virol.* **24**:129.

Dubois-Dalcq, M., and Barbosa, L. H., 1973, Immunoperoxidase stain of measles antigen in tissue culture, *J. Virol.* **12**:909.

Dunnebacke, T. H., Levinthal, J. D., and Williams, R. C., 1969, Entry and release of poliovirus as observed by electron microscopy of cultured cells, *J. Virol.* **4**:505.

Enders, J. F., and Peebles, T. C., 1954, Propagation in tissue cultures of cytopathogenic agents from patients with measles, *Proc. Soc. Exp. Biol. Med.* **86**:277.

Enegren, B. J., and Burness, A. T. H., 1977, Chemical structure of attachment sites for viruses on human erythrocytes, *Nature (London)* **268**:536.

Fan, D. P., and Sefton, B. M., 1978, The entry into host cells of Sindbis virus, vesicular stomatitis virus and Sendai virus, *Cell* **15**:985.

Farber, F. E., and Eberle, R., 1977, Effects of cytochalasin and alkaloid drugs on the biological expression of herpes simplex virus type 2 DNA, *Exp. Cell Res.* **103**:15.

Fazekas de St. Groth, S., 1948, Viropexis, the mechanism of influenza virus infection, *Nature (London)* **162**:294.

Fenger, T. W., and Howe, C., 1979, Isolation and characterization of erythrocyte receptors for measles virus, *Proc. Soc. Exp. Biol. Med.* **162**:299.

Fenger, T. W., Smith, J. W., and Howe, C., 1978, Analysis of immunoprecipitated surface glycoproteins in measles virions and in membranes of infected cells, *J. Virol.* **28**:292.

Fidgen, K. J., 1975, The action of *Vibrio cholerae* and *Corynebacterium diphtheriae* neuraminidases on the Sendai virus receptor of human erythrocytes, *J. Gen. Microbiol.* **89**:49.

Fraser, K. B., and Martin, S. J., 1978, Measles virus and its biology, in: *Experimental Virology* (T. W. Tinsley and F. Brown, eds.), Academic Press, London.

Gallagher, M. R., and Flanagan, T. D., 1976, Replication of measles virus in continuous lymphoid cell lines, *J. Immunol.* **116**:1084.

Gallaher, W. R., and Howe, C., 1976, Identification of receptors for animal viruses, *Immunol. Commun.* **5**:535.

Gallaher, W. R., Levitan, D. B., Kirwin, K. S., and Blough, H. A., 1979, Molecular and biological parameters of membrane fusion, in: *Cell Membranes and Viral Envelopes* (H. A. Blough and J. M. Tiffany, eds.), p. 395, Academic Press, London.

Glaser, R., De The, G., Lenoir, G., and Ho, J. H., 1976, Superinfection of epithelial nasopharyngeal carcinoma cells with Epstein-Barr virus, *Proc. Natl. Acad. Sci. USA* **73**:960.

Gould, E. A., Ratcliffe, N. A., Basarab, O., and Smith, H., 1972, Studies of the basis of localization of influenza virus in ferret organ cultures, *Br. J. Exp. Pathol.* **53**:31.

Gould, E. A., Cosby, S. L., and Shirodaria, P. V., 1976, Salt-dependent haemagglutinating measles virus in S.S.P.E., *J. Gen. Virol.* **33**:139.

Granados, R. R., 1973, Entry of an insect poxvirus by fusion of the virus envelope with the host cell membrane, *Virology* **52**:305.

Granados, R. R., 1978, Early events in the infection of *Heliothis zea* midgut cells by a baculovirus, *Virology* **90**:170.

Graves, M. C., Silver, S. M., and Choppin, P. W., 1978, Measles virus polypeptide synthesis in infected cells, *Virology* **86**:254.

Hardwick, J. M., and Bussell, R. H., 1978, Glycoproteins of measles virus under reducing and nonreducing conditions, *J. Virol.* **25**:687.

Haywood, A. M., 1975, "Phagocytosis" of Sendai virus by model membranes, *J. Gen. Virol.* **29**:63.

Heine, J. W., and Schnaitman, C. A., 1969, Fusion of vesicular stomatitis virus with the cytoplasmic membrane of L cells, *J. Virol.* **3**:619.

Heine, J. W., and Schnaitman, C. A., 1971, Entry of vesicular stomatitis virus into L cells, *J. Virol.* **8**:786.

Helenius, A., Morein, B., Fries, E., Simons, K., Robinson, P., Schirrmacher, V., Terhorst, C., and Strominger, J. L., 1978, Human (HLA-A and HLA-B) and murine (H-2K and H-2D) histocompatibility antigens on cell surface receptors for Semliki Forest virus, *Proc. Natl. Acad. Sci. USA* **75**:3846.

Hennache, B., and Boulanger, P., 1977, Biochemical study of KB-cell receptor for adenovirus, *Biochem. J.* **166**:237.

Holmes, I. H., Rodger, S. M., Schnagl, R. D., Ruck, B. J., Gust, I. D., Bishop, R. F., and Barnes, G. L., 1976, Is lactase the receptor and uncoating enzyme for infantile enteritis (Rota) viruses? *Lancet* **1**:1387.

Homma, M., Shimizu, K., Shimizu, Y. K., and Ishida, N., 1976, On the study of Sendai virus hemolysis. I. Complete Sendai virus lacking in hemolytic activity, *Virology* **71**:41.

Howe, C., and Bächi, T., 1973, Localization of erythrocyte membrane antigens by immune electron microscopy, *Exp. Cell Res.* **76**:321.

Howe, C., and Lee, L. T., 1972, Virus-erythrocyte interactions, *Adv. Virus Res.* **17**:1.

Howe, C., and Morgan, C., 1969, Interactions between Sendai virus and human erythrocytes, *J. Virol.* **3**:70.

Howe, C., Bächi, T., and Hsu, K. C., 1974, Application of immunoferritin techniques for the detection of viral and cellular antigens, in: *Viral Immunodiagnosis* (E. Kurstak and R. Morisset, eds.), pp. 215–234, Academic Press, New York.

Hummeler, K., Tomassini, N., and Zajac, B., 1969, Early events in herpes simplex virus infection: An autoradiographic study, *J. Virol.* **4**:67.

Hummeler, K., Tomassini, N., and Sokol, F., 1970, Morphological aspects of the uptake of simian virus 40 by permissive cells, *J. Virol.* **6**:87.

Jackson, R. L., Segrest, J. P., Kahane, I., and Marchesi, V. T., 1973, Studies on the major sialoglycoprotein of the human red cell membrane. Isolation and characterization of tryptic glycopeptides, *Biochemistry* **12**:3131.

Johnson, G. S., Friedman, R. M., and Pastan, I., 1971, Analysis of fusion of XC cells induced by homogenates of murine leukemia virus-infected cells and by purified murine leukemia virus, *J. Virol.* **7**:753.

Kawanishi, C. Y., Summer, M. D., Stolz, D. B., and Arnott, H. J., 1972, Entry of an insect virus *in vivo* by fusion of viral envelope and microvillus membrane, *J. Inverteb. Pathol.* **20**:104.

Kennedy, S. I. T., 1974, The effect of enzymes on structural and biological properties of Semliki Forest virus, *J. Gen. Virol.* **23**:129.

Knutton, S., 1977, Studies of membrane fusion. II. Fusion of human erythrocytes by Sendai virus, *J. Cell Sci.* **28**:189.

Knutton, S., and Bächi, T., 1980, The role of cell swelling and haemolysis in Sendai virus-induced cell fusion and in diffusion of incorporated viral antigens, *J. Cell Sci.* **42**:153.

Koch, G., and Koch, F., 1978, The use of cytochalasins in studies on the molecular biology of virus-host cell interactions, in: *Cell Surface Reviews: Cytochalasins: Biochemical and Cell Biological Aspects* (S. W. Tanenbaum, ed.), Chap. 15, pp. 475–498, Elsevier/North-Holland Biomedical Press, Amsterdam.

Lakshmi, M. V., and Schulze, I. T., 1978, Effects of sialylation of influenza virions on their interactions with host cells and erythrocytes, *Virology* **88**:314.

Levanon, A., and Kohn, A., 1978, Changes in cell membrane microviscosity associated with adsorption of viruses. Differences between fusing and non-fusing viruses, *FEBS Lett.* **85**:245.

Levanon, A., Kohn, A., and Inbar, M., 1977, Increase in lipid fluidity of cellular membranes induced by adsorption of RNA and DNA virions, *J. Virol.* **22**:353.

Linser, P., Bruning, H., and Armentrout, R. W., 1978, Uptake of minute virus of mice into cultured rodent cells, *J. Virol.* **31**:537.

Linser, P., Bruning, H., and Armentrout, R. W., 1977, Specific binding sites for a parvovirus, minute virus of mice, on cultured mouse cells, *J. Virol.* **24**:211.

Lonberg-Holm, K., and Philipson, L., 1969, Early events of virus-cell interaction in an adenovirus system, *J. Virol.* **4**:323.

Lonberg-Holm, K., and Philipson, L., 1974, Early interaction between animal viruses and cells, Monographs in Virology No. 9 (J. L. Melnick, ed.), S. Karger, Basel.

Lonberg-Holm, K., and Philipson, L., 1979, Molecular aspects of virus receptors and cell surfaces, in: *Cell Membranes and Viral Envelopes* (H. A. Blough and J. M. Tiffany, eds.), Academic Press, London.

Lonberg-Holm, K., Crowell, R. L., and Philipson, L., 1976a, Unrelated animal viruses share receptors, *Nature (London)* **259**:679.

Lonberg-Holm, K., Gosser, L. B., and Shimshick, E. J., 1976b, Interaction of liposomes with subviral particles of poliovirus type 2 and rhinovirus type 2, *J. Virol.* **19**:746.

Loyter, A., Ben-Zaquen, R., Marash, R., and Milner, Y., 1977, Dephosphorylation of human erythrocyte membranes induced by Sendai virus, *Biochemistry* **16**:3903.

Lutz, H. U., von Däniken, A., and Bächi, T., 1978, Segregation of glycophorin from other integral membrane proteins, Experientia 34/7 July, 1978, Union of Swiss Societies of Experimental Biology, Abstracts of 10th Annual Meeting, p. 22.

Lutz, H. U., von Däniken, A., Semenza, G., and Bächi, T., 1979, Glycophorin-enriched vesicles obtained by a selective extraction of human erythrocyte membranes with a non-ionic detergent, *Biochim. Biophys. Acta* **552**:262.

Lyles, D. S., and Landsberger, F. R., 1976, Virus and lectin agglutination of erythrocytes: Spin label study of membrane lipid-protein interactions, *Proc. Natl. Acad. Sci. USA* **73**:3497.

Lyon, M., Chardonnet, Y., and Dales, S., 1978, Early events in the interaction of adenoviruses with HeLa cells. V. Polypeptides associated with the penetrating inoculum, *Virology* **87**:81.

Mackay, R. L., and Consigli, R. A., 1976, Early events in polyoma virus infection: Attachment, penetration and nuclear entry, *J. Virol.* **19**:620.

Mandel, B., 1967a, The interaction of neutralized poliovirus with HeLa cells. I. Adsorption, *Virology* **31**:238.

Mandel, B., 1967b, The interaction of neutralized poliovirus with HeLa cells. II. Elution, penetration, uncoating, *Virology* **31**:248.

Manservigi, R., Spear, P. G., and Buchan, A., 1977, Cell fusion induced by herpes simplex virus is promoted and suppressed by different viral glycoproteins, *Proc. Natl. Acad. Sci. USA* **74**:3913.

Marchesi, V. T., Furthmayr, H., and Tomita, M., 1976, Molecular features of a sialoglycoprotein of the human erythrocyte membrane which carries influenza virus receptors, in: *Cell Membrane Receptors for Viruses, Antigens and Antibodies, Polypeptides and Small Molecules* (R. E. Beers, Jr., and E. G. Bassett, eds.), Raven Press, New York.

Maul, G. D., Rovera, G., Vorbrodt, A., and Abramezuk, J., 1978, Membrane fusion as a mechanism of simian virus 40 entry into different cellular compartments, *J. Virol.* **28**:936.

McGrath, M. S., Declève, A., Lieberman, M., Kaplan, H. S., and Weissman, I. L., 1978, Specificity of cell surface virus receptors on radiation leukemia virus and radiation-induced thymic lymphomas, *J. Virol.* **28**:819.

Menezes, J., Seigneurin, J. M., Patel, P., Bourkas, A., and Lenoir, G., 1977, Presence of Epstein-Barr virus receptors, but absence of virus penetration, in cells of an Epstein-Barr virus genome-negative human lymphoblastoid T line (MOLT 4), *J. Virol.* **22**:816.

Milner, Y., Ben-Zaquen, R., and Loyter, A., 1978, A possible correlation between the fusogenic activity of Sendai virus and its ability to dephosphorylate membrane proteins, *Proceedings of the 12th Annual Meeting, FEBS* (S. Rapport, ed.), Pergamon Press (in press).

Miyamoto, K., and Gilden, R. V., 1971, Electron microscopic studies of tumor viruses. I. Entry of murine leukemia virus into mouse embryo fibroblasts, *J. Virol.* **7**:395.

Miyamoto, K., and Morgan, C., 1971, Structure and development of viruses as observed in the electron microscope. VI. Entry and uncoating of Herpes simplex virus, *J. Virol.* **8**:910.

Moldow, C. F., McGrath, M., and Van Santen, L., 1976, Avian tumor virus interactions with chicken fibroblast plasma membranes, *J. Supramol. Struct.* **4**:497.

Moldow, C. F., McGrath, M., and Peterson, C., 1977*a*, Solubilization of initial attachment site activity for avian tumor viruses with lithium diiodosalicylate, *Proc. Soc. Exp. Biol. Med.* **154**:201.

Moldow, C. F., Volberding, P., McGrath, M., and Lee, J. L., 1977*b*, Avian tumor virus interactions with chicken fibroblast membranes: Partial characterization of initial attachment site activity, *J. Gen. Virol.* **37**:385.

Mooney, J. J., Dalrymple, J. M., Alving, C. R., and Russell, P. K., 1975, Interaction of Sindbis virus with liposomal model membranes, *J. Virol.* **15**:225.

Moore, N. F., Patzer, E. J., Shaw, J. M., Thompson, T. E., and Wagner, R. R., 1978, Interaction of vesicular stomatitis virus with lipid vesicles: Depletion of cholesterol and effect on virion membrane fluidity and infectivity, *J. Virol.* **27**:320.

Morgan, C., and Howe, C., 1968, Structure and development of viruses as observed in the electron microscope. IX. Entry of parainfluenza I (Sendai) virus, *J. Virol.* **2**:1122.

Morgan, C., and Rose, H. M., 1968, Structure and development of viruses as observed in the electron microscope. VIII. Entry of influenza virus, *J. Virol.* **2**:925.

Morgan, C., Rose, H. M., and Mednis, B., 1968, Electron microscopy of herpes simplex virus. I. Entry, *J. Virol.* **2**:507.

Morgan, C., Rosenkranz, H. S., and Mednis, B., 1969, Structure and development of viruses as observed in the electron microscope. X. Entry and uncoating of adenovirus, *J. Virol.* **4**:777.

Morrison, T. G., and McQuain, C. O., 1978, Assembly of viral membranes: Nature of the association of vesicular stomatitis virus proteins to membranes, *J. Virol.* **26**:115.

Okada, Y., Koseki, I., Kim, J., Maeda, Y., and Hashimoto, T., 1975, Modification of cell membranes with viral envelopes during fusion of cells with HVJ (Sendai virus), *Exp. Cell Res.* **93**:368.

Örvell, C., and Norrby, E., 1977, Immunological properties of purified Sendai virus glycoproteins, *J. Immunol.* **119**:1882.

Palese, P., and Compans, R. W., 1976, Inhibition of influenza virus replication in tissue culture by 2-deoxy-2, 3-dehydro-*N*-trifluoroacetylneuraminic acid (FANA): Mechanism of action, *J. Gen. Virol.* **33**:159.

Palese, P., Tobita, K., Ueda, M., and Compans, R. W., 1974, Characterization of temperature sensitive influenza virus mutants defective in neuraminidase, *Virology* **61**:397.

Payne, L. G., and Norrby, E., 1978, Adsorption and penetration of enveloped and naked vaccinia virus particles, *J. Virol.* **27**:19.

Periés, J. R., and Chany, C., 1962, Studies on measles virus hemagglutination, *Proc. Soc. Exp. Biol. Med.* **110**:477.

Philipson, L., Lonberg-Holm, K., and Pettersson, M., 1968, Virus-receptor interaction in an adenovirus system, *J. Virol.* **2**:1064.

Philipson, L., Everitt, E., and Lonberg-Holm, K., 1976, Molecular aspects of virus-receptor interaction in the adenovirus system, in: *Cell Membrane Receptors for Viruses, Antigens and Antibodies, Polypeptide Hormones and Small Molecules* (R. F. Beers, Jr., and E. G. Bassett, eds.), pp. 203–216, Raven Press, New York.

Pierce, J. S., Strauss, E. G., and Strauss, J. H., 1974, Effects of ionic strength on the binding of Sindbis virus to chick cells, *J. Virol.* **13**:1030.

Piraino, F., 1967, The mechanism of genetic resistance of chick embryo cells to infection with Rous sarcoma virus—Bryan strain (BS-RSV), *Virology* **32**:700.

Poste, G., and Waterson, A. P., 1975, Cell fusion by Newcastle disease virus, in: *Negative Strand Viruses*, Vol. 2 (B. W. J. Mahy and R. D. Barry, eds.) pp. 905–922, Academic Press, New York.

Robertson, M. A., Etchison, J. R., Robertson, J. S., and Summers, D. F., 1978, Specific changes in the oligosaccharide moieties of VSV grown in different lectin-resistant CHO cells, *Cell* **13**:515.

Roesing, T. G., Toselli, P. A., and Crowell, R. L., 1975, Elution and uncoating of Coxsackievirus B3 by isolated HeLa cell plasma membranes, *J. Virol.* **15**:654.

Sarkar, M. H., Lasfargues, E. Y., and Moore, D. H., 1970, Attachment and penetration of mouse mammary tumor virus in mouse embryo cells, *J. Microsc. (Paris)* **9**:477.

Sarmiento, M., Haffey, M., and Spear, P. G., 1979, Membrane proteins specified by Herpes simplex viruses. III. Role of glycoprotein VP7(B_2) in virion infectivity, *J. Virol.* **29**:1149.

Scheid, A., 1978, Studies on the structure and function of paramyxovirus glycoproteins, in: *Negative Strand Viruses and the Host Cell* (B. W. J. Mahy and R. D. Barry, eds.), pp. 181–193, Academic Press, New York.

Scheid, A., and Choppin, P. W., 1974, Identification of biological activities of paramyxovirus glycoproteins, *Virology* **57**:475.

Schloemer, R. H., and Wagner, R. R., 1975, Cellular adsorption function of the sialoglycoprotein of vesicular stomatitis virus and its neuraminic acid, *J. Virol.* **15**:882.

Schluederberg, A. E., and Nakamura, M., 1967, A salt-dependent hemagglutinating particle from measles infected cells, *Virology* **33**:297.

Schnebli, H. P., and Bächi, T., 1975, Reactions of lectins with human erythrocytes. I. Factors governing the agglutination reaction, *Exp. Cell Res.* **91**:175.

Sekiguchi, K., and Asano, A., 1978, Participation of spectrin in Sendai virus-induced fusion of human erythrocytes, *Proc. Natl. Acad. Sci. USA* **75**:1740.

Sharom, F. J., Barratt, D. G., Thede, A. E., and Grant, C. W. M., 1976, Glycolipids in model membranes. Spin label and freeze-etch studies, *Biochim. Biophys. Acta* **455**:484.

Shimizu, K., Shimizu, Y. K., Kohama, T., and Ishida, N., 1974, Isolation and characterization of two distinct types of HVJ (Sendai virus) spikes, *Virology* **62**:90.

Shimizu, Y. K., Shimizu, K., Ishida, N., and Homma, M., 1976, On the study of Sendai virus hemolysis. II. Morphological study of envelope fusion and hemolysis, *Virology* **71**:48.

Shirodaria, P. V., Dermott, E., and Gould, E. A., 1976, Some characteristics of salt-dependent haemagglutinating measles viruses, *J. Gen. Virol.* **33**:107.

Shotton, D., Thompson, K., Wofsy, L., and Branton, D., 1978, Appearance and distribution of surface proteins of the human erythrocyte membrane, *J. Cell Biol.* **76**:512.

Silverstein, S. C., and Dales, S., 1968, The penetration of reovirus RNA and initiation of its genetic function in L-strain fibroblasts, *J. Cell Biol.* **36**:197.

Simpson, R. W., Hauser, R. E., and Dales, S., 1969, Viropexis of vesicular stomatitis virus by L cells, *Virology* **37**:285.

Smith, H., 1977, Host and tissue specificities in virus infections of animals, in: *Virus Infection and the Cell Surface*, Cell Surface Reviews (G. Poste and G. L. Nicolson, eds.), Vol. 2, pp. 1–46, North-Holland, Amsterdam.

Tomita, M., and Marchesi, V. T., 1975, Amino-acid sequence and oligosaccharide attachment sites of human erythrocyte glycophorin, *Proc. Natl. Acad. Sci. USA* **72**:2964.

Tooze, J. (ed.), 1973, The molecular biology of tumor viruses. Chapter 10, The RNA tumor viruses: morphology, composition and classification, pp. 502–584.

Toyoshima, K., Hata, S., and Miki, T., 1960, Virological studies on measles virus. IV. The effect of active and inactivated measles virus on cultured cells, *Biken J.* **3**:281.

Tyrrell, D. A. J., and Norrby, E., 1978, Structural polypeptides of measles virus, *J. Gen. Virol.* **39**:219.

Valdirmarsson, H., Agnarsdottir, G., and Lachmann, P. J., 1975, Measles virus receptor on human T lymphocytes, *Nature (London)* **255**:554.

Volsky, D. J., and Loyter, A., 1978, Role of Ca^{2+} in virus-induced membrane fusion, *J. Cell Biol.* **78**:465.

Wainberg, M. A., and Howe, C., 1973, Infection-mediated resistance to cell fusion by inactive Sendai virus, *Proc. Soc. Exp. Biol. Med.* **142**:981.

Waite, M. R. F., Brown, D. T., and Pfefferkorn, E. R., 1972, Inhibition of Sindbis virus release by media of low ionic strength: An electron microscope study, *J. Virol.* **10**:537.

Wassilewa, L., 1977, Cell receptors for paramyxoviruses, *Arch. Virol.* **54**:299.

Weiner, H. L., Ramig, R. F., Mustoe, T. A., and Fields, B. N., 1978, Identification of the gene coding for the hemagglutinin of reovirus, *Virology* **86**:581.

Wilson, T., Papahadjopoulos, D., and Taber, R., 1977, Biological properties of poliovirus encapsulated in lipid vesicles: Antibody resistance and infectivity in virus-resistant cells, *Proc. Natl. Acad. Sci. USA* **74**:3471.

Yamamoto, K., Inoue, K., and Suzuki, K., 1974, Interaction of paramyxovirus with erythrocyte membranes modified by concanavalin A, *Nature (London)* **250**:511.

Yefenof, E., Klein, G., Jondal, M., and Oldstone, M. B., 1976, Surface markers on human B and T-lymphocytes. IX. Two-color immunofluorescence studies on the association between EBV receptors and complement receptors on the surface of lymphoid cell lines, *Int. J. Cancer* **17**:693.

Yefenof, E., Klein, G., and Kvarnung, K., 1977, Relationships between complement activation, complement binding, and EBV absorption by human hematopoietic cell lines. *Cell. Immunol.* **31**:225.

CHAPTER 2

Viral Persistence: Evolution of Viral Populations

Julius S. Youngner and Olivia T. Preble

Department of Microbiology
School of Medicine
University of Pittsburgh
Pittsburgh, Pennsylvania 15261

1. INTRODUCTION

There is an extensive literature dealing with persistent infections established by a wide variety of animal viruses. Several mechanisms have been suggested that may be involved in the establishment and maintenance of persistent infection by a normally virulent, cytolytic virus. One of these mechanisms, which involves defective-interfering (DI) virus particles in the initiation and regulation of some persistent infections, is discussed in Chapter 3 of this volume. This chapter will concentrate on another aspect of persistent viral infection, namely, the evolution of virus populations in infections initiated by virulent viruses in cell culture model systems or in immunologically competent animals. A comprehensive survey of the findings with many different groups of viruses will be followed by a discussion of the patterns of virus evolution during persistent infection and the implications of these changes in systems in which cytolytic viral infections are converted to more temperate host–virus interactions. Persistent infections in which the evolution of the virus population has not been studied will be mentioned but are outside the main focus of this review.

2. EVOLUTION OF VIRUS IN PERSISTENCE OF RNA VIRUSES

2.1. Paramyxoviruses

2.1.1. Newcastle Disease Virus (NDV)

Henle *et al.* (1959) demonstrated that persistent infection of mouse L cells could be readily established with the Victoria strain of NDV. The virus reisolated from the persistently infected cultures differed from the parental virus used to initiate persistence in plaque type in permissive chick embryo (CE) cells (Henle *et al.*, 1959) and in virulence for L cells (Rodriguez *et al.*, 1967). Thacore and Youngner (1969) found that within a short time after initiation of persistent infection at 37°C in L cells with Herts NDV (NDV_0) the virus population contained predominantly stable small-plaque mutants. These mutants (NDV_{pi}) differed from parental NDV_0 in several other characteristics, as shown in Table 1. NDV_{pi} mutants had reduced lethality for embryonated eggs, grew more slowly, and produced fewer progeny than NDV_0 in permissive CE cells at 37°C, and did not elute from chicken red blood cells after adsorption. However, NDV_{pi} replicated more efficiently in L cells than NDV_0, which produced a covert infection in L cells (Thacore and Youngner, 1970).

Although the infectivity of NDV_{pi} was labile at 50°C, the hemagglutinin (HA) and neuraminidase (NA) activities of NDV_{pi} particles were thermostable compared to the HA and NA of NDV_0. Additional experiments measured the NA activity of NDV_0 and NDV_{pi} using a soluble substrate and tested the thermal stability of enzyme activity from disrupted virions (Thacore and Youngner, 1971). The results

TABLE 1

Comparison of Properties of Wild-Type Herts NDV (NDV_0) and Virus (NDV_{pi}) Recovered from Persistently Infected L Cells

Property	NDV_0	NDV_{pi}
Lethality for embryonated eggs (10^4 PFU)	100% at 48 hr	65–70% at 48 hr
Plaque size in chick embryo cells (3 days, 37°C)	Large (2–3 mm)	Small (<1 mm)
Stability of infectivity at 50°C	Stable	Unstable
Stability of hemagglutinin at 50°C	Unstable	Stable
Interferon production in L cells	Yes	Yes
Replication in L cells at 37°C	Covert infection	Productive infection
Replication in chick embryo cells at 42–43°C	Yes	No

showed that there probably was a structural difference between NDV_{pi} and NDV_0 in the way the NA polypeptide was incorporated into the viral envelope. The HA of both intact and disrupted NDV_{pi} was more resistant to thermal inactivation than that of NDV_0. These differences probably represent alterations in the structural proteins of the NDV_{pi} mutants which evolved during persistence; however, detailed analyses of virion polypeptides will be required to determine the nature of the changes.

Further studies showed that the NDV_{pi} viruses were spontaneously selected temperature-sensitive (*ts*) mutants (Preble and Youngner, 1972); NDV_{pi} virus clones isolated from carrier L-cell lines maintained at 37°C were unable to replicate in either CE or canine kidney (MDCK) cells at 42–43°C, whereas NDV_0 replicated efficiently at the elevated temperature (Table 1). The cutoff temperature of the NDV_{pi} mutants was between 41°C and 42°C, and optimal virus yields were produced at 34–37°C, in contrast to 39–40°C for NDV_0.

When L_{NDV} cultures were transferred to 32°C after reaching confluency or were subcultured and maintained at 32°C, the level of infectious virus in the cultures rose 50- to 200-fold, and remained at a high level for several months. The virus released from the L_{NDV} cultures at 32°C was temperature sensitive. Virus production in the L_{NDV} cultures at 32°C gradually returned to its former low level, with the concurrent evolution of virus with an even lower optimum temperature than NDV_{pi} (Preble, unpublished data). During the entire period of incubation at 32°C the L_{NDV} cell cultures continued to produce interferon at the same low level found in cell cultures incubated at 37°C and were completely resistant to challenge with either NDV_0 or VSV (Preble, unpublished).

Characterization of various NDV_{pi} virus clones showed that all of the *ts* mutants had RNA$^-$ phenotypes; none of the NDV_{pi} clones were able to direct the synthesis of significant amounts of virus-specific RNA at the nonpermissive temperature in either infected CE or MDCK cells (Preble and Youngner, 1973*a*). Temperature-shift experiments suggested that two different *ts* defects in RNA synthesis at 43°C, both associated with RNA polymerase, might be present in different NDV_{pi} clones. Evolution of very similar *ts* RNA$^-$ NDV_{pi} clones also occurred in mouse L cells persistently infected with two additional strains of NDV, Kansas-Man and Texas GB (Preble and Youngner, 1973*b*) and in hamster (BHK) and canine (MDCK) cell lines persistently infected with Herts NDV (Youngner and Quagliana, 1975). When measured by an *in vitro* assay system, purified virions of NDV_{pi} contained less RNA polymerase activity per unit of virus protein than purified virions of NDV_0 (Stanwick and Hallum, 1976). It was also reported that purified preparations of NDV_{pi} obtained from L_{NDV} cells and amplified in the allantoic sac of embryonated eggs contained an RNA-directed DNA polymerase activity not found in purified NDV_0 grown under the same conditions (Furman and Hallum, 1973). This finding has not been confirmed.

There was a progressive evolution of the NDV_{pi} isolated from persistently infected L cells. Two years after establishment of persistence, virus clones isolated from L_{NDV} cell cultures produced smaller plaques in CE cells, had more thermostable HA and NA, and were less virulent for embryonated eggs than virus clones which were isolated within a few months of initiation of the persistent infection (Preble and Youngner, unpublished). These results suggested that evolution of virus within the persistent infection was continuous and that selection of multiple mutants probably occurred. Furthermore, the plaque size, virulence, and thermostability properties of NDV_{pi} were independent of but coselected with the *ts* marker (Preble and Youngner, 1973*b*); *ts*⁺ revertants of NDV_{pi} retained the other biological properties characteristic of NDV_{pi}, whereas nitrous-acid-induced *ts* mutants of NDV_0 were still "NDV_0-like" except for the ability to replicate at 43°C. The importance of selection of *ts* virus mutants during the establishment of NDV persistence in L cells was emphasized by experiments which used the $NDV_{pi}ts$⁺ revertants to initiate persistence. Virus reisolated from these persistently infected cultures at the eighth cell passage was again *ts* (Preble and Youngner, 1973*b*).

Attempts were made to genetically group NDV_{pi} mutants isolated at various times (from < 1 month to > 3 years) after initiation of L_{NDV} cultures (Preble and Youngner, 1972) or recovered from BHK_{NDV} cultures (Youngner and Quagliana, 1975). Several different methods of complementation analysis at the nonpermissive temperature were used. In each case interference between pairs of NDV_{pi} mutants in mixed infections was noted (Preble and Youngner, 1973*a*). Also, none of the NDV_{pi} mutants tested complemented with four *ts* mutants of NDV_0 induced by nitrous acid.

The reason for the selection of *ts*RNA⁻ mutants in persistently infected cultures is not clear. The L_{NDV} cultures always produced a low level of interferon. Although some NDV_{pi} clones were better inducers of interferon in L cells than NDV_0, the NDV_{pi} clones were no more resistant than NDV_0 to the action of interferon (Hallum *et al.*, 1970; Preble and Youngner, unpublished data). However, NDV_{pi} clones interfered with the replication of NDV_0 at the level of RNA synthesis at both permissive and nonpermissive temperatures (Preble and Youngner, 1973*b*). Interference with wild-type virus replication may be a mechanism by which virus mutants are selected and maintained during persistent infection. This possibility is considered in more detail in Section 4.4.

Other cell cultures persistently infected with NDV were studied by Fraser *et al.* (1976) when NDV appeared "accidentally" in established cell lines of pig, ox, and sheep kidney maintained routinely at 37°C. Virus particles released from the cultures were not infectious but could be quantitated by their ability to agglutinate red blood cells. Similar to the NDV$_{pi}$ mutants released from persistently infected L cells (Thacore and Youngner, 1970), the virus released from the accidentally contaminated carrier cultures did not elute from agglutinated erythrocytes (Fraser *et al.*, 1976). Also, more HA was released from persistently infected cultures incubated at 31°C than at 37°C, and incubation of the cultures at 41°C resulted in a marked reduction in the release of viral HA. Further studies suggested that a defect in virus maturation caused an accumulation of defective nucleocapsids (McNulty *et al.*, 1977). The maturation defect was due to a lack of synthesis of the matrix (M) protein (Louza and Bingham, 1978) essential for correct alignment of virus nucleocapsids with appropriate areas of plasma membrane in preparation for virion bud formation.

Finally, Sato *et al.* (1978*b*) reported the recovery of NDV$_{pi}$ variants from BHK21/WI2 cells persistently infected with NDV and maintained at 34°C. The NDV$_{pi}$ virus carried structural antigens of a latent virus of the BHK21/WI2 cells as a result of phenotypic mixing between NDV and the latent virus. NDV$_{pi}$ was neutralized by rabbit antiserum against the latent virus and by antiserum prepared against wild-type NDV, whereas wild-type NDV was neutralized only by homologous serum. NDV$_{pi}$ also formed minute plaques on BHK21/WI2 monolayers at 34°C, but did not plaque in these cells at 43°C. This suggests that the NDV$_{pi}$ variants are *ts*, although no data are given for the plaquing efficiency of wild-type NDV at 43°C in BHK21/WI2 cells. Sato *et al.* (1976) previously reported that variants released from BHK21/WI2 cells persistently infected with rubella virus appear to be stable genetic hybrids between rubella and the latent virus, which is also *ts* (Sato *et al.*, 1976). In order to investigate whether the *ts* NDV$_{pi}$ variants were hybrid viruses, the variants were passaged in embryonated eggs. Both the *ts* and plaque size markers and the antigenic properties of the NDV$_{pi}$ reverted to those of wild-type virus after one passage in embryonated eggs, indicating that the variants probably

resulted from phenotypic mixing. The role of the interaction between
NDV_{pi} and the latent virus in maintenance of the persistence will
require further study.

2.1.2. Measles Virus (MV)

The evolution of measles virus (MV) during persistent infection
has been studied in several different host cell systems. HeLa cells
infected with the Edmonston strain of MV initially developed extensive
cytopathology which was followed by outgrowth of surviving cells (Rustigian, 1962). These cells (termed K11 cells) could be subcultured and
they continued to shed infectious MV at 37°C. Following prolonged
cultivation in the presence of antiviral serum, the persistently infected
cultures (K11A) no longer released infectious virus, although viral
antigens were still present in the cells. Later studies showed that the
virus released from the K11 cultures differed from parental Edmonston
MV; the K11 virus produced delayed cytopathic effects (CPE) in HeLa
cells, and the progression of CPE once it began was also slower (Rustigian, 1966a). This difference in virulence between K11 virus and the
parental Edmonston MV became more pronounced with increasing
time of persistence. Further studies showed that, although the K11 virus
produced a lytic infection of two monkey kidney cell lines, Vero and
BSC1, infection of either HeLa or WI38 human cell lines resulted in
persistent infection (Rustigian, personal communication). These results
suggested the K11 virus may be a host range mutant of the parental
Edmonston MV.

A similar pattern of virus evolution was seen when HeLa cells were
infected with the Toyoshima strain of MV (Minagawa, 1971). Virus
recovered from the persistently infected HeLa cells had a longer latent
period and slower growth rate and produced lower yields in both HeLa
and Vero cells than the parental MV used to initiate persistence. In
addition, the carried virus produced "delayed" plaques on Vero cells.
Minagawa (1971) concluded that the carrier state was maintained by a
slowly replicating variant virus which had been selected from the
standard virus population.

Detailed studies have been made of the virus populations released
from K11 persistently infected HeLa cell cultures maintained at 37°C
and of the virus rescued at that temperature from K11A nonyielder cultures by cocultivation with Vero cells. Both K11 and K11A viruses were
ts in CV1 and Vero monkey kidney cell lines at 40.3–40.6°C (Wechsler
et al., personal communication); the efficiency of plating (EOP) of K11

or K11a virus at the elevated temperature was at least a thousandfold lower than that of wild-type Edmonston MV. In yield experiments, K11 and K11A viruses replicated more slowly in CV1 cells than wild-type MV at 33°C, and no infectious virus was produced at 40.3°C; wild-type MV produced approximately 1 log less virus at 40.3°C than at 33°C. However, incubation at 33°C neither induced virus release from K11A nonyielder cultures nor increased the efficiency of virus rescue during co-cultivation of K11A cells with Vero cells (Rustigian, personal communication). K11 and K11A viruses could also be distinguished from wild-type Edmonston MV by analysis of virus-specific proteins. The matrix (M) protein in purified K11 and K11A viruses was slightly smaller than that in wild-type MV (Wechsler *et al.*, personal communication). Smaller M protein was also found in CV1 or Vero cells undergoing lytic infection with K11 virus and in the K11 persistently infected HeLa cell cultures. The roles of the aberrant M protein and of temperature sensitivity in either establishment or maintenance of the persistently infected HeLa cell cultures are still under investigation.

Armen *et al.* (1977) also studied HeLa cells persistently infected with Edmonston MV. The virus (MV_{pi}) released from the $HeLa_{pi}$ virus carrier cultures produced small plaques on Vero cells, was approximately tenfold more resistant to thermal inactivation than wild-type Edmonston virus, and was less virulent for HeLa cells than the parental virus. The EOP (39°C/33°C) of MV_{pi} from $HeLa_{pi}$ culture fluids was 10^{-4}–10^{-5} compared to an EOP of 1.0 for wild-type Edmonston virus, indicating that MV_{pi} was a *ts* virus population. MV_{pi} virus therefore appeared to be very similar to the K11 virus, which was also derived from persistently infected HeLa cells (Rustigian, 1962, 1966a, and personal communication). When persistently infected HeLa cell cultures were shifted from 37°C to 33°C, the yield of infectious virus was increased fiftyfold, even though no CPE was observed. A similar result was reported previously when human lung (Lu106) cells persistently infected with MV were incubated at 33°C (Norrby, 1967). Further characterization of the virus released from Lu106 cells at 33°C suggested that it might differ in neuropathogenicity from wild-type MV (Norrby and Kristensson, 1978); no additional properties were studied.

Measles virus persistence in another human cell line (HEp2) has also been investigated (Gould, 1974; Gould and Linton, 1975). Virus released from the persistently infected HEp2 cultures produced small syncytial plaques on Vero cell monolayers and was *ts* in Vero cells at 39.5°C; the 39.5°C/33°C EOP of wild-type Edmonston virus was 0.56, while the EOP of virus in culture fluids from persistently infected HEp2 cell cultures was < 0.01. The cutoff temperature of the *ts* virus was between 39°C and 39.5°C (Gould and Linton, 1975). When the persistently infected HEp2 cultures were serially propagated at 39.5°C, the expression of virus-specific antigens (as measured by surface fluorescence and hemadsorption) ceased in the first cell passage, and virus-specific antigens were lost from the cytoplasm by the fifth cell passage. There was considerable heterogeneity in the properties of the virus used to initiate the persistence (Gould, 1974), and it was concluded that the *ts* virus from the carrier HEp2 cell line may have been selected from variants present in the parental virus pool (Gould and Linton, 1975).

Since persistence of measles virus variants in lymphoid as well as nervous tissue has been implicated in the etiology of subacute sclerosing panencephalitis (SSPE), several laboratories have investigated model systems of MV persistence in human lymphoblastoid cell lines at 37°C. Minagawa *et al.* (1976) studied human lymphoid cells (NC37) persistently infected with attenuated measles vaccine viruses (Schwarz and AIKC strains), with the TYCSA neurovirulent strain of measles virus, or with the Mantooth or Hallé strains of SSPE virus. In each case virus released from persistently infected cells had a lower EOP at 39.5°C than the parental virus strain used to initiate the persistence. However, the proportion of *ts* mutants in the populations was not determined. No differences were found in either plaque morphology or thermal inactivation rates when MV_{pi} and parental viruses were compared. Because no increase in the production of infectious virus occurred when the virus–carrier cultures were shifted to 33°C, it was concluded that, although *ts* variants may be selected during initiation of the persistent infections, they may not play a role in maintenance (Minagawa *et al.*, 1976). However, in persistently infected HeLa cells, virus rescued from nonyielder cultures by cocultivation at 37°C was *ts* even though no increase in virus release was obtained when the cells were incubated at 33°C (Rustigian, personal communication).

Bloom and his colleagues studied persistence of Edmonston MV in two different human lymphoblastoid cell lines (Ju *et al.*, 1978; Ju, personal communication). The persistently infected cells produced low levels of interferon, and no defective virus particles were detectable after three serial undiluted passages of culture fluids in Vero cells. Although the EOP at 39.5°C of uncloned virus recovered from these cell cultures was the same as that of wild-type MV virus, analysis of clonal virus isolates revealed a high proportion of *ts* virus mutants in the persistent virus population (Ju *et al.*, 1978). The high degree of sensitivity of clonal analysis for determining the proportion of *ts* mutants in a virus population had been noted previously during analysis of the evolution of virus in mouse L cells persistently infected with vesicular stomatitis virus (Youngner et al., 1976). Of 70 measles virus clones isolated from four different persistently infected lymphoid cell lines, 51 (73%) were ts, whereas none of 21 clones of wild-type MV was ts. The EOP (39.5°C/33°C) of the 70 clonal isolates from carrier cultures varied from 0.1 to < 10^{-4}. However, the clones were serially passed twice in Vero cells to yield working stocks of virus before testing for temperature sensitivity, and evidence from other systems suggests that this procedure may result in an accumulation of ts^{+} revertants in stocks of unstable or leaky mutants (Youngner et al., 1976, 1978a). A prospective study showed that as early as the second cell passage (33 days after initiation of persistence) the EOP at 39.5°C. of uncloned virus in culture fluids was lower than that of wild-type MV and that 33% of the virus clones isolated at that time were ts. The ts MV isolates also produced small plaques on Vero cell monolayers, but the plaque size of a given mutant did not necessarily correlate with its EOP at 39.5°C. Based on the synthesis of virus-specific antigens in Vero cells infected at 39.5°C, both early (antigen-negative) and late (antigen-positive) mutants were found. Further analysis showed that the ts mutants isolated from the persistently infected cultures represented at least four of the five known measles virus complementation groups (Ju, personal communication). The data also indicated that many of the mutants were probably multiple mutants since most of them did not map unambiguously in any one group. Finally, ts MV clones isolated from persistently infected cultures also interfered with the replication of wild-type MV at 31°C, 37°C, and 39.5°C (Ju, personal communication). The significance of this inhibition will be discussed in more detail in Section 4.4.

   Persistent infection with measles virus has also been studied using cell cultures from other animal species. Hamster embryo fibroblast (HEF) cell cultures persistently infected with the Schwarz attenuated vaccine strain of MV at 37°C progressed through three distinct phases (Knight et al., 1972). Prior to cell passage 19, no infectious virus was detected in the cultures. Virus could be recovered between cell passages 19 and 45 either by reducing the incubation temperature to 33°C or by cocultivating with BSC1 monkey kidney cells (Haspel et al., 1973). During this stage of persistence, a hundredfold more virus was produced if the cultures were incubated at 33°C instead of 37°C, and virus maturation was completely suppressed by incubation at 39°C. The virus released by temperature reduction was ts and produced smaller plaques on Vero cell monolayers than parental Schwarz virus. However, the virus released by cocultivation with BSC1 cells was ts^+ and produced large plaques on Vero cells. After cell passage 45, the persistently infected cultures entered a third phase in which virus release could still be enhanced by incubation at 33°C, but the virus released by temperature shift was identical to that released after cocultivation with BSC1 cells (Haspel *et al.*, 1975). Virus particles released from persistently infected HEF cells during the third phase possessed all of the normal measles virus structural proteins, although proportionately there was less G, VP2, and NP protein than in the Hallé SSPE measles strain used as the standard (Fisher and Rapp, 1979). There also appeared to be a relatively high proportion of non infectious, low-density interfering particles released from persistently infected HEF cells at passages 89–95. It was concluded that the MV virus variants in the persistent infection were unable to replicate normally in the carrier HEF cells.

The temperature-shift data also suggested that a temperature-dependent host cell function may be necessary for virus maturation. A host-cell function was probably also involved in the temperature-dependent maturation of measles virus from persistently infected RN2-2 rat cells (Lucas *et al.*, 1978). These RN2-2/MV cells stopped producing virus after 2–3 days at 39.5°C, although the virus produced at 32.5°C did not appear to be *ts* (as determined by EOP at 39.5°C). Further work showed that this cell line could support both lytic and persistent infections with MV at 32.5°C but failed to allow replication of even wild-type Edmonston MV at 39.5°C. Consideration of host-cell factors which may be involved in the limitation of virus replication in persistent virus infections is beyond the scope of this chapter.

Chiarini *et al.* (1978) established a latent MV infection in Vero cells by infecting the cells with a small-plaque clone of Edmonston MV derived from serial undiluted passages of the virus. Virus released from persistently infected Vero cells maintained at 37°C was *ts* at 39.5°C compared to the parental virus used to initiate persistence. The authors concluded that a *ts* persistent virus was therefore responsible for or selected during the establishment of latency. In contrast, BGM monkey kidney cells persistently infected with the Hallé strain of SSPE measles virus did not produce *ts* virus (Wild and Dugre, 1978). No difference was found in the amount of virus produced by persistently infected cultures at 33°C, 37°C, or 39.5°C, and the EOP at 39.5°C of culture fluids from persistently infected cells was no different from that of cloned Hallé virus or cloned Edmonston wild-type MV. However, virus released from persistently infected BGM cells was able to establish persistent infection in Vero cells, whereas the parental Hallé virus produced only lytic infection in this cell line, results reminiscent of those obtained with virus recovered from HeLa cells persistently infected with MV (Minagawa, 1971).

Another type of measles virus persistent infection is characterized by failure of the cultures to release infections virus even though a large proportion of the cells contains viral antigens and viral nucleocapsids are visible by electron microscopy. In some cases such as the K11A HeLa cell nonyielder cultures described previously (Rustigian, 1966*b*) and the phase 1 HEF persistent infection (Knight *et al.*, 1973), infectious virus can be rescued from the persistently infected cultures by cocultivation with permissive cells. More often, the persistent infection appears to be maintained by defective virus variants which are not rescuable using a variety of methods (Menna *et al.*, 1975; Burnstein *et al.*, 1974; Dubois-Dalcq *et al.*, 1976; Kratzch *et al.*, 1977). Since no direct studies of the properties of the carried virus have been done, it is not clear whether evolution of the virus, the host, or both, occurs in these systems. Persistent infections maintained by defective virus may be useful *in vitro* models of the defective virus replication which occurs in SSPE.

A comparison of SSPE-derived and wild-type measles virus strains suggests that evolution of the virus also occurs during persistent infections *in vivo*. Since SSPE is considered in detail elsewhere in this volume, only a brief discussion is presented here. Payne and Baublis (1973) compared six isolates of SSPE virus to both the Edmonston and Schwarz strains of measles virus using cross-neutralization and neutralization kinetics. All six SSPE isolates were less reactive with homologous antisera than the laboratory-adapted viruses. This suggested either a qualitative or a quantitative change in the surface antigens of the SSPE viruses. The SSPE viruses in this study could also be distinguished from wild-type MV by plaque morphology. However, others found no consistent differences in the infectivity and antigenicity of two SSPE strains and wild-type Edmonston MV (Hamilton *et al.*, 1973; Thormar *et al.*, 1978).

Wild and Dugre (1978) reported no difference between the EOP at 39.5°C of the Hallé strain of SSPE virus and wild-type Edmonston MV. However, Hodes (1979) found that higher viral yields were produced at 32°C instead of 37°C or 39°C. In addition, ten out of 16 Hallé subclones were *ts* at 39°C, while none of the 16 clones of wild-type Edmonston MV tested was *ts*. It is clear that additional studies are necessary in order to determine whether or not evolution of MV mutants occurs during persistent infections of humans *in vivo*.

Recent studies suggested that the virus-specific M protein in cells infected with SSPE viruses is slightly larger than wild-type M protein

(Wechsler and Fields, 1978; Hall *et al.*, 1978). However, Rima *et al.* (1979) claim that the size of the M protein depends more on the degree of adaptation of the virus to cell cultures than on the origin of the virus; more recent isolates of MV had a larger M protein than laboratory-adapted strains which had been passed many times in cell cultures. Furthermore, addition of a chymotrypsin inhibitor to the growth medium of the virus-infected cells blocked conversion of the larger M protein to the smaller form (Rima, personal communication).

Two groups of workers have used immunoprecipitation to study the proteins of several different measles and SSPE virus strains (Hall *et al.*, 1979; Wechsler *et al.*, 1979). Both groups report a relative lack of antibodies to the nonglycosylated viral membrane protein (M) in the sera of patients with SSPE. In contrast, the sera from these patients contain a high level of antibodies to other viral proteins. These results were not due to the existence of a large number of antigenically unique M proteins; other hyperimmune human or rabbit sera precipitated M protein as well as the other viral proteins. These results suggest that in patients with SSPE the synthesis of M protein is diminished; alternatively, the M Protein may not be recognized normally by the immune system in SSPE patients. In either case, an abnormality in M protein may be involved in the pathogenesis of SSPE. Although differences in electrophoretic mobility of the M proteins and several other viral proteins were observed among different SSPE and measles strains, there was no pattern characteristic of SSPE strains, nor could these strains be distinguished by peptide mapping (Hall *et al.*, 1979).

2.1.3. Sendai Virus (Hemagglutinating Virus of Japan)

The evolution of Sendai virus in persistently infected BHK cells (BHK-HVJ cells) was described by Nagata *et al.* (1972). Initially, no infectious virus was detected in the carrier (BHK-HVJ) cell culture maintained at 34°C, although the release of virus particles capable of hemagglutination was increased at 31°C and suppressed at 37°C; wild-type Sendai virus grew equally well in BHK cells at 31°C or 37°C. Fluorescent antibody studies suggested that virus maturation was *ts* because of a defect in the insertion of virus-specific proteins into the plasma membrane at the higher temperature.

Additional experiments showed that infectious virus (HVJ-pB) could be recoverd from the BHK-HVJ cultures if medium from cultures incubated at 32°C was inoculated into embryonated eggs also maintained at 32°C (Kimura *et al.*, 1975). No virus grew in eggs incubated at 38°C, indicating that HVJ-pB was temperature sensitive. HVJ-pB was less thermostable and less cytocidal in BHK and L cells than wild-type Sendai virus (Kimura *et al.*, 1975). HVJ-pB produced small plaques on monkey kidney cell monolayers at the permissive tempera-ture, and specifically interfered with the replication of wild-type Sendai virus at both 32°C and 38°C (Kimura *et al.*, 1976). Although the interfering activity in HVJ-pB preparations cosedimented in sucrose gradients with infectious particles, the presence of DI particles was not rigorously excluded. Roux and Holland (1979) suggested that DI parti-cles may play a role in either establishment or maintenance of persistent infections with Sendai virus in BHK and other cell lines, although evolution of virus mutants in the persisting virus populations was not studied.

At a later phase of virus persistence in the BHK-HVJ cultures described above, virus released at 32°C could not be grown directly in embryonated eggs at 32°C, but was infectious for BHK and L cells at this temperature (Nishiyama *et al.*, 1976). The virus (HVJ_{pi}) passed in BHK or L cells was then infectious for eggs. HVJ_{pi} was similar to the HVJ-pB isolated previously; both viruses were *ts*, thermolabile, and less cytopathogenic for several types of cell cultures. Analysis of the polypeptide composition of HVJ_{pi} and of wild-type Sendai virus grown in BHK cells suggested that HVJ_{pi} had a smaller M protein, less glyco-protein F, and more of the precursor glycoprotein, F_0, than the wild-type virus (Nishiyama *et al.*, 1976). The dependence of infectivity of Sendai virus on conversion of precursor F_0 to F by proteolytic activity has been demonstrated (Homma and Ohuchi, 1971; Ohuchi and Homma, 1976). The relationship between HVJ_{pi} and the earlier HVJ-pB isolates is not clear, although the difference in host range of the two viruses suggests a continuing evolution of the virus population in BHK-HVJ cells.

A Sendai-like virus (6/94 virus) was isolated from persistently infected cell cultures obtained after using lysolecithin to fuse brain cells derived from a multiple sclerosis patient with CV1 monkey kidney cells (ter Meulen *et al.*, 1972). The 6/94 virus proved to be a parainflu-enza type 1 virus which was very closely related to Sendai virus (Lewandowski *et al.*, 1974; Kolakofsky *et al.*, 1974). Although Sendai virus grew equally well at 33°C and 37°C, 6/94 virus yields were sig-nificantly enhanced at 33°C; virus-specific hemadsorption by the CV1/MS cell cultures at 37°C was also only 1–10% of that seen in cul-tures incubated at 33°C. These results suggest that, whatever its origin,the 6/94 virus isolated from the persistently infected cells is *ts*, although the role of the virus in human disease remains in doubt.

2.1.4. Respiratory Syncytial Virus

Simpson and Iinuma (1975) established persistent infection with respiratory syncytial (RS) virus in bovine embryonic kidney (BEK) and human HEp2 cells. The presence of an infectious proviral DNA copy of the RSV genomic RNA in these cell cultures (Simpson and Iinuma, 1975) has not been confirmed (Pringle *et al.*, 1978; Simpson, personal communication). The HEp2/RS cell line has continued to shed infectious RS virus during more than 3 years of continuous cultivation. Clones of virus released from both early- and late-passage cells do not appear to be *ts* (Simpson, personal communication). However, some nude mice persistently infected with RS virus yield virus with a *ts* phenotype. Further analysis of virus from these *in vivo* and *in vitro* systems is necessary to determine the evolutionary patterns in persistent RS virus infections.

Infection of BSC1 monkey kidney cells with certain *ts* mutants of RS virus defective in late functions, followed by cultivation of the infected cells at 39°C (the nonpermissive temperature), resulted in virus persistence (Pringle *et al.*, 1978). After cell passage 21, the persistently infected RS *ts*1/BSC1 cells were shifted to and maintained at 37°C; low levels of infectious virus were shed at this temperature. The released virus formed small plaques on BSC1 cell monolayers at both 31°C and 39°C, but no quantitative data were given concerning either plaquing or replication efficiency of the carried virus at the nonpermissive temperature.

A persistent infection of HeLa cells was established by cultivating cells which survived cytolytic infection with the Long strain of RS virus (Peeples and Levine, personal communication). Virus released from the persistently infected HeLa/RS cells was neutralized by antiserum prepared against wt RS virus. However, the RS_{pi} virus produced small plaques on HeLa cell monolayers; RS_{pi} also was less cytopathogenic and produced lower viral yields in HeLa cells than wt RS virus. Since the yield of progeny virus was the same when RS_{pi}-infected HeLa cells were incubated at 33°C, 37°C, or 39°C, it was concluded that RS_{pi} was not *ts*. Although no evidence was found for the presence of DI particles of RS virus, RS_{pi} passed once in HeLa cells at very low MOI inhibited the replication of wt RS (Peeples and Levine, personal communication). These results suggest that persistent infection of HeLa cells with RS virus resulted in the selection of virus with a slower growth rate and lowered cytopathogenicity and yield, and which interfered with the replication of wild-type virus. Preliminary results also indicated that the GP2 protein of RS_{pi} may differ from the corresponding protein found in wild-type virus (Peeples and Levine, personal communication).

2.1.5. Mumps Virus

Walker and Hinze (1962) studied human conjunctival cells persistently infected with mumps virus. Virus isolated after about 30 cell passages was less cytopathogenic for several types of cells including various human and monkey cell lines. No CPE was observed when the persistently infected cell cultures were incubated at various temperatures above or below 37°C. Although additional investigations were carried out of the persistence of mumps virus in these systems, no further information on the properties of the virus populations was reported.

More recently, persistent infection of BHK21 cells by mumps virus was described by Truant and Hallum (1977*a*). Virus (MuV_{pi}) isolated from the carrier cultures did not differ from wild-type mumps virus (MuV_0) in plaque morphology but was less able than MuV_0 to replicate at 39°C in BHK and HeLa cells. Five of six clones of MuV_{pi} were *ts*, while only one of six clones of MuV_0 was *ts*; the cutoff temperature for *ts* virus yield appeared to be between 37°C and 39°C. However, when BHK_{pi} cells were incubated at 33°C, no increase occurred in CPE, virus production, hemadsorption, or mumps antigens detectable by fluorescent antibody. When the persistently infected BHK cells were cloned, both uninfected and latently infected nonvirus yielder clones were obtained (Truant and Hallum, 1977*b*). The latter cell clones could be induced to release virus by incubation at 33°C. The virus released under these conditions (MuV_{LI}) produced the same yield in HeLa cells at both 33°C and 39°C, and the EOP at 39°C of uncloned virus stocks was similar to that of wild-type MuV_0. The situation is reminiscent of the two Sendai virus mutants (HVJ-pB and HVJ_{pi}) released from persistently infected BHK cells under different conditions (Kimura *et al.*, 1975; Nishiyama *et al.*, 1976). The relationship between MuV_{pi} and MuV_{LI} is not yet clear.

2.1.6.   Parainfluenza Virus, Type 3

Tsai (1977) investigated persistence of para-3 virus in alveolar macrophages (AM) isolated from calves infected *in vivo* or in AM cells infected in culture. Transfer of infected AM cells from 37°C to 32°C resulted in increased virus synthesis. Virus produced at 32°C was *ts* when tested in bovine kidney (MDBK) cells at 37°C; wild-type para-3 was able to replicate at both temperatures. In contrast, Hodes *et al.* (personal communication) established a persistent infection in Vero cells using the third undiluted passage of para-3. In order to look for mutants in the persistent virus population, Vero cells were productively infected at different temperatures with wild-type para-3 or with para-3$_{pi}$ from the sixth passage of the persistently infected cells. Viral yields at 32°C, 37°C, and 39°C were the same with both viruses. Cloned virus preparations were not evaluated, and virus isolated at later times after initiation of the persistence was not tested.

2.2.   Orthomyxoviruses: Influenza Virus

The WSN strain of influenza virus A was able to establish a persistent infection in pig embryo kidney (RES) cells (Gavrilov *et al.*, 1972). Virus isolated after 16 subcultures (WSN/RES$_{16}$) had approximately the same virulence for mice as the original WSN virus but was more cytopathogenic for RES, Vero, and human lung cells. WSN/RES$_{16}$ virus reestablished persistence in pig embryo kidney cells with difficulty (Perekrest *et al.*, 1974). A nonhemagglutinating variant of influenza WSN, which has not been further characterized, was isolated from one subline of persistently infected RES cells.

2.3.   Rhabdoviruses

2.3.1.   Vesicular Stomatitis Virus

The selection of virus mutants in persistent infections with VSV was reported by Mudd *et al.* in 1973. Using wild-type VSV (Indiana), persistent infections were established at 28°C in a line of cells from the fruit fly, *Drosophila melanogaster*. The cells showed no cytopathic effects but continued to produce low levels of infectious virus which were detectable by plaque assay on the BHK21 hamster cell line. By 50 days after initiation of the carrier culture (fourth cell passage at 28°C), the virus isolated in BHK21 cells exhibited a small-plaque morphology and an altered ability to replicate at 37°C, although the parental wild-type VSV replicated equally well in BHK21 cells at both temperatures. Clonal isolates of virus from the carrier cells retained the *ts* phenotype during serial passage in BHK21 cells, indicating that the viruses were not phenotypic variants modified by the *D. melanogaster* host cells. A representative mutant clone (G) isolated from the persistent infection 9 weeks after initiation had a small-plaque morphology, was *ts*, and had an RNA⁻ phenotype at 37°C. Whether the defect in RNA synthesis was due to an alteration of virion polymerase or secondary RNA synthesis was not determined. Study of revertant clones selected in infected BHK21 cells at 37°C showed that the small-plaque and *ts* markers seemed to vary independently.

Very similar virus mutants were isolated from *Aedes albopictus* and *Aedes aegypti* mosquito cell lines persistently infected with the Cocal strain of VSV (Artsob and Spence, personal communication). There was a fairly rapid selection of an altered virus population which was *ts*, produced small plaques, and had a reduced virulence for adult mice. Printz (1970) had previously observed the evolution of a VSV population of *ts* small-plaque virus during serial *in vivo* passages of VSV (Indiana) in the fruit fly, *D. melanogaster*. Virus progeny which produced small plaques were observed in the virus population harvested from infected flies by the third to fifth passages. By the fifth to tenth passages *in vivo*, *ts* mutants were evident.

These experiments demonstrate that *ts* small-plaque virus populations evolve when VSV is passed serially in fruit flies and when persistent infections with this virus are established in cell lines of fruit fly and mosquito origin. In both situations the virus was selected at 28°C, the optimum temperature for insect cells. The question arises whether the viruses which evolve should be considered "cold adapted" rather than "temperature sensitive." The term "cold adapted" might be more appropriate if the selection was for viruses which could replicate efficiently at the temperature optimum of the insect cells. Unfortunately, studies have not been done with VSV passed serially at 28°C in BHK21 or some other mammalian cell line with a temperature optimum of 37°C. The roles played by the species of host cell and the ambient temperature might be distinguished by such an experiment.

A more comprehensive picture of the evidence that the selection of virus mutants plays an important role in the establishment and maintenance of persistent infections with VSV is provided by a series of papers published by Youngner et al. (1976, 1978a,b). Attempts to establish persistent infections in mouse L cells at 37°C with a large-plaque strain of wild-type VSV (Indiana) essentially free of defective interfering (DI) particles were unsuccessful. However, when the technique of Holland and Villarreal (1974) was used, that is, when L cells were infected with wild-type infectious B particles in the presence of a thousandfold excess of DI particles, persistent infections were readily established. At 84 days after initiation of the persistently infected cell line (L_{VSV}), the properties of the virus (VSV_{pi}) present in the persistently infected cells were determined. The wild-type virus (VSV_0) had been completely replaced by a population of *ts* small-plaque virus. VSV_{pi} plaques after 3 days at 32°C were < 1–1.5 mm in diameter compared to 2–3 mm for plaques of VSV_0.

A prospective study was done to determine more precisely the rate at which *ts* mutants appeared during the establishment of persistently infected L_{VSV} cell cultures at 37°C (Youngner *et al.*, 1976). Table 2 shows the details of this prospective study. Clonal analysis revealed that the frequency of spontaneous *ts* mutants in the inoculum used to initiate the persistent infection was 4.4%. By 10 days after initiation of persistence there was a statistically significant increase in the frequency (17.8%) of *ts* mutants in the fluids harvested from L_{VSV} cells. By 63 days all 29 clones isolated from L_{VSV} cells were temperature sensitive. This persistently infected cell line was maintained for over 3 years without the appearance of ts^+ revertants in the virus population. It is important to note the limiations of relying solely on the efficiency of plating method to determine the presence or absence of *ts* mutants in a given population. As shown in Table 2, the virus from P2, 11-day fluid had an EOP (0.18) not significantly different from that of the wild-type

TABLE 2

Prospective Study: Appearance of *ts* Mutants in L Cells Persistently Infected with VSV_0[a]

Cell passage	Days after initiation	EOP[b] (39.5/32°C)	Number of clones isolated	Number of *ts*	Percent *ts*
Inoculum[c]		0.27	90	4	4.4
P-1	7	0.55	59	5	8.4
P-1	10	0.46	56	10	17.8
P-2	11	0.18	56	41	73.2
P-2	17	0.088	61	52	85.2
P-8	63	0.001	29	29	100

[a] From Youngner *et al.* (1976).
[b] Infectivity assays in primary chick embryo cells. PFU/ml at 32°C ranged from 1.1×10^3 to 3.7×10^5.
[c] Third undiluted passage of VSV_0 in BHK21 cells at 37°C.

VSV_0 (0.27); however, clonal analysis revealed that *ts* mutants composed 73.2% of the virus population.

All of the *ts* virus clones isolated from 84-day fluid were defective in their ability to synthesize virus-specific RNA in infected cells at the nonpermissive temperature (39.5°C) and were classified as having an RNA^- phenotype. In addition, the *ts* RNA^- clones all belonged to VSV complementation group I, which is associated with a defect in the virion-associated transcriptase (Pringle, 1977). This genetic uniformity is not surprising since Flamand (1970) reported that 81.7% of spontaneous mutants present in VSV (Indiana) populations were classed as group I mutants. If the *ts* mutants that maintain the persistently infected state were selected from those spontaneously present in the wild-type population, there is a strong possibility that they would belong to group I.

A *ts* mutant (*ts* pi 364) isolated from the 7-day fluid of the persistent infection summarized in Table 2 was able to establish persistent infection in L cells at 37°C in the absence of DI particles. It is interesting that Wagner *et al.* (1963) had previously reported that persistent infection of L cells could be established only with a small-plaque mutant of VSV (Indiana).

Additional evidence of a role for *ts* mutants in the maintenance of the persistent infection was provided by temperature-shift experiments. When L_{VSV} cell cultures were shifted from 37°C to 32°C, there was complete cell destruction and a significant increase in the amount of virus present in the culture fluids. In marked contrast, the shift of L_{VSV} cells to 39.5°C resulted in progressively diminished virus production until no virus was detectable after 30 days. Cocultivation of the "cured" cells with chick embryo or BHK21 cells at 37°C did not reactivate virus production.

Representative *ts* mutants from L_{VSV} cells were tested for a mutation in a viral function (P) for inhibition of protein synthesis in infected cells (Stanners *et al.*, 1977). A group I mutant of VSV (T1026), derived from the HR strain, contains a second non-*ts* mutation in addition to its *ts* transcriptase mutation. Whereas wild-type VSV is P^+ and effectively shuts off protein synthesis in infected cells, T1026 and its ts^+ revertants are phenotypically P^-. Rates of total protein synthesis in cells infected with these P^- viruses are equal to or greater than in uninfected cells. Seventeen *ts* mutants from L_{VSV} cells were unequivocally P^+ and were able to inhibit protein synthesis of infected L cells at 37°C as well as wild-type VSV (Youngner *et al.*, 1978b). It was concluded that the *ts* mutants which evolve in L_{VSV} cell cultures do not appear to lose the P function.

Another approach to the establishment of persistent VSV infections of L cells was offered by Nishiyama (1977), Nishiyama *et al.* (1978), and Ramseur and Friedman (1977). Instead of mediation by DI particles, these workers used pretreatment of L cells with interferon to minimize the cytolytic effects of wild-type VSV. Under these conditions persistent or prolonged infections at 35°C or 37°C were readily established. Studies of the virus present in carrier cultures established in this manner also revealed the emergence of a population of *ts* small-plaque virus. In Nishiyama's (1977) experiments, small-plaque viruses completely replaced the large-plaque parental population by the nineteenth cell passage, and as early as the tenth passage *ts* virus was detected by reduced efficiencies of plating at 38°C. At the fortieth cell passage medium- (MP) and small- (SP) plaque-size clones were isolated from the culture fluid (Nishiyama *et al.*, 1978). One-step growth curves in L cells revealed that the MP and SP clones replicated more slowly than the parental wild-type virus, giving maximum yields in 12 hr rather than in 6 hr. Both MP and SP viruses induced low levels of interferon at 35°C but not at 38°C; the wild-type virus did not produce interferon at either temperature. in agreement with Youngner *et al.* (1976), the *ts* mutant (SP) was also able to establish persistent infection at low MOI in L cells in the absence of interferon pretreatment or coinfection with DI particles. Ramseur and Friedman (1977, 1978) also showed that *ts* virus emerged as early as 10 days after initiation of infection of L cells pretreated with IF; by 17 days they noted a hundredfold decrease in the plaquing efficiency at 39°C compared to 32°C. All of the *ts* viruses isolated had a small-plaque phenotype. No further characterization of the viruses was reported.

The above evidence indicates that prolonged infections with VSV in L cells were probably due to the emergence of *ts* mutants and to endogenous interferon production rather than to DI particles. Endogenous interferon was implicated in these experiments not by the detection of the inhibitor in fluids from the infected cells but by the enhancement of virus replication and cell destruction after treatment of persistently infected cell cultures with antimouse interferon antibody (Ramseur and Friedman, 1977, 1978; Youngner *et al.*, 1978a). This approach had been used previously to elucidate the role of endogenous interferon in persistent infections of L cells with Sindbis virus (Inglot *et al.*, 1973).

It was suggested that interferon activity present in L_{VSV} cell cultures might exert pressure for the selection of *ts* mutants during viral persistence (Ramseur and Friedman, 1978). To test this possibility, six-times-cloned wild-type VSV was serially passed at low MOI in L cells which had been pretreated with mouse interferon (Youngner *et al.*, 1978*a*); parallel serial passages were made in L cells treated with medium alone. After the sixth serial passage, the 39.5°C/33°C plating efficiency of the virus harvested from interferon-treated or control cell cultures was not different from the plating efficiency of the wild-type inoculum. Clonal analyses of the sixth serial passages revealed that replication in L cells pretreated with interferon did not increase the frequency of *ts* virus above that spontaneously present in the wild-type inoculum (2–5%).

Holland and his co-workers have extensively studied persistent infections initiated with VSV (Indiana) in BHK21 and other cell lines. They described in detail the major role played by DI particles in the establishment and maintenance of persistent infections of BHK21 cells (Holland and Villarreal, 1974; Villarreal and Holland, 1976; Holland *et al.*, 1976*a,b*, 1978). In regard to the evolution of virus populations in persistently infected BHK21 cells, it was reported that after a year of persistence the cultures shed small-plaque mutant virus that was "slightly" temperature sensitive (Holland *et al.*, 1976*b*). After 4 years of persistence, these carrier cultures shed temperature-sensitive mutants which were "very slow growing" (Holland *et al.*, 1978). No quantitative data were given dealing with the phenotypic expression of the mutants at different temperatures, but it was reported that the carrier cells were stable when shifted from 37°C to 25°C or 32°C. Since BHK21 cells are defective interferon producers (Taylor-Papadimitriou and Stoker, 1971), it is apparent that this viral inhibitor probably plays no role in the long-term maintenance of persistence in these cells. Holland *et al.* (1979) reported that changes in the oligonucleotide map of the persisting virus accumulated over a 5-year period; over 100 mutations could be present according to the changes observed. The oligonucleotide map patterns of wild-type VSV serially passed in different cell lines were very stable (Clewley *et al.*, 1977; Kang *et al.*, 1978; Holland *et al.*, 1979). Further work will be necessary in order to determine how many of the multiple changes in oligonucleotide patterns are reflected in changes in virion polypeptides and which virion proteins are involved.

Holland and Villarreal (1974) reported that the B virions purified from BHK21 carrier cells showed greatly reduced levels of virion transcriptase activity. The particular carrier line involved was initiated using *ts*G31, which belongs to complementation group III (M protein defect). Although no further details are given, it is possible that the carrier BHK21 cells had evolved mutants with an RNA synthesis defect, akin to the drift to group I (virion transcriptase defect) virus identified in L$_{VSV}$ cells (Youngner *et al.*, 1976).

Holland *et al.* (1978) also established persistent infections with VSV in a line of HeLa cells defective in its ability to produce DI particles. A carrier line was initiated using wild-type VSV (Indiana) plus large numbers of DI particles. After persistence was established, it was found that the virus population in the HeLa$_{VSV}$ line consisted of *ts* small-plaque mutants. No DI particles or immature DI ribonucleoproteins were detectable in the carrier cell line. The *ts* virus which had evolved was capable of initiating persistent infection in HeLa cells at low MOI in the absence of added DI particles. No further characterization of the evolved virus was given.

As detailed previously, the persistent infections initiated in L cells with VSV$_0$ in the presence of large numbers of DI particles showed a rapid selection of *ts* viruses with RNA$^-$ phenotypes belonging to VSV complementation group I (Youngner *et al.*, 1976). To investigate the possible selective advantage of RNA$^-$ VSV mutants in persistence, infections were initiated in L cells with *ts*023, an RNA$^+$ mutant belonging to complementation group III (Youngner *et al.*, 1978a). The clonal analysis summarized in Table 3 revealed that 29 of 30 clones (97%) of *ts*023 parental virus showed an RNA$^+$ phenotype, but by 2 days after infection the frequency of RNA$^-$ mutants had risen to 10%. At 37 days the frequency of RNA$^-$ mutants was 68%; and by 198 days RNA$^-$ mutants composed 81% of the virus population. The results obtained with individual clones, displayed graphically in Fig. 1, reveal that, in addition to the increasing frequency of RNA$^-$ clones in the population, the RNA synthesis defect became progressively more pronounced with time. Essentially similar results were obtained when

TABLE 3

Appearance of RNA$^-$ Phenotype in Persistent Infections of L Cells Initiated With a Group III (RNA$^+$) *ts* Mutant of VSV (*ts*023)[a]

Cell passage	Days after initiation	Number of clones *ts*/ number isolated	Number of clones with RNA$^-$ phenotype[b]
Parental virus (*ts*023)	—	30/30	1 (3%)
P-0	2	30/30	3 (10%)
P-8	37	28/28	19 (68%)
P-18	75	29/29	21 (72%)
P-44	198	26/26	21 (81%)

[a] From Youngner *et al.* (1978a).
[b] RNA$^-$ phenotype = 39.5/33°C ratio of RNA synthesis in BHK21 cells by the cloned virus divided by the 39.5/33°C ratio of wild-type virus in infected cells is 0.2 or less.

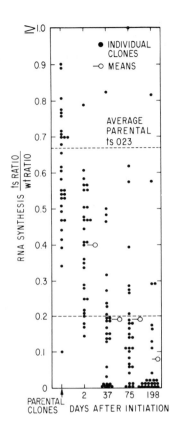

Fig. 1. Efficiency of RNA synthesis (39.5°C/33°C ratio) of *ts* virus clones isolated at different intervals from persistent infection of L cells initiated with *ts*023, a group III RNA⁺ mutant of VSV. Time on abscissa not to scale. From Youngner *et al.* (1978*a*).

the experiment was repeated using as inoculum a subclone of *ts*023 (III) which had been plaque-purified six times in CE cells and amplified at low MOI in MDBK cells which are poor producers of DI particles.

Persistent infection was also begun by infecting L cells with VSV *ts*045 (V), another RNA⁺ mutant (Youngner *et al.*, 1978*a*). In addition to reduced viral replication at 39.5°C, *ts*045 has another phenotypic marker: the virion G protein is defective and renders the virion heat labile (*hl*) at 50°C (Pringle, 1977). This marker enabled further characterization of the evolution of virus in persistent VSV infections of L cells. At 7 days after infection the carried virus was very similar to parental *ts*045. At 16 and 21 days after initiation of persistence the high EOP at 39.5°C of uncloned culture fluids was explained by the presence of a large number (17–37%) of non-*ts* (*ts*⁺), apparently wild-type revertant clones in the virus populations. By 36 days the virus population was again predominantly (85%) *ts*, and from 49 days on all virus clones were *ts*. Concurrent with these changes in the virus population, the heat lability of the *ts* virus clones changed dramatically. Figure 2 displays graphically the evolution of heat-resistant (hr) virus clones during persistent infection with *ts*045 (V). Of 26 stable *ts* hr clones isolated between 16 and 235 days after initiation, 22 (84.6%) had an RNA⁻ phenotype, indicating evolution of RNA⁻ viruses from the RNA⁺ *ts*045 mutant used to initiate the persistent infection. Attempts to carry out complementation analysis of the RNA⁻ clones isolated from persistent infections initiated with group III or group V RNA⁺ mutants were unsuccessful because of the leakiness of these mutants when used at high MOI in complementation analyses.

The findings summarized above demonstrate that, when persistent infections are initiated in L cells with RNA⁺ VSV mutants representing complementation groups III and V, the viruses which evolve are quite different from the parental viruses (Youngner *et al.*, 1978*a*). While

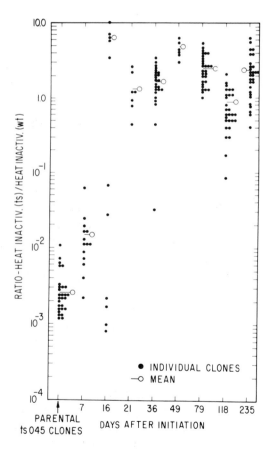

Fig. 2. Evolution of *ts* virus clones isolated at different intervals from persistent infection of L cells with *ts*045 (F-4), a six-times-cloned VSV group V RNA⁺ mutant. Inactivation of infectivity (compared to wild-type virus) after heating at 50°C for 10 min. Virus samples were diluted 1:100 in phosphate-buffered saline (pH 7.2) prior to heating. From Youngner *et al.* (1978*a*).

there was a long-term maintenance of the *ts* marker, a selection of viruses with RNA⁻ phenotypes occurred. The *ts* phenotype itself was not sufficient to stabilize the virus population since infections initiated with *ts* RNA⁺ mutants did not continue to produce virus with *ts* RNA⁺ phenotypes. Instead, there seemed to be a strong selective advantage for RNA⁻ viruses. The *ts* mutants isolated from persistent infections initiated with *ts*023 and *ts*045 were tested for P function; none differed from wild-type virus in ability to inhibit host protein synthesis in L cells at 37°C (Youngner *et al.*, 1978*b*). Furthermore, the mutants selected in these persistent infections did not differ significantly from their parental *ts* virus in induction of or sensitivity to interferon in L cells at 37°C (Preble and Youngner, unpublished data).

The lack of selective advantage of a "late" defect in a structural protein is emphasized by the results obtained in the case of persistent infection established with *ts*045, a group V mutant. The *ts hl* RNA⁺ parental *ts*045 inoculum evolved into a virus population that was *ts hr* RNA⁻. On the basis of this finding it appears that a defect in the G protein provides no selective advantage during persistence, in contrast to the *ts hr* RNA⁻ phenotype which does.

2.3.2. Rabies Virus

The evolution of virus populations during persistent infection of BHK cells with the HEP-Flury strain of rabies virus has been studied by Kawai *et al.* (1975). They found that large-plaque (LP) wild-type virus was replaced in a stepwise fashion by a small-plaque (SP) virus; after 22 cell transfers, the SP virus completely supplanted the LP parental virus. In the carrier cell cultures, the SP virus produced significant numbers of DI particles in a cyclic manner, and these defective particles effectively suppressed the cytopathic effect of standard LP parental virus. Cyclic production of DI particles in the persistently infected BHK cells was demonstrated by this inhibition test. The SP virus had the capacity to produce DI particles even during the first passage in BHK cells, regardless of the MOI (Kawai and Matsumoto, 1977). Previous work had shown that clonal isolates from the HEP-Flury strain of rabies virus generated DI particles in BHK cells at a significantly more rapid rate than VSV (Holland *et al.*, 1976*b*).

Kawai and Matsumoto (1977) demonstrated that rabies virus also produced a defective particle which showed no CPE-suppressing or interfering activity against standard virus. These defective noninterfering (DNI) particles, as well as conventional defective interfering (DI) particles, were generated by serial passage of SP virus in persistent infection in which SP virus predominated. Further investigation showed that the DNI particles lacked projecting spikes and contained little if any G protein (Matsumoto and Kawai, 1978). The spikeless particles contained low-molecular-weight material (12,000 mol. wt.) which comigrated in polyacrylamide gels with a similar fragment from infectious viruses which had been treated with trypsin to cleave the G protein (Matsumoto, personal communication).

Interestingly, DI particles generated by SP virus interfered with the growth of infective B virions of both SP and LP viruses; on the other hand, DI particles generated by LP virus interfered only with the replication of infective LP virions. The stepwise replacement of LP parental virus by SP virus in the rabies carrier line of BHK cells may be explained by this rather unique situation. In rabies persistence, the rapid generation of CPE-suppressing particles by SP virus may be a mechanism for cell sparing in a cell system (BHK) in which interferon is not produced. Villarreal and Holland (1976) also found that rabies virus persistence in BHK21 cells could be readily established using cloned wild-type virus in the absence of added DI particles; this was in marked contrast to the requirement for DI particles to establish persistent infections with VSV.

The possibility that the HEP-Flury as well as fixed rabies viruses can be classed as spontaneously occurring *ts* mutants (Clark and Wiktor, 1972) raises some interesting questions. The ease with which rabies viruses can establish persistent infections (Wiktor and Clark, 1972; Kawai *et al.*, 1975; Holland *et al.*, 1976*b*) may in part depend on this characteristic, as well as on the ability of rabies virus to generate CPE-suppressing DI particles with great rapidity (Kawai and Matsumoto, 1977). However, detailed phenotypic analysis of rabies viruses from persistent infections has not yet been done.

2.4. Togaviruses

2.4.1. Alphaviruses

2.4.1a. Western Equine Encephalitis (WEE) Virus

Cloned WEE virus was used to initiate persistent infection at 37°C in a line (Frukto) of mouse sarcoma cells (Simizu and Takayama, 1969). After 4 months of persistence two kinds of stable plaque-size mutants, large (LP) and small (SP), were present. The SP mutant was avirulent for adult mice, whereas the LP mutant was as virulent as the parental WEE virus. Temperature optimum studies showed that the SP mutant was unable to replicate at 42°C in CE cells, whereas the wild-type virus replicated as efficiently at 42°C as at 37°C, and temperature-shift experiments revealed that the SP virus had a defect late in the replication cycle (Simizu and Takayama, 1971). Non-*ts* (*ts*⁺) revertants of SP mutants, selected by passage at 41°C, did not regain their neurovirulence. Conversely, neurovirulent revertants retained the *ts* phenotype (Simizu and Takayama, 1971), indicating that the mutations to avirulence and to temperature sensitivity during the persistent infection probably were independent.

Persistent infection of *Aedes albopictus* mosquito cells with WEE virus at 28°C was also investigated (Maeda *et al.*, 1979). Most *ts* and SP mutants isolated early (< 30 days) after infection were leaky when tested in CE cells by plating or yield efficiency (41.5°C/34°C ratios); three of four stable *ts* mutants isolated early in the persistence had RNA⁺ phenotypes. By 80 days 100% of the population had converted to a *ts* RNA⁻ phenotype; by 170 days the *ts* RNA⁻ mutants were stable and showed no significant leakiness at 41.5°C. The infectivity of the *ts* RNA⁻ mutants was much more labile at 50°C than the infectivity of the parental virus, indicating that the *ts* lesion might be in a structural protein. Complementation analysis of 24 stable *ts* mutants from the persistent infection classified the clones into three groups. All four mutants from early phases of the persistence (3 RNA⁺, 1 RNA⁻) complemented as single-site mutants. All 20 RNA⁻ mutants from later phases of persistence were multiple mutants; 19 were double mutants, while one clone was a triple mutant.

2.4.1b. Sindbis Virus

A detailed study of the evolution of virus in persistent infections initiated by Sindbis virus in insect cell lines was made by Stollar and his colleagues (Shenk *et al.*, 1974; Stollar *et al.*, 1974; Igarashi *et al.*, 1977). Mosquito cells (*A. albopictus*) infected with Sindbis virus at 28°C exhibited no cytopathic effects. However, assay of the fluids from the infected mosquito line at 34°C in CE cells revealed that small-plaque variants of Sindbis virus were seen as early as 4–6 weeks, and small-plaque virus predominated by 10 weeks after initiation. Although parental Sindbis virus plaqued with equal efficiency at 34°C, 37°C, and

39.5°C, virus released from carrier cultures as early as 8 weeks after infection was *ts* at 39.5°C. By 20 weeks plaque formation was also inhibited at 37°C. Cloned virus isolates remained *ts* after several serial passages in BHK21 cells, ruling out the possibility of a host-induced modification of the virus.

Of 20 *ts* clones tested for RNA synthesis in BHK21 cells at 39.5°C, 19 were classed as RNA$^+$ and one as RNA$^-$ (Shenk *et al.*, 1974). In addition all the *ts* clones were more heat labile at 60°C than the parental virus. One clone (SVC2) which was RNA$^-$ at 39.5°C was also heat labile, suggesting at least two genetic lesions, one affecting RNA synthesis, the other affecting a structural protein. The appearance of similar *ts* RNA$^+$ mutants during persistent Sindbis infection of *A. albopictus* cells has also been noted by Eaton (personal communication). In additional studies of the evolution of *ts* mutants during persistent infections with Sindbis virus, a greater proportion of RNA$^-$ mutants was seen (Stollar, personal communication). The RNA$^-$ mutants have not been characterized further. Attempts to complement *ts* mutants from the persistent infection with each other were unsuccessful; neither RNA$^+$ × RNA$^+$ nor RNA$^+$ × RNA$^-$ crosses showed any complementation. In contrast, RNA$^+$ and RNA$^-$ *ts* mutants obtained by chemical mutagenesis showed significant complementation under the same conditions. Although it was concluded that the lack of complementation was additional evidence that the *ts* mutants contain more than one mutation (Shenk *et al.*, 1974), no data were presented dealing with crosses of the mutants from the persistent infection with mutagenized *ts* mutants.

Viral RNA synthesis in persistently infected *A. albopictus* cells was also studied in detail (Igarashi *et al.*, 1977). During acute infections and during the early stages of persistence, only one species of virus-specific double-stranded (ds) RNA, sedimenting at 22 S, was noted. At 10 weeks after initiation of persistence, a clear peak of ds RNA at 12–15 S was detected in addition to the 22 S ds RNA. It was concluded that the small ds RNA species reflected the presence of Sindbis virus DI genomes in the carrier line. This finding is a bit paradoxical since, under conditions of serial undiluted passages, *A. albopictus* cells do not generate DI particles of Sindbis virus; in addition, these cells do not respond to DI particles generated in CE or BHK21 cells (Eaton, 1975; Igarashi and Stollar, 1976). The explanations of these puzzling findings are not yet available.

When persistent Sindbis virus infections were established at 28°C in a mosquito line from *Aedes aegypti*, a similar pattern of virus evolution resulted (Stollar *et al.*, 1974). The wild-type Sindbis inoculum was replaced during persistence by a *ts* small-plaque RNA$^+$, heat-labile population. Interestingly, the 12–15 S ds RNA species detected in persistently infected lines of *A. albopictus* cells was not detected in the *A. aegypti* carrier lines.

2.4.1c. Other Alphaviruses

There have been other reports of the evolution of alphaviruses during persistent infection of mammalian and insect cell lines, but the viral properties studied have been limited to plaque size and virulence for mice. Persistence established by Semliki Forest virus in *A. albopictus* cells at 26°C (Davey and Dalgarno, 1974) and Venezuelan equine encephalitis virus in *A. aegypti* cells at 28°C (Carreño and Esparza, 1977) resulted in the evolution of a population with small-plaque morphology and reduced virulence for mice. In mammalian cells, carrier infections initiated with Ross River virus in primary mouse muscle cells at 37°C gave rise to virus populations with small-plaque morphology (Eaton and Hapel, 1976). No other virus properties were reported.

2.4.2. Flaviviruses: Japanese Encephalitis Virus

Japanese encephalitis virus (JEV) persistence in a continuous line of suckling mouse brain cells was established by Gavrilov *et al.* (1974, 1975). The virus recovered after many cell passages at 36.5°C differed from the parental JEV in several interesting characteristics. The virus from the carrier lines was sensitive to pancreatic ribonuclease and was highly resistant to 4 M urea compared to wt JEV; both of these properties reverted to wild-type after two passages in suckling mice. Also, the evolved virus, in contrast to parental JEV, had no hemagglutinating activity and was not neutralized by antibody against wild-type JEV (Gavrilov *et al.*, 1974).

Further studies of this system showed that the JEV virus recovered from persistently infected suckling mouse brain cells was *ts* in CE cells at 42°C; conditions at 37°C were considered semipermissive (Gavrilov *et al.*, 1975). The *ts* marker of the carrier virus was stable after passage in suckling mice, in contrast to RNAse sensitivity and urea resistance phenotypes which reverted to wild-type JEV patterns.

2.4.3. Rubiviruses: Rubella Virus

Evolution of unusual rubella virus mutants was described in detail by Sato *et al.* (1976). When a line of BHK21 cells was persistently infected with wild-type rubella virus (strain M33) and maintained at 34°C, the parental virus was replaced by a population of small-plaque *ts* mutants which appeared to be hybrids between rubella virus and a latent retrovirus found in many BHK21 cell lines (Shipman *et al.*, 1971; Mayo *et al.*, 1973). This latent virus also was *ts* since it was released from uninfected BHK21 cells at 34°C but not at 39.5°C.

Antirubella serum inhibited the hemagglutinating activity of the mutants and wild-type rubella virus, but neutralized the plaque-forming ability of only wild-type virus. The infectivity of the *ts* virus from the carrier cultures was neutralized by antiserum against the latent virus, whereas the wild-type parental rubella virus was not affected by the same serum (Sato *et al.*, 1976). A five- to tenfold increase in virus production by the persistently infected BHK cells in the presence of 5-bromodeoxyuridine or mitomycin C suggested that the rubella genome might be present in a proviral DNA form (Sato *et al.*, 1977). However, no additional analytic evidence such as hybridization data was presented to support this conclusion. In contrast to these results a provirus DNA copy was not detected in a line of monkey kidney cells (LLCMK$_2$) persistently infected with rubella virus; the methods used included filter hybridization, *in situ* hybridization, and treatment of the cells with mitomycin C, actinomycin D, or 5-bromodeoxyuridine (Norval, 1979). However, the presence of defective virus particles in these cell cultures was suggested by a peak of virus RNA which sedimented at 12 S, in addition to 40 S RNA typical of fully infectious virus.

Another difference between wild-type rubella virus and the *ts* mutant from the carrier cultures was that concanavalin A inactivated the infectivity of the wild-type virus but had little effect on the *ts* mutants (Urade *et al.*, 1978). It was concluded that the carbohydrate configuration or content of the envelope glycoproteins of the evolved hybrid viruses was different from that of the wild-type virus. Clones resistant to the lectin were isolated from the wild-type rubella virus stock, indicating that rubella–latent virus hybrids present in the parental population used to initiate the persistent infection may be the source of the hybrid viruses selected during persistence. Since the *ts* phenotype of the virus clones resistant to concanavalin A was not tested, it is difficult to draw a firm conclusion concerning this possibility.

Virus clones which resembled the hybrids from persistent infection were also isolated after about 50 serial passages of rubella virus in BHK21 cells (Sato *et al.*, 1978*a*). The putative hybrids were clearly rubella by complement-fixation tests and also reacted with antilatent virus serum in hemagglutination-inhibition and neutralization tests. However, unlike the hybrids from the carrier cultures, the serial passage hybrid virus was *ts*⁺ and did not contain reverse transcriptase activity. Virions of the high-passage hybrids may have a reverse transcriptase which is unstable or may lack a primer required for DNA synthesis (Sato *et al.*, 1978*a*). Additional studies will be necessary to clarify these problems.

2.5. Picornaviruses

2.5.1. Coxsackie Virus

Takemoto and Habel (1959) found that prolonged cultivation of HeLa cells persistently infected with Coxsackie A9 virus tended to select for virus with altered properties as well as for cells with increased resistance to A9 virus infection. Virus recovered from persistently infected cultures lacked virulence for mice, had increased virulence for HeLa cells, was "slow" to produce plaques on permissive monkey kidney cell monolayers, and could be distinguished antigenically from parental virus. The change in the mouse virulence marker occurred between cell passages 8 and 10. The difference in antigenicity between parental Coxsackie virus and persistent virus was analyzed using cross-neutralization and neutralization kinetics. Virus from persistent infection was neutralized three- to eightfold less efficiently than wild-type virus by antibody against wild-type A9 virus. In addition, neutralization kinetics confirmed that each virus was most efficiently neutralized by homologous antibody. Since the carrier cultures were maintained in medium containing 10% human serum, it is possible that a very low level of antiviral antibody was present, which would favor antigenic drift of the carried virus. Further characterization of the persistent virus was not reported.

2.5.2. Foot-and-Mouth Disease Virus

Foot-and-mouth disease virus (FMDV) may persist for long periods of time in the oropharynx of carrier cattle in the presence of specific neutralizing antiviral antibody (Van Bekkum *et al.*, 1959; Sutmoller and Gaggero, 1965; Burrows, 1966). *In vitro* and *in vivo* simulation of the conditions in carrier cattle was obtained by performing serial passages of FMDV in cell cultures in the presence of antiviral sera (Hyslop, 1965) or in partially immunized animals (Hyslop and Fagg, 1965). In each case, antigenic variants were accumulated in the serially propagated virus populations. The role of antigenic drift in chronic infections with other viruses, as well as with nonviral infectious agents, will be discussed in detail in Section 4.1.

Since both *in vitro* and *in vivo* model systems suggested that passage of FMDV in the presence of antiviral antibody led to evolution of virus with properties different from those of the original virus, the biological characteristics of virus isolated from carrier cattle was studied in more detail. Virus isolated from carrier cattle at various times after infection with strain A or strain O of FMDV was examined for the following characteristics: ability to replicate at various temperatures; resistance to pH 6.5, heat, and UV light; and neutralization by homologous and heterologous antisera (Fellowes and Sutmoller, 1970). Viruses isolated from carrier cattle often showed a progressive increase in resistance to UV light and/or mild acid treatment, although this was not seen with all carrier virus isolates. Several steers were infected with strain A, then superinfected with strain O 4 weeks later while type A virus was still present; the type A viruses isolated at 14 and 28 days after the first infection were more resistant to acid and UV than the original type A virus, while subsequent type O virus isolates tended to be less UV resistant than the parental type O virus used for superinfection. Type O virus isolates obtained from animals with a previous type A persistence also were partially neutralized by anti-A serum. Since additional evidence indicated that this cross-neutralization was not due to viral aggregates, the possibility was suggested that recombination had occurred between the resident type A virus population and the superinfecting type O virus, but this has not been confirmed.

Type A carrier isolates resembled the original type A virus in their ability to replicate at 30°C and 37°C but not at 42°C. In contrast, type O virus isolated from carrier cattle as early as 7 days after infection had lost the ability to replicate at 42°C, although original type O virus could replicate well at 30°C, 37°C, and 42°C (Fellowes and Sutmoller, 1970). Later virus isolates had an even more restricted temperature range and could not replicate at either high (42°C) or low (30°C) temperatures; virus isolated from carrier cattle 106 days after infection could replicate only at 37°C.

These results were complicated by the prior infection with type A FMDV, apparently a naturally occurring temperature-sensitive virus strain. However, a similar evolution of virus with reduced ability to replicate at high temperatures was also found in carrier cattle persistently infected with FMDV type C (Straver and van Bekkum, 1972). Initial studies of FMDV type C carrier isolates showed that most were more sensitive to both heat and low pH than prototype FMCV type C, and also produced smaller plaques than isolates from acutely infected cattle (Straver *et al.*, 1970). Further investigation showed that vesicular isolates produced plaques in BHK cells at 41°C, whereas both the number and diameter of plaques produced by carrier virus isolates were inhibited at temperatures above 37°C (Straver and van Bekkum, 1972). Conversely, carrier isolates from cows on one farm plaqued better at 30°C than vesicular isolates from acutely infected animals from the same area. Carrier viruses isolated later after infection produced smaller plaques in BHK cells at 37°C than carrier virus isolated previously from the same animal. The authors do not specifically use the term "temperature sensitive," although the carrier virus isolates plaqued at 41°C with an efficiency at least a hundredfold less than wild-type FMDV. The small-plaque property was evident in early isolates which still retained a high efficiency of plating at 41°C, suggesting that the small-plaque marker of the carrier isolates was independent from, but coselected with, restricted replication at 41°C. In addition, preliminary evidence showed that some of the later *ts* small-plaque FMDV carrier isolates had reduced virulence in cattle (Straver and van Bekkum, 1972). This pattern of virus evolution toward *ts* virus which forms small plaques and has reduced virulence during a naturally occurring persistent infection with FMDV *in vivo* is very similar to the pattern in several different model systems of *in vitro* persistent infection discussed elsewhere in this chapter.

2.6. Coronaviruses: Mouse Hepatitis Virus

Persistence of mouse hepatitis virus (MHV) strain JHM in mouse neuroblastoma cells (N_J cells) was accompanied by virus-specific cytopathic effects which were demonstrable at each cell passage, and virus isolated at various times between the twentieth and fortieth subcultures was no different from wild-type virus in plaquing behavior (Stohlman and Weiner, 1978). More than 200 virus clones isolated during this interval were also tested for EOP at 32°C, 37°C, and 39°C; no evidence of *ts* virus mutants was found. MHV reisolated from N$_J$ cell cultures did not differ from parental MHV in ability to cause demyelination in susceptible mice inoculated intracerebrally. There was no evidence to suggest that defective or defective-interfering virus particles were being produced in the persistently infected cells and, although the N$_J$ cells were resistant to superinfection with MHV, no interferon was detectable in the culture fluids. The mechanism by which virus persists in N$_J$ cell cultures is therefore still unclear.

When persistently infected N$_j$ cells were cloned in the presence of antiviral antibody, both antigen-positive and antigen-negative cell clones were obtained. None of the cell clones produced infectious virus at 32°C, 37°C, or 39°C (Stohlman *et al.*, personal communication). Infectious virus was rescued from cell clones only after fusion with permissive cells using polyethylene glycol. Rescued virus clones exhibited temperature-dependent inhibition of growth at 32°C and were classified as cold sensitive (*cs*). The *cs* mutants replicated more efficiently at 39°C than the parental MHV but produced fiftyfold less virus at 32°C.

Further characterization of *cs* mutants, performed using virus cloned in the DBT mouse cell line showed that the *cs* virus clones were also more thermostable than the parental MHV (Stohlman *et al.*, personal communication). The *cs* mutation and the thermostability markers appeared to be independent but coselected, since serial passage of *cs* virus in DBT cells resulted in a decrease in the thermal stability of the virus with no change in *cs* phenotype. All of the *cs* mutants were defective in virus-specific RNA synthesis at 32°C, and the *cs* block in replication occurred prior to 6 hr after infection; infected cell cultures shifted to 32°C later than 6 hr after infection produced normal viral yields. When the *cs* mutants were used in mixed infections for complementation analysis at 32°C, only eight out of 37 crosses yielded complementation indexes greater than 1. Mixed infections at 32°C with *cs* mutants and parental MHV resulted in a slight decrease in the yields of both the *cs* and parental viruses similar to the interference reported between *ts* mutants and other wild-type viruses (see Section 4.4). The significance of the selection of *cs* mutants in neuroblastoma cells latently infected with MHV is not known.

In contrast to the sudies decribed above, Lucas *et al.* (1978) reported the persistence of prototype mouse hepatitis virus (MHV3) and the JHM strain in a variety of continous cell lines of neural and nonneural origin. The persistently infected cultures were initiated and maintained at 32.5°C. To determine whether selection of *ts* virus mutants had occurred, cultures producing virus at 32.5°C were shifted to 39.5°C. This temperature shift resulted in a rapid inhibition of virus synthesis. However, the restriction of virus production at 39.5°C appeared to be due to a host factor since lytic infection of these cell lines with either strain of MHV was also inhibited at 39.5°C. Virus produced from the persistently infected cultures at 32.5°C was able to plaque with equal efficiency at 39.5°C on monolayers of fully permissive L cells (Lucas *et al.*, 1978). The role of temperature-dependent host factors in virus maturation from persistently infected cells has also been discussed with respect to measles virus persistence (see Section 2.1.2).

2.7. Arenaviruses

2.7.1. Lymphocytic Choriomeningitis Virus

Lymphocytic choriomeningitis (LCM) virus establishes a lifelong persistence in infected mice, and continuous virus production occurs in the presence of antiviral antibody; deposition of virus/antibody complexes in the tissues results in polyarteritis and glomerulonephritis (Hotchin, 1962; Pfau, 1978). In order to better understand LCM infection *in vivo*, several laboratories have studied model systems of persistence of LCM in cell cultures. Persistent LCM virus infection in mouse L cells, established in the absence of either antiviral antibody or interferon, was accompanied by little or no cytopathogenicity (Lehmann-Grube, 1967). There was a regular and extensive fluctuation in the amount of infectious virus released into the medium of the persistently infected cultures; the amplitude of the cyclic changes in virus production decreased with time after initiation of persistence. Further studies showed that L cells persistently infected with the Armstrong strain of LCM release virus particles which were neutralizable with anti-LCM serum, immunized but did not kill mice, and were not infectious for normal L cells or for primary monkey kidney cells (Lehmann-Grube *et al.*, 1969).

Similar variants of LCM with low cytopathogenicity (LPV) were isolated from L cells and BHK cells persistently infected with the WE strain of LCM virus (Hotchin and Sikora, 1973). The LPV did not produce plaques in LCM-susceptible cell cultures and lacked neurovirulence for mice. LPV variants were not found in persistently infected L-cell lines established with a turbid-plaque viscerotropic variant of LCM (Hotchin *et al.*, 1971). Since LPV was isolated only when persistent infection was initiated with a clear plaque-producing neurotropic variant of LCM, these results suggest that evolution of the LPV variants was associated with persistence.

The selection of clear-plaque and turbid-plaque variants in different tissues of persistently infected mice first described by Hotchin *et al.* (1971) was studied by Popescu and Lehmann-Grube (1976). Virus isolated from brains of persistently infected mice produced clear lytic plaques on L-cell monolayers, whereas virus isolated from spleens of the same mice produced turbid plaques. Cloned virus pools of one variant were never entirely free of the other plaque variant. Both clear- and turbid-plaque variants were able to establish persistence in newborn mice. When newborn mice were infected with clear-plaque virus, titers of both clear-plaque virus and LCM defective-interfering (DI) particles peaked within a few days and then rapidly declined; within 1 month after infection, the concentrations of both types of virus particles were at most 1% of their former levels. Regardless of the plaque characteristics of the inoculated virus, by 6 months after infection blood and viscera of carrier mice contained predominantly turbid-plaque variants, while brain homogenates contained predominantly clear-plaque virus. However, by 1 year after infection the level of turbid-plaque variants had also increased in the brains of persistently infected mice (Popescu and Lehmann-Grube, 1977). The turbid-plaque variant was reported to produce fewer defective-interfering particles in infected L cells than the clear-plaque virus. Pfau (1978) has suggested that, during the early stages of infection, DI virus may be necessary to limit the cell-killing activity of wt LCM (Dukto and Pfau, 1978) to a specific subpopulation of T lymphocytes, but that, later in infection, selection of DI-resistant virus mutants may actually occur.

Pfau and his colleagues found that a previously undescribed "stubborn-plaque" (SP) variant of LCM may play an indispensable role in the establishment and maintenance of persistent infection of LCM in the MDCK line of canine kidney cells (Jacobson *et al.*, 1979). The SP virus was detectable only by plaque assay on MDCK cells. This virus was isolated from persistently infected L cells which were also synthesizing DI virus and was present in all previously prepared stocks of LCM DI particles which were tested. Cloned SP virus was resistant to inhibition by standard DI virus and was able to convert self-curing infections of standard LCM in MDCK cells into persistent infections in which both SP and DI virus were produced. SP virus had a lower efficiency of plating at 39.5°C than standard LCM (Jacobson *et al.*, 1979); clonal analysis of SP virus to determine whether it is temperature sensitive is in progress (Pfau, personal communication). Evolution of SP-like virus in persistent infection of neonatally infected mice is also under study (Pfau, personal communication). The properties of SP and its presence in stocks of LCM DI particles may warrant reevaluation of the role of DI particles in LCM persistence.

2.7.2.   Other Arenaviruses

Another arenavirus, Junin virus (JV), was used to establish a persistent infection at 37°C in the Vero line of monkey kidney cells (Damonte and Coto, 1979). A low level of infectious virus was released from the persistently infected (JV) cells in a somewhat cyclical pattern, and the cell cultures were resistant to challenge with Junin virus or the related arenavirus, Tacaribe virus. Virus (JV_{pi}) isolated from the persistently infected cultures produced plaques like those of wild-type JV on Vero cells, did not differ from wild-type JV in lethality for mice, and was neutralized by antibody made against wild-type virus. However, the JV_{pi} recovered from the persistently infected cells did not replicate in Vero cells at 39°C; in contrast, wild-type JV replication was unaffected by incubation at 39°C. Replication of JV_{pi} at 33°C was slower than that of wild-type JV, and JV_{pi} was more thermolabile between 37°C and 50°C than parental virus. These characteristics are consistent with a pattern of evolution of *ts* mutants with altered properties in Junin virus infections.

The same workers have also studied persistent infection of Vero cells with Tacaribe virus (Coto, personal communication). Virus isolated from supernatant fluids of the persistently infected cultures was thermolabile and *ts*. Virus from carrier cell cultures showed a progressive loss with time in ability to replicate at 40°C. At 5 days after infection, the virus plaqued with about equal efficiency at 40°C and 33°C; 62 days after initiation (passage 8), virus from persistently infected culture fluids had an EOP (40°C/33°C) of approximately 10^{-3} More detailed analysis of the virus which evolved is not yet available.

2.8.   Reoviruses

Temperature-sensitive mutants of reovirus have been associated with chronic degenerative brain disease induced in laboratory rats (Fields, 1972). Wild-type reovirus inoculated intracerebrally into newborn rats produced an acute encephalitis with a high fatality rate. When animals were infected with mutants with a *ts* defect which maps in group B, the majority appeared to be healthy for several weeks or months, after which slowly progressive hydrocephalus became apparent (Fields, 1972; Fields and Raine, 1972). It was postulated that *ts* virus mutants may also be involved in similar chronic degenerative diseases of human central nervous system.

Spandidos and Graham (1976) reported the evolution of reovirus DI particles in a persistent infection of rats. Two-day-old rats were infected subcutaneously with wild-type reovirus type 3 or with B or C class *ts* mutants. The viruses multiplied rapidly in the brain and other tissues and reached a peak by 10 days after infection, after which the virus titers rapidly declined. Defective virus could be demonstrated during the acute phase of the infection, and the defective population contained almost exclusively virions with the L_1 segment of the genome deleted. During progression of the chronic disease, infectious virus disappeared from the brain; no infectivity was demonstrable by 80 days after infection. By 30 days after infection, a fraction of the defective virions contained multiple deletions in addition to those with only the L_1 deletion. Some brain samples contained a mixed population of defective virus particles. The possibility was raised that a population containing a mixture of defective virions with various genomic segments deleted might be able to replicate through mutual complementation even in the absence of infectious virus. This circumstance could explain the chronic degenerative effects of some viral infections, late effects which occur long after the detectable infectious virus has disappeared from the host or is difficult to demonstrate.

Persistent reovirus infections in L and Vero cells were established by Ahmed and Graham (1977) with class C and E *ts* mutants provided a large excess of defective virions were present in the viral inoculum. By the sixth cell passage of the infected cells the original *ts* parental virus had been replaced by a small-plaque mutant with a *ts*+ phenotype. This virus population, when free of defective particles, was unable to establish persistent infection in L cells.

Fields and his associates (1978) analyzed *ts*+ clones isolated from the persistently infected L-cell line initiated by Ahmed and Graham (1977) to determine if these *ts*+ mutants were true- or pseudorevertants (Ramig and Fields, 1977, 1979; Ramig *et al.*, 1977). Of seven *ts*+ clones analyzed by backcrossing to the wild-type parent, two were clearly shown to be pseudorevertants containing a suppressor mutation. When the *ts* progeny of these backcrosses were grouped by standard two-factor crosses with prototype *ts* mutants, one *ts*$^+$ clone from the persistent infection contained three distinct *ts* lesions. Therefore, viral mutation occurred coincident with the establishment and maintenance of the reovirus persistent infection. The developing ability to map biological functions to specific genes should provide important leads to the mechanisms involved in persistence of reovirus and other viral agents.

2.9. Retroviruses

The viruses which cause visna and equine infectious anemia (EIA) resemble RNA C-type retroviruses in structure and replication patterns. In permissive cells both visna virus (Haase and Varmus, 1973) and EIA virus (Crawford *et al.*, 1978) effect a complete transfer of genetic information from RNA to DNA by a virion reverse transcriptase during the viral eclipse period, and some of the viral DNA is covalently integrated into host DNA. Both visna and EIA viruses are representative of so-called exogenous RNA retroviruses: proviral DNA is added to the genetic complement of a cell that previously lacked nucleotide sequences homologous to the virus. These viruses and other agents referred to as "lentiviruses" form a closely related and distinct group of retroviruses that are not related to the RNA viruses that cause tumors or latent infections in animals (Stowring *et al.*, 1979). Both visna and EIA viruses produce chronic diseases in animals which illustrate interesting patterns of viral evolution.

2.9.1. Visna Virus

Visna is an inflammatory demyelinating disease of the central nervous system of sheep. The disease is a prototype of "slow virus infections" with incubation periods of several months or years. More details concerning visna virus infections will be found in Chapter 6 of this volume.

An interesting facet of visna is the persistence of the viral agent in sheep which show significant neutralizing antibody responses (Thormar and Palsson, 1967). This can partially be explained by the sequestration of proviral DNA which has been demonstrated by *in situ* hybridization in the nuclei of brain cells from infected animals (Haase *et al.*, 1977). It has also been suggested that recurrent inflammatory episodes leading to slow progression of clinical disease may be the result of evolution of antigenically distinct mutants of visna virus during the prolonged infection (Narayan *et al.*, 1977*a,b*). Hampshire lambs inoculated intracerebrally with plaque-purified visna virus (strain 1514) were studied for prolonged periods. Visna virus was isolated from peripheral blood leukocytes (PBL) using indicator sheep choroid plexus cells (Narayan *et al.*, 1977*a*). Within 6 months, all infected sheep showed good serum neutralizing antibody titers against the parental strain (1514) of visna virus, but not against a serologically distinct but related strain (D1-2). Interestingly, viruses isolated from sheep almost 2 years after infection were neutralized poorly if at all by serum from the sheep from which they were recovered, although all of the sera neutralized the parental strain 1514 virus. The recovered viruses were all clearly visna virus when tested by neutralization with goat hyperimmune sera made against strains 1514 and D1-2. The antigenic drift from the parental strain 1514 was not apparent prior to the development of antibody in the infected sheep.

Sheep from the above study were followed for 3½ years (Narayan *et al.*, 1978). The virus underwent progressive antigenic drift over the years concomitant with the development of antibody to preexisting strains of virus. The mutants were (1) stable antigenically after plaque purification, (2) virulent in cell culture and when inoculated into sheep, and (3) elicited antibody which cross-reacted with the parental virus (strain 1514) from which they were derived.

The selection of antigenic variants under antibody pressure was reproduced in sheep choroid plexus cell cultures infected with plaque-purified strain 1514 and maintained in the continuous presence of immune sheep serum (Narayan *et al.*, 1977*a,b*). Viruses obtained after five cell passages in antibody were then cultivated in antibody-free medium and compared to the original parent virus by neutralization tests. The viruses passaged in the presence of antibody showed significant antigenic differences from the parental strain. Further testing with additional sheep sera and hyperimmune goat serum suggested that the viruses derived in the presence of antibody also differed from one another. These results, contrasted with the antigenic homogeneity of clonal isolates of parental strain 1514, suggested that the antigenic variants which evolved arose *de novo* (Haase *et al.*, 1978).

Variants which are antigenically distinct from the parental virus by neutralization tests cannot be distinguished from the parental virus by complement fixation tests. Preliminary examination of the variants by peptide mapping of the structural polypeptides revealed significant differences between the antigenic variants and the parental virus only in the virion glycoprotein, gP135, the envelope antigen which elicits a neutralizing antibody response (Haase *et al.*, 1978).

Further analysis of the antigenic variants and the parental visna virus by restriction endonuclease mapping showed that strain 1514 and an antigenic variant from persistently infected sheep, LV1-1, could not be distinguished by BAM I endonuclease digestion (Clements *et al.*, 1978). However, differences between LV1-1 and 1514 were seen with Taq I endonuclease which cleaves visna cDNA at several sites. These changes have not yet been localized on the endonuclease map of visna virus.

2.9.2. Equine Infectious Anemia (EIA) Virus

EIA is an exogenous retrovirus infection of horses which is expressed as an immunologically mediated destruction of red blood cells. Cycles of virus replication in macrophages originate from an unknown site of persistence and lead to anemia and clinical disease (Henson and McGuire, 1974). The evolution of antigenic variants of EIA virus in horses had been reported by Kono *et al.* (1973). Horses experimentally infected with cloned EIA virus showed a chronic disease with periodic relapses of fever accompanied by increased viremia. Viruses isolated at successive stages of the chronic disease were not susceptible to previously formed neutralizing antibody but reacted with antibodies produced some weeks later. In addition, isolates from late in the disease differed antigenically from one another when tested by neutralization, an observation which strongly suggested that the EIA virus underwent antigenic drift during the course of the chronic infection. Similar to the visna virus mutants described above, the EIA antigenic variants which were differentiated by neutralization tests could not be distinguished by complement fixation. This suggested that a modification of a surface glycoprotein antigen may have occurred.

Antigenic variants derived from the chronically infected animals retained a high level of infectivity for horses and were antigenically stable after ten serial passages in equine leukocyte cultures (Kono *et al.*, 1973). This genetic stability ruled out phenotypic mixing as an explanation of the antigenic differences observed. The most plausible assumption concerning the origin of these variants is that they evolved as a result of the selection pressure of antibody in the infected horses. The evolution of variants which are antigenically different and not susceptible to antibody formed previously may be the explanation of the periodic febrile relapses and the persistence of viremia in horses. Further discussion of the evolution of viruses and other agents by antigenic drift is present in more detail in Section 4.1.

3. EVOLUTION OF VIRUS IN PERSISTENCE OF DNA VIRUSES

3.1. Herpesviruses

It has been amply documented that members of the herpesvirus group commonly establish persistent infections in normal individuals (Rapp and Jerkofsky, 1973). Herpes simplex type 1 (HSV1) or cytomegaloviruses can be recovered from a significant proportion of healthy persons, most of whom continually excrete virus even in the presence of circulating antibody, although some have latent infections in which infectious virions can only be recovered during reoccurrences of overt disease. The state of the virus genome during these silent periods is not well understood; however, many different stimuli may activate latent infections with herpesviruses, and it is well known that debilitated patients or those with compromised immunological responses are at special risk.

Although there have been many studies of the persistence of herpesviruses *in vivo* and *in vitro*, there is a very limited understanding of the mechanisms involved. Some evidence has been reported of the evolution of herpes simplex virus type 1 (HSV1) in persistent infections of humans and in cell culture models. HSV1 persistence was established in various human cell lines maintained in medium which contained low levels of antibody derived from screened human sera (Hoggan and Roizman, 1959; Hinze and Walker, 1961). There was an evolution of the virus in the carrier cells to small-plaque variants which also produced an altered type of cell destruction. Instead of the cytolytic effect produced by the parental HSV, the virus from the carrier lines caused a proliferative type of lesion which was characterized by the formation of cell foci and large syncytial aggregates. If the viruses which evolved were passaged in the absence of anti-HSV serum, the cell damage reverted to the cytolytic parental type. Further studies of the variants which evolved showed that they had a much reduced virulence for mice, with little or no capacity for replication in mouse brain, in contrast to virulent parental virus; in addition, there was no gross change in the antigenicity of the variants when tested by neutralization with HSV antibody (Hinze and Walker, 1961).

More recently, HSV1 infections were initiated at 37°C in a rat central nervous system tumor cell line which continued to produce infectious HSV1 particles for 20–57 cell passages (Doller *et al.*, 1979). Preliminary evidence indicated that several sublines of the carrier cells maintained at 37°C produced significantly more virus when shifted to 31°C and assayed at the lower temperature. These findings suggest that *ts* virus was evolved in this system; however, no further characterization of the altered virus was reported. A preliminary study has been made of the ability of wild-type HSV1 and five chemically induced *ts* mutants to establish latent infection in mice (Lofgren *et al.*, 1977). The results showed that the wild-type and four *ts* mutants were able to latently infect mouse brain. One mutant (*ts*I) failed to produce a latent infection.

Antigenic drift of HSV1 has been reported in persistent infections of humans (Ashe and Scherp, 1965). Thirteen strains of HSV1 were isolated from recurrent herpes labialis in four persons. Kinetic analysis of neutralization by rabbit antisera against a range of strains showed that successive isolates from the same person varied antigenically but not in a regular manner. The variations observed could not be correlated with the sequence or temporal proximity of the recurrences. Neutralization kinetic analysis of the reactions of eight HSV1 strains from two subjects were made with five samples of their own sera. The results showed that successive isolates from the same individual were not identical. It is puzzling that these serological relationships did not correlate with those established by rabbit antisera and varied with different serum samples from the same person.

Hampar and Keehn (1967) studied persistent infection of a line of Chinese hamster cells (MAL) with HSV1; the carrier culture was established and maintained in the absence of specific antibody. Reciprocal neutralization kinetic analysis was carried out using virus isolated from 17 to 132 weeks after initiation of the persistence. The sera against each virus were prepared by immunization of rabbits. With time, the viruses recovered from the persistently infected cells acquired new antigenic determinants while still retaining the determinants of the antecedent virus. Neutralization kinetics, determined using plaque-purified virus isolated 17 and 23 weeks after initiation of the persistence, revealed that the antigenic variations were not due to fortuitous responses of heterogeneous virus populations. Further studies of this cell culture system by Hampar and Burroughs (1969) led them to postulate that a genetically determined cell–virus equilibrium may serve to maintain localized infections at a low level during periods of remission, with a concomitant slow rate of change in the virus and perhaps the cells. The progressive evolution of antigenic variants of HSV1 in the presence of antibody in humans (Ashe and Scherp, 1965) and in a cell culture system maintained without antibody (Hampar and Keehn, 1967) lends credence to this idea.

3.2. Parvoviruses: Aleutian Disease Virus

Aleutian disease is a common and economically important persistent virus infection of mink which results in severe hypergamma-globulinemia with associated immune complex arteritis and glomerulonephritis (Porter *et al.*, 1969, 1973). Recent evidence suggests that Aleutian disease virus (ADV) may be a naturally selected *ts* virus. Virus was isolated from tissues of diseased mink by infecting a continuous line of feline renal cells (CRFK); ADV replication occurred only when the CRFK cells were incubated at 31.8°C and not when the cultures were kept at 37°C or 39°C (Porter *et al.*, 1977). Five strains of ADV tested were all *ts* in CRFK cells at 37–39°C. Serial passage of ADV in CRFK cells at 37°C selected a virus population capable of optimal replication at 37°C. However, when this virus was used to infect mink, virus could be reisolated from the infected animals in CRFK cells incubated at 31.8°C but not at 37°C. These results strongly suggest that persistent infection *in vivo* favors evolution of a *ts* variant of ADV, although the possibility of a temperature-dependent host-cell factor necessary for ADV replication in CRFK cells has not been excluded. Detailed discussion of ADV is the subject of Chapter 5 of this volume.

4. PATTERNS OF EVOLUTION OF VIRUS PROPERTIES IN PERSISTENT INFECTION

4.1. Antigenic Drift

A significant body of information has accumulated which deals with the evolution of antigenic variants as a mechanism of viral persistence. In an infected animal such an alteration would allow the viruses to escape from neutralization by antibody, thus perpetuating the virus infection in an immunologically competent host. Evidence for the selection of antigenic variants with time has been reported in humans persistently infected with herpes simplex virus, type 1 (Ashe and Scherp, 1965), in sheep carrying visna virus (Narayan *et al.*, 1977*a,b*, 1978), and in horses suffering from equine infectious anemia (Kono *et* *al.*, 1973). In addition, there is some evidence that the viruses isolated from patients with SSPE, a delayed neurological disease caused by measles virus, are antigenically different from viruses from acute measles disease (Payne and Baublis, 1973). Details of these systems have been presented in the appropriate sections of this chapter.

A representative schematic pattern for what occurs in visna is described in Fig. 3. Antigenically distinct mutants of visna virus which arise in an infected animal allow the virus to replicate and spread. Immunological controls are reestablished by antibody production to the new antigenic variant which is not neutralized by the preexisting antibody. As successive virus variants appear, the infectious process is advanced until the host produces antibody to the newest variant.

Selection of antigenic variants has also been demonstrated in cell culture models of viral persistence of HSV1 and visna virus. In the case of HSV1 this was accomplished in the absence of specific antibody in the culture medium (Hampar and Keehn, 1967). With visna virus, persistently infected cells were maintained in the continuous presence of antiviral antibody in the medium (Narayan *et al.*, 1977*a*). There is also evidence that antigenic variants of coxsackie A9 virus were selected in persistent infections of cell cultures (Takemoto and Habel, 1959). In the *in vivo* and *in vitro* systems studied the antigenic mutants which appeared sequentially were stable. Clonal isolates passaged in the absence of antibody maintained their unique antigenic properties and retained the virulence characteristics of the parental wild-type virus.

The ability of viruses to alter their antigenic properties when serially passed in the presence of antibody has been well documented

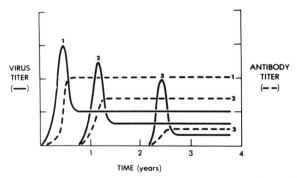

Fig. 3. Theoretical scheme of the role of antigenic drift in the spread of visna virus. Curve 1 (———) represents the increase in titer of the inoculum strain of virus and fall in titer with the appearance of neutralizing antibody to virus 1 (– – –1); spread of virus 1 is limited until antigenic variants 2 and 3 arise which reproduce and spread until restricted by antibodies in the manner described for virus 1. From Haase *et al.* (1978).

for influenza A virus (Laver and Webster, 1968; Webster and Laver, 1975). The interplay of viral mutability and immunological selection was evidenced by the gradual drift which occurred with influenza A subtypes in human populations and in laboratory model systems. In the latter, antigenic variants were produced by serially propagating influenza virus in the presence of sublimiting amounts of antibody and in animals which were partially immune. There is no doubt that such mutants have a distinct advantage in regard to replication in the presence of the antibody used in the selection process. The antigenic mutants selected *in vitro* in the presence of antibody showed changes from parental influenza A virus in peptide maps and amino acid sequences of the hemagglutinin subunits (Laver and Webster, 1968).

Stable antigenic variants of foot-and-mouth disease virus (FMDV) were produced by serial passages in partly immunized cattle (Hyslop and Fagg, 1965) and in cell cultures containing antiviral sera (Hyslop, 1965). The modifications of antigenic structure of FMDV were demonstrable by both neutralization and complement-fixation tests. As reported for other virus systems, e.g., HSV1, visna, and influenza A viruses, the homogeneity of the antigenic specificity of cloned parental virus seemed to rule out the selection of variants from a heterogeneous population of viruses. Instead, the antigenic drift seemed to be caused by the selection of mutant viruses under the pressure of the presence of specific antibody.

Antigenic drift is a phenomenon which occurs in chronic infections with agents other than viruses. As early as 1928 it was reported that *Borrelia* recovered from patients with relapsing fever or from animals with experimentally transmitted disease showed altered antigenicity in successive relapses (Meleney, 1928). In addition, chronic malarial infections with *Plasmodium knowlesi* in rhesus monkeys were maintained by a succession of antigenically distinct parasite populations, each of which was able to stimulate a specific agglutinin response (Brown *et al.*, 1968). Vickerman (1974), studying tsetse-fly-transmitted sleeping sickness, reported that the ability of the trypanosome population to change its surface antigen seemed to be the principal mechanism by which the organisms survived in the immunologically competent host. In the case of complex organisms such as *Borrelia*, *Plasmodia*, or *Trypanosoma*, it is likely that each parasite is capable of expressing a range of surface antigens, but normally only one subset of antigens at a time is evident in response to selection in the presence of antibody. With viruses, on the other hand, genetic mutation which involves the specificity of surface antigens is the likely mechanism involved in antigenic drift.

4.2. Selection of Virus Mutants

Although selection of antigenically distinct virus variants may be favored during virus persistence in immune animals or in cell culture model systems maintained in the presence of antiviral antibody, evolution of other specific types of virus mutants commonly occurs in persistently infected virus carrier cultures propagated in the absence of specific antibody. Data summarized in the preceding sections overwhelmingly indicates that virus evolved in persistently infected cell cultures often differs from parental virus in (1) virulence markers, including cytopathogenicity, growth rate, and plaque type in permissive cells, and pathogenicity for experimental animals; (2) host range in cell culture; (3) virion properties such as thermal stability; and (4) ability to replicate at elevated temperatures.

The selective advantage in persistent infection of virus mutants which are less cytopathic, thereby allowing survival of the host cells, is obvious. Since noncytopathic mutants may replicate more slowly and produce fewer progeny per cell, it is understandable that such mutants may produce small or delayed plaques in permissive cells. Selection of virus mutants partially deficient in a viral function, P, necessary for inhibition of host cell protein synthesis may occur during persistence of VSV in L cells (Stanners *et al.*, 1977; Francoeur *et al.*, personal communication). In addition, infection with noncytopathic virus mutants may allow the host cell to produce interferon; this would then limit the progression of infection (Sekellick and Marcus, 1979).

In those instances in which the biological properties of the persisting virus have been characterized, the virus has most often been shown to be a mutant that produces small plaques and is temperature sensitive. Evolution of *ts* small-plaque mutants occurs in cells of many different species persistently infected with herpesvirus, paramyxoviruses, rhabdoviruses, togaviruses, arenaviruses, and coronaviruses; many of these *ts* mutants also have an RNA$^-$ phenotype at the nonpermissive temperature. In addition, the evolution of *ts* mutants may also occur during *in vivo* persistence of FMDV, ADV, and SSPE measles viruses in natural hosts. Although attenuation, small-plaque morphology, and temperature sensitivity are often co-selected in the virus population during persistent infection, several studies have shown that these changes are due to independent mutations (Simizu and Takayama, 1971; Straver and van Bekkum, 1972; Preble and Youngner, 1973*b*; Youngner *et al.*, unpublished data). The association between attenuation, small-plaque morphology, and temperature sensitivity has been noted previously. For example, attenuated strains of poliovirus developed for use as oral vaccine are unable to replicate at elevated temperatures (Sabin, 1961). The relationship between small-plaque phenotype and lack of virulence for both animals and cell cultures has also been demonstrated with measles virus (Rapp, 1964) and NDV (Schloer and Hanson, 1968; Reeve and Poste, 1971). Furthermore, replication of some lentogenic (avirulent) strains of NDV may be inhibited at 42°C, as compared with velogenic (virulent) strains (Jones and Hanson, 1976).

The selective advantage in persistence of a *ts* phenotype is not immediately obvious. Most often, persistent infection at 37°C results in selection of virus which is unable to replicate at 39–40°C, but which retains some ability to replicate at 37°C. The conditions under which persistence is maintained, i.e., 37°C, are therefore semipermissive for virus growth. Presumably, enough "leak" occurs at this semirestrictive temperature to allow perpetuation of virus without rapid cell killing. Two alternative mechanisms which might allow *ts* virus to become amplified and then maintain its dominance in the persisting virus population are discussed below (Sections 4.3 and 4.4).

Finally, the selective advantage in several systems of *ts* mutants with RNA$^-$ phenotypes (Preble and Youngner, 1973a; Youngner et al., 1976, 1978a) remains to be clarified. Since the majority of spontaneous *ts* mutants of VSV (Flamand, 1970) and NDV (Youngner and Quagliana, unpublished data) occur in genes coding for polymerase function, preexisting spontaneous RNA$^-$ mutants may be selected in persistent infections initiated with these viruses. However, persistent infections initiated using cloned RNA$^+$ *ts* mutants of VSV also evolved until RNA$^-$ *ts* mutants predominated in the virus population (Youngner et al., 1978a,b). Since a *ts* defect in an early function would "mask" a *ts* defect in a later function, the possibility exists that the mutants which evolved during persistence were really double mutants. In this case a second spontaneously occurring group I *ts* defect in polymerase function would be superimposed on the original group III (M protein) or group V (G protein) defect. However, in the case of persistence initiated with VSV *ts*045 (V), thermal inactivation (Youngner et al., 1978a,b) and temperature shift experiments (Preble, unpublished) suggest that the RNA$^-$ mutants which evolve during persistence do not retain the original G protein defect and are not double mutants.

The selective advantage of the RNA$^-$ phenotype *per se* may be explained by the limited ability of RNA$^-$ *ts* mutants to produce virus-specific RNA and cytotoxic proteins at the semi-restrictive temperature at which persistence is maintained. In fact, noncytopathic mutants of NDV have been found which are defective in secondary transcription at 37°C and 41.8°C, even though significant viral yields were obtained at both temperatures (Madansky and Bratt, 1978, and personal communication). However, other evidence exists which contradicts the idea that RNA⁻ mutants inherently allow greater cell survival at semipermissive temperatures and also raises doubts about the necessity of P⁻ mutants in persistence: VSV *ts* RNA⁻ mutants isolated from persistently infected cells inhibited host cell macromolecular synthesis at 37°C almost as efficiently as wild-type VSV (Youngner *et al.*, 1978*b*).

Although a combination of temperature sensitivity, attenuation, and small-plaque morphology occurred in virus evolved during persistence in most of the well-characterized virus/host systems described in this chapter, there were also many exceptions. For example, virus recovered from some cell cultures persistently infected with wild-type respiratory syncytial virus (Simpson, personal communication) or with measles virus (Wild and Dugre, 1978) was not *ts*. Persistent infection of L or Vero cells initiated using certain *ts* mutants of reovirus (Ahmed and Graham, 1977) resulted in the evolution of *ts*⁺ pseudorevertants, in which the original *ts* mutation was suppressed by additional extragenic mutations (Fields *et al.*, 1978). Finally, virus rescued from nonproducer cells persistently infected with mouse hepatitis virus was cold sensitive and unable to replicate or synthesize virus-specific RNA at 32°C, although its growth at 37°C was unimpaired (Stohlman *et al.*, personal communication). The mechanisms of persistence and the evolution of other genetic characteristics of the viruses in these situations remain to be elucidated.

Virus recovered from persistently infected cell cultures also often differs from parental virus in properties associated with structural proteins; the carried virus may be more or less resistant to inactivation by heat, pH, UV light, or chemical agents, or may have altered hemagglutinating activity. These changes may reflect mutations in structural proteins with multiple functions in the virus replication cycle; the alteration may therefore affect virus-specific RNA and protein synthesis as well as virion integrity and infectivity. Choppin *et al.* (1975) have discussed the possibility that persistent paramyxovirus infections characterized by an intracellular accumulation of defective nucleocapsids may be the result of lack of cleavage of a virus glycoprotein precursor, F_0, to the biologically active form in the persistently infected host cells. Conversely, emergence of virus mutants more resistant to proteolytic cleavage by the enzymes present in a particular host cell

(Scheid and Choppin, 1976) might also play a role in virus evolution in chronic infections.

4.3. Interaction between Selection of Virus Mutants and the Interferon System

It has been proposed that initiation and maintenance of persistent infection in cell cultures competent for the interferon system involves evolution of either special defective-interfering (DI) particles or virus mutants with an increased capacity to induce interferon in the infected cells (Sekellick and Marcus, 1978, 1979). Two lines of evidence led to this hypothesis: (1) the recent demonstration that [±] DI particles of VSV, which contain covalently linked message [+] and antimessage [−] RNA genome (Lazzarini *et al.*, 1975; Perrault, 1976; Perrault and Leavitt, 1978), were able to induce interferon in aged chick embryo cells *in vitro* (Marcus and Sekellick, 1977; Sekellick and Marcus, 1978); and (2) the use of antiinterferon serum to demonstrate the role of this inhibitor in L cells persistently infected with VSV (Nishiyama, 1977; Ramseur and Friedman, 1977; Youngner *et al.*, 1978*a,b,*). Further investigations showed that many *ts* mutants of VSV induced interferon in aged chick embryo cells at 40.5°C (Sekellick and Marcus, 1979), whereas conventional [−] RNA DI particles and infectious B particles of wild-type VSV did not induce interferon under the same conditions. DI 011, a [±] RNA-containing DI particle, and the *ts* mutants also induced lower levels of interferon in L cells at 37°C (Sekellick and Marcus, 1979).

Detailed analysis of 29 temperature-sensitive virus clones isolated at various times from four different persistently infected L-cell cultures established independently with wild-type VSV or with VSV *ts* mutants showed that there was no uniformity in the ability of these clones to induce interferon in L cells at 37°C, i.e., under the conditions of virus persistence (Preble and Youngner, unpublished data). In addition, serial passage of VSV in the presence of low concentrations of interferon did not result in the evolution of *ts* mutants (Youngner *et al.*, 1978*a*). Furthermore, 22 *ts* virus clones isolated from several L-cell lines persistently infected with VSV did not differ from wild-ype VSV in their sensitivity to interferon in L cells at 37°C. Similar results were obtained with *ts* virus clones isolated from L cells persistently infected with Newcastle disease virus (NDV) (Hallum *et al.*, 1970; Preble and Youngner, unpublished data).

Attempts were made to establish persistent infection by infecting L cells with a small-plaque variant (s_2) of VSV (Indiana) which induces high levels of interferon in L cells at 37°C (Wertz and Youngner, 1970). These attempts were uniformly unsuccessful; in each case high levels of interferon were produced and the infection "cured" itself (Youngner, unpublished data). However, persistence in L cells at 37°C was readily established with cloned VSV $ts023$ (III) or VSV $ts045$ (V) (Youngner et al., 1978a), both of which were classified as interferon-forming-particle-negative (ifp⁻) (Sekellick and Marcus, 1979). In such L-cell cultures persistently infected with $ts023$ and $ts045$ (both ts RNA⁺ mutants), there was a rapid selection of ts RNA⁻ mutants (Youngner et al., 1978a); many of the virus clones which evolved were among those found negative for interferon induction in the experiments summarized above. It is possible that some ts mutants previously characterized as interferon-negative might actually induce very low levels of interferon in competent cells recognizable by the failure of virus plaques to enlarge on such cell monolayers (Francoeur et al., personal communication). Such virus mutants were found to be "weakly" P⁻ at 37°C, a semipermissive temperature for the mutants.

On the basis of their study of productive infections, Sekellick and Marcus (1978) proposed that the evolution of special [±] DI particles capable of inducing interferon may play a role in the maintenance of persistent infections. However, the DI particles of VSV amplified from persistently infected L cells by serial undiluted passages in BHK 21 cells were not more efficient inducers of interferon than DI particles from wild-type VSV (Frey et al., 1979). In addition, the RNA from DI particles amplified from persistently infected L cells lacked the self-annealing characteristics of [±] "snap-back" RNA found in DI 011.

It is difficult to invoke the interferon system in the case of cell lines which are defective interferon producers. Despite this deficiency these cell lines (Vero or BHK21) have been persistently infected with a variety of viruses. In these instances, evolution of either special DI particles or virus mutants may play a role in maintenance of persistence.

4.4. Interference with Wild-Type Virus Replication by ts Mutants

The dominance of the replication of ts virus over that of wild-type virus has been reported for a wide variety of RNA viruses. These include NDV (Preble and Youngner, 1973b), Sendai (Kimura et al.,

1976), measles (Ju and Bloom, personal communication), Sindbis (Stollar *et al.*, 1974; Peleg and Stollar, 1974), Semliki Forest (Keränen, 1977), VSV (Youngner and Quagliana, 1976), and reovirus (Chakraborty *et al.*, 1979). The interference of *ts* mutants with wild-type virus replication can be demonstrated most readily at the temperature non-permissive for the mutant, but with some viruses *ts* dominance can be shown at the permissive temperature as well (Stollar *et al.*, 1974; Youngner and Quagliana, 1976; Ju and Bloom, personal communication). No distinction seems to exist between the interfering ability of *ts* mutants obtained by mutagenesis and those selected in persistent infection (Youngner and Quagliana, 1976).

The biochemical basis of the dominance of *ts* mutant replication over that of the wild type is not completely understood. In the case of VSV (Youngner and Quagliana, 1976; Youngner, unpublished data) and reovirus type 3 (Chakraborty *et al.*, 1979), *ts* mutants with RNA⁻ and RNA⁺ phenotypes are able to interfere with *ts*⁺ virus replication. With Semliki Forest virus, only one *ts* RNA⁻ mutant was tested at the nonpermissive temperature (Keränen, 1977). In the case of Sindbis virus, interference by a *ts* RNA⁺ mutant at both the permissive and nonpermissive temperatures was reported (Stollar *et al.*, 1974). With RNA⁻ mutants of NDV (Preble and Youngner, 1973*b*), VSV (Youngner, unpublished data), and Semliki Forest virus (Keränen, 1977), the interference seems to be at the level of RNA transcription by the *ts*⁺ virus.

An interesting finding with VSV was that inhibition of wild-type virus replication at 37°C and 39.5°C was accompanied by a significant enhancement of the coinfecting *ts* RNA⁻ mutants (Youngner and Quagliana, 1976). In this respect the *ts* mutants were acting as conditionally defective interfering particles which can interfere with and be rescued by wild-type virus. These phenomena of interference were also seen with RNA⁺ VSV mutants representing complementation groups III and V (Youngner, unpublished data).

The dominance of the replication of *ts* virus over that of the wild-type at 37°C must be considered a rationale for the spontaneous selection and maintenance of *ts* mutants in persistently infected cell lines. The ability of the *ts* mutants to interfere with the replication of wild-type virus at 37°C would provide an answer to the question, "Why don't revertants replace the *ts* population at 37°C, a temperature not optimum for the *ts* mutants?" Since the mutants present in a persistent infection can inhibit the replication of wild-type virus, revertants would be prevented from providing a significant portion of the virus population. In this way, a *ts* virus population selected during a persistent infection could maintain its mutant character.

5. REFERENCES

Ahmed, R., and Graham, A. F., 1977, Persistent infections in L cells with temperature-sensitive mutants of reovirus, *J. Virol.* **23**:250.

Armen, R. C., Evermann, J. F., Truant, A. L., Laughlin, C. A., and Hallum, J. V., 1977, Temperature-sensitive mutants of measles virus produced from persistently infected HeLa cells, *Arch. Virol.* **53**:121.

Ashe, W. K., and Scherp, H. W., 1965, Antigenic variations in herpes simplex virus isolants from successive recurrences in herpes labialis, *J. Immunol.* **94**:385.

Brown, I. N., Brown, K. N., and Hills, L. A., 1968, Immunity to malaria: The antibody response to antigenic variation by *Plasmodium knowlesi, Immunology* **14**:127.

Burnstein, T., Jacobsen, L. B., Zeman, W., and Chen, T. T., 1974, Persistent infection of BSC-1 cells by defective measles virus derived from subacute sclerosing panencephalitis, *Infect. Immun.* **10**:1378.

Burrows, R., 1966, Studies on the carrier state of cattle exposed to foot-and-mouth disease virus, *J. Hyg.* **64**:81.

Carreño, G., and Esparza, J., 1977, Induction of Venezuelan equine encephalitis (Mucambo) virus by iododeoxyuridine in chronically infected "cured" cultured mosquito cells, *Intervirology* **8**:193.

Chakraborty, P. R., Ahmed, R., and Fields, B. N., 1979, Genetics of reovirus: The relationship of interference to complementation and reassortment of temperature-sensitive mutants at nonpermissive temperature, *Virology* **94**:119.

Chiarini, A., Ammatuna, P., di Stefano, R., and Sinatra, A., 1978, Latent measles virus infection depending on a temperature-sensitive phenomenon, *Arch. Virol.* **56**:263.

Choppin, P. W., Scheid, A., and Mountcastle, W. E., 1975, Paramyxoviruses, membranes and persistent infections, *Neurology* **25**:494.

Clark, H. F., and Wiktor, T. J., 1972, Temperature-sensitivity characteristics distinguishing substrains of fixed rabies virus: Lack of correlation with plaque size markers or virulence for mice, *J. Infect. Dis.* **125**:637.

Clements, J. E., Narayan, O., and Griffin, D. E., 1978, The proviral DNA of visna virus: Synthesis and physical maps of parental and antigenic mutant DNA, in: *Persistent Viruses* (J. G. Stevens, G. J. Todaro, and C. F. Fox, eds.), *ICN-UCLA Symp. Mol. Cell. Biol.*, Vol. 11, pp. 275–283, Academic Press, New York.

Clewley, J. P., Bishop, D. H. L., Kang, C. Y., Coffin, J., Schnitzlein, W. M., Reichmann, M. E., and Shope, R. E., 1977, Oligonucleotide fingerprints of RNA species obtained from rhabdoviruses belonging to the vesicular stomatitis virus subgroup, *J. Virol.* **23**:152.

Crawford, T. B., Cheevers, W. P., Klevjer-Anderson, P., and McGuire, T. C., 1978, Equine infectious anemia: Virion characteristics, virus-cell interaction and host responses, in *Persistent Viruses* (J. G. Stevens, G. J. Todaro, and C. F. Fox, eds.), *ICN-UCLA Symp. Mol. Cell. Biol.*, Vol. 11, pp. 268–314, Academic Press, New York.

Damonte, E. B., and Coto, C. E., 1979, Temperature sensitivity of the arenavirus Junin isolated from persistently infected Vero cells, *Intervirology* **11**:282.

Davey, M. W., and Dalgarno, L., 1974, Semliki Forest virus replication in cultured *Aedes albopictus* cells: Studies on establishment of persistence, *J. Gen. Virol.* **24**:453.

Doller, D., Aucker, J., and Weissbach, A., 1979, Persistence of herpes simplex virus type 1 in rat neurotumor cells, *J. Virol.* **29**:43.

Dubois-Dalcq, M., Reese, T. S., Murphy, M., and Fucillo, D., 1976, Defective bud formation in human cells chronically infected with subacute sclerosing panencephalitis virus, *J. Virol.* **19**:579.

Dukto, F. J., and Pfau, C. J., 1978, Arenavirus defective interfering particles mask the cell-killing potential of standard virus, *J. Gen. Virol.* **38**:195.

Eaton, B. T., 1975, Defective-interfering particles of Semliki Forest virus do not interfere with viral RNA synthesis in *Aedes albopictus* cells, *Virology* **68**:534.

Eaton, B. T., and Hapel, A. J., 1976, Persistent noncytolytic togavirus infection of primary mouse muscle cells, *Virology* **72**:266.

Fellowes, O. N., and Sutmoller, P., 1970, Foot-and-mouth disease virus: Biological characteristics of virus from bovine carriers, *Arch. Gesamte Virusforsch.* **30**:173.

Fields, B. N., 1972, Genetic manipulation of reovirus—A model for modification of disease? *N. Engl. J. Med.* **287**:1026.

Fields, B. N., and Raine, C. S., 1972, Altered disease in rats due to mutants of reovirus type 3, *J. Clin. Invest.* **51**:30a.

Fields, B. N., Weiner, H. L., Ramig, R. F., and Ahmed, R., 1978, Genetics of reovirus: Aspects related to virulence and viral persistence, in: *Persistent Viruses* (J. G. Stevens, G. J. Todaro, and C. F. Fox, eds.), *ICN-UCLA Symp. Mol. Cell. Biol.*, Vol. 11, pp. 389–398, Academic Press, New York.

Fisher, L. E., and Rapp, F., 1979, Role of virus variants and cells in maintenance of persistent infection by measles virus, *J. Virol.* **30**:64.

Flamand, A., 1970, Etude génétique du virus de la stomatite vésiculaire: Classement de mutants thermosensibles spontanés en groups de complémentation, *J. Gen. Virol.* **8**:187.

Fraser, G., Edwards, H. H., McNulty, M. S., and Ruben, J. M. S., 1976, Accidental persistent infection of cell lines by Newcastle disease virus, showing three unusual features—Defective neuraminidase, temperature sensitivity and intranuclear inclusions, *Arch. Virol.* **50**:147.

Frey, T. K., Jones, E. V., Cardamone, J. J., Jr., and Youngner, J. S., 1979, Induction of interferon in L cells by defective-interfering (DI) particles of vesicular stomatitis virus: Lack of correlation with content of [±] snapback RNA, *Virology* **99**:95.

Furman, P. A., and Hallum, J. V., 1973, RNA-dependent DNA polymerase activity in preparations of a mutant of Newcastle disease virus arising from persistently infected L cells, *J. Virol.* **12**:548.

Gavrilov, V. I., Asher, D. M., Vyalushkina, S. D., Ratushkina, L. S., Smieva, R. G., and Tumyan, B. G., 1972, Persistent infection of a continuous line of pig kidney cells with a variant of the WSN strain of influenza A_0 virus, *Proc. Soc. Exp. Biol. Med.* **140**:109.

Gavrilov, V. I., Deryabin, P. G., Lozinsky, T. F., Loghinova, N. V., Karpova, E. F., and Zhdanov, V. M., 1974, Continuous mouse brain cell lines chronically infected with Japanese encephalitis virus, *J. Gen. Virol.* **24**:293.

Gavrilov, V. I., Deryabin, P. G., and Loghinova, N. V., 1975, Temperature-sensitive mutants of Japanese encephalitis virus isolated from chronically infected suckling mouse brain cells, *Vopr. Virusol.* **4**:282.

Gould, E., 1974, Variants of measles virus, *Med. Microbiol. Immunol.* **160**:211.

Gould, E. A., and Linton, P. E., 1975, The production of a temperature-sensitive persistent measles virus infection, *J. Gen. Virol.* **28**:21.

Haase, A. T., and Varmus, H. E., 1973, Demonstràtion of a DNA provirus in the lytic cycle of visna virus, *Nature (London) New Biol.* **245**:237.

Haase, A. T., Stowring, L., Narayan, O., Griffin, D. E., and Price, D., 1977, Slow persistent infection caused by visna virus: Role of host restriction, *Science* **195**:175.

Haase, A. T., Brahic, M., Carroll, D., Scott, J., Stowring, L., Traynor, B., Ventura, P., and Narayan, O., 1978, Visna: An animal model for studies of virus persistence, in: *Persistent Viruses* (J. G. Stevens, G. J. Todaro, and C. F. Fox, eds.), *ICN-UCLA Symp. Mol. Cell. Biol.*, Vol. 11, pp. 643–654, Academic Press, New York.

Hall, W. W., Kiessling, W., and ter Meulen, V., 1978, Membrane proteins of subacute sclerosing panencephalitis and measles viruses, *Nature (London)* **272**:460.

Hall, W. W., Lamb, R. A., and Choppin, P. W., 1979, Measles and subacute sclerosing panencephalitis virus proteins: Lack of antibodies to the M protein in patients with subacute sclerosing panencephalitis, *Proc. Natl. Acad. Sci. USA* **76**:2047.

Hallum, J. V., Thacore, H. R., and Youngner, J. S., 1970, Factors affecting the sensitivity of different viruses to interferon, *J. Virol.* **6**:156.

Hamilton, R., Barbosa, L., and DuBois, M., 1973, Subacute sclerosing panencephalitis measles virus: Study of biological markers, *J. Virol.* **12**:632.

Hampar, B., and Burroughs, M. A. K., 1969, Mechanism of persistent herpes simplex virus infection *in vitro*, *J. Natl. Canc. Inst.* **43**:621.

Hampar, B., and Keehn, M. A., 1967, Cumulative changes in the antigenic properties of herpes simplex virus from persistently infected cell cultures, *J. Immunol.* **99**:554.

Haspel, M. V., Knight, P. R., Duff, R. G., and Rapp, F., 1973, Activation of a latent measles virus infection in hamster cells, *J. Virol.* **12**:690.

Haspel, M. V., Duff, R., and Rapp, F., 1975, The isolation and preliminary characterization of temperature-sensitive mutants of measles virus, *J. Virol.* **16**:1000.

Henle, G., Deinhardt, F., Bergs, V. V., and Henle, W., 1959, Studies on persistent infections of tissue cultures. I. General aspects of the system, *J. Exp. Med.* **108**:537.

Henson, J. B., and McGuire, T. C., 1974, Equine infectious anemia, *Prog. Med. Virol.* **18**:143.

Hinze, H. C., and Walker, D. L., 1961, Variation of herpes simplex virus in persistently infected tissue cultures, *J. Bacteriol.* **82**:498.

Hodes, D. S., 1979, Temperature sensitivity of subacute sclerosing panencephalitis virus and its ability to establish persistent infection, *Proc. Soc. Exp. Biol. Med.* **161**:407.

Hoggan, M. D., and Roizman, B., 1959, The isolation and properties of a variant of herpes simplex producing multinucleated gaint cells in monolayer cultures in the presence of antibody, *Am. J. Hyg.* **70**:208.

Holland, J. J., and Villarreal, L. P., 1974, Persistent noncytocidal vesicular stomatitis virus infections mediated by defective T particles that suppress virion transcriptase, *Proc. Natl. Acad. Sci. USA* **71**:2956.

Holland, J. J., Villarreal, L. P., Breindl, M., Semler, B. L., and Kohne, D., 1976*a*, Defective interfering virus particles attenuate virus lethality *in vivo* and *in vitro*, in: *Animal Virology* (D. Baltimore, A. S. Huang, and C. F. Fox, eds.), *ICN-UCLA Symp. Mol. Cell. Biol.*, Vol. 4, pp. 773–786, Academic Press, New York.

Holland, J. J., Villarreal, L. P., Welsh, R. M., Oldstone, M. B. A., Kohne, D., Lazzarini, R., and Scolnick, E., 1976b, Long term persistent vesicular stomatitis and
rabies virus infection of cells *in vitro*, *J. Gen. Virol.* **33**:193.

Holland, J. J., Semler, B. L., Jones, C., Perrault, J., Reid, L., and Roux, L., 1978,
Role of DI, virus mutation, and host response in persistent infections by enveloped
RNA viruses, in: *Persistent Viruses* (J. G. Stevens, G. Todaro, and C. F. Fox,
eds.), *ICN-UCLA Symp. Mol. Cell. Biol.*, Vol. 11, pp. 57–73, Academic Press,
New York.

Holland, J. J., Grabau, E. A., Jones, C. L., and Semler, B. L., 1979, Evolution of
multiple genome mutations during long-term persistent infection by vesicular stomatitis virus, *Cell* **16**:495.

Homma, M., and Ohuchi, M., 1971, Trypsin action on the growth of Sendai virus in
tissue culture cells. III. Structural difference of Sendai viruses grown in eggs and
tissue culture cells, *J. Virol.* **12**:1457.

Hotchin, J., 1962, The biology of lymphocytic choriomeningitis infection: Virus-induced
immune disease, *Cold Spring Harbor Symp. Quant. Biol.* **27**:479.

Hotchin, J., and Sikora, E., 1973, Low-pathogenicity variant of lymphocytic choriomeningitis virus, *Infect. Immun.* **7**:825.

Hotchin, J., Kinch, W., and Benson, L., 1971, Lytic and turbid-plaque type mutants of
lymphocytic choriomeningitis virus as a cause of neurological disease or persistent
infection, *Infect. Immun.* **4**:281.

Hyslop, N. S. G., 1965, Isolation of variant strains from foot-and-mouth disease virus
propagated in cell cultures containing antiviral sera, *J. Gen. Microbiol.* **41**:135.

Hyslop, N. S. G., and Fagg, R. H., 1965, Isolation of variants during passage of a
strain of foot-and-mouth disease virus in partly immunized cattle, *J. Hyg.* **63**:357.

Igarashi, A., and Stollar, V., 1976, Failure of defective interfering particles of Sindbis
virus produced in BHK or chick cells to affect viral replication in *Aedes albopictus*
cells, *J. Virol.* **19**:398.

Igarashi, A., Koo, R., and Stollar, V., 1977, Evolution and properties of *Aedes
albopictus* cell cultures persistently infected with Sindbis virus, *Virology* **82**:69.

Inglot, A. D., Albin, M., and Chudzio, T., 1973, Persistent infections of mouse cells
with Sindbis virus: Role of virulence of strains, autointerfering particles and
interferon, *J. Gen. Virol.* **20**:105.

Jacobson, S., Dukto, F. J., and Pfau, C. J., 1979, Determinants of spontaneous
recovery and persistence in MDCK cells infected with lymphocytic choriomeningitis virus, *J. Gen. Virol.* **44**:113.

Jones, T., and Hanson, R. P., 1976, Competition between non plaquing and plaquing
strains of Newcastle disease virus as affected by temperature, *Avian Dis.* **20**:293.

Ju, G., Udem, S., Rager-Zisman, B., and Bloom, B. R., 1978, Isolation of a
heterogeneous population of temperature sensitive mutants of measles virus from
persistently infected human lymphoblastoid cell lines, *J. Exp. Med.* **601**:1637.

Kang, C. Y., Glimp, T., Clewley, J. P., and Bishop, D. H. L., 1978, Studies on the
generation of vesicular stomatitis virus (Indiana sertotype) defective interfering
particles, *Virology* **84**:142.

Kawai, A., and Matsumoto, S., 1977, Interfering and noninterfering defective particles
generated by a rabies small plaque variant virus, *Virology* **76**:60.

Kawai, A., Matsumoto, S., and Tanabe, K., 1975, Characterization of rabies viruses
recovered from persistently infected BHK cells, *Virology* **67**:520.

Keränen, S., 1977, Interference of wild-type virus replication by an RNA negative temperature-sensitive mutant of Semliki Forest virus, *Virology* **80**:1.

Kimura, Y., Ito, Y., Shimokata, K., Nishiyama, Y., Nagata, I., and Kitoh, J., 1975, Temperature-sensitive virus derived from BHK cells persistently infected with HVJ (Sendai virus), *J. Virol.* **15**:55.

Kimura, Y., Norrby, E., Nagata, I., Ito, Y., Shimokata, K., and Nishiyama, Y., 1976, Homologous interference induced by a temperature-sensitive mutant derived from an HVJ (Sendai virus) carrier culture, *J. Gen. Virol.* **33**:333.

Knight, P., Duff, R., and Rapp, F., 1972, Latency of human measles virus in hamster cells, *J. Virol.* **10**:995.

Knight, P., Duff, R., Glaser, R., and Rapp, F., 1973, Characteristics of the release of measles virus from latently infected cells after co-cultivation with BSC-1 cells, *Intervirology* **2**:287.

Kolakofsky, D., Spahr, P.-F., and Koprowski, H., 1974, Comparison of 6/94 virus and Sendai virus RNA by RNA-RNA hybridization, *J. Virol.* **13**:935.

Kono, Y., Kobayashi, K., and Fukunaga, Y., 1973, Antigenic drift of equine infectious anemia virus in chronically infected horses, *Arch. Gesamte Virusforsch.* **41**:1.

Kratzch, V., Hall, W. W., Nagashima, K., and ter Meulen, V., 1977, Biological and biochemical characterization of a latent SSPE virus infection in tissue culture, *J. Med. Virol.* **1**:139.

Laver, W. G., and Webster, R. G., 1968, Selection of antigenic mutants of influenza viruses. Isolation and peptide mapping of their hemagglutinating proteins, *Virology* **34**:193.

Lazzarini, R. A., Weber, G. H., Johnson, L. D., and Stamminger, G. M., 1975, Covalently linked message and anti-message (genomic) RNA from a defective vesicular stomatitis virus particle, *J. Mol. Biol.* **97**:289.

Lehmann-Grube, F., 1967, A carrier state of lymphocytic choriomeningitis virus in L cell cultures, *Nature (London)* **213**:770.

Lehmann-Grube, F., Slenczka, W., and Tees, R., 1969, A persistent and inapparent infection of L cells with the virus of lymphocytic choriomeningitis, *J. Gen. Virol.* **5**:63.

Lewandowski, L. J., Lief, F. S., Verini, M. A., Prenkowski, M. M., ter Meulen, V., and Koprowski, H., 1974, Analysis of a viral agent isolated from multiple sclerosis brain tissue: Characterization as a parainfluenza virus type 1, *J. Virol.* **13**:1037.

Lofgren, K. W., Stevens, J. G., Marsden, H. S., and Subak-Sharpe, J. H., 1977, Temperature-sensitive mutants of herpes simplex virus differ in the capacity to establish latent infections in mice, *Virology* **76**:440.

Louza, A. C., and Bingham, R. W., 1978, A defect in viral protein synthesis in cells persistently infected with Newcastle disease virus, *FEMS Microbiol. Lett.* **3**:1.

Lucas, A., Coulter, M., Anderson, R., Dales, S., and Flintoff, W., 1978, *In vivo* and *in vitro* models of demyelinating diseases. II. Persistence and host-regulated thermosensitivity in cells of neural derivation infected with mouse hepatitis and measles viruses, *Virology* **88**:325.

Madansky, C. H., and Bratt, M. A., 1978, Noncytopathic mutants of Newcastle disease virus, *J. Virol.* **26**:724.

Maeda, S., Hashimoto, K., and Simizu, B., 1979, Complementation between temperature-sensitive mutants isolated from *Aedes albopictus* cells persistently infected with Western equine encephalitis virus, *Virology* **92**:532.

Marcus, P. I., and Sekellick, M. J., 1977, Defective interfering particles with covalently linked [±] RNA induce interferon, *Nature (London)* **266**:815.

Matsumoto, S., and Kawai, A., 1978, Characterization of rabies defective viruses, in: *Negative Strand Viruses and the Host Cell* (B. W. J. Mahy and R. D. Barry, eds.), pp. 591–597, Academic Press, New York.

Mayo, J., Lombardo, J. L., Klein-Szanto, A. J. P., Conti, C. J., and Moreira, J. L., 1973, An oncogenic virus carried by hamster kidney cells, *Cancer Res.* **33**:2273.

McNulty, M. S., Gowans, E. J., Louza, A. C., and Fraser, G., 1977, An electron microscopic study of MDBK cells persistently infected with Newcastle disease virus, *Arch. Virol.* **53**:185.

Meleney, H. E., 1928, Relapse phenomena of Spironema recurrentis, *J. Exp. Med.* **48**:65.

Menna, J. H., Collins, A. R., and Flanagan, T. D., 1975, Characterization of an *in vitro* persistent-state measles virus infection: Establishment and virological characterization of the BGM/MV cell line, *Infect. Immun.* **11**:152.

Minagawa, T., 1971, Studies on the persistent infection with measles virus in HeLa cells. II. The properties of the carried virus, *Jpn. J. Microbiol.* **15**:333.

Minagawa, T., Sakuma, T., Kuwajima, S., Yamamoto, T. K., and Iida, H., 1976, Characterization of measles virus in establishment of persistent infections in human lymphoid cell line, *J. Gen. Virol.* **33**:361.

Mudd, J. A., Leavitt, R. W., Kingsbury, D. T., and Holland, J. J., 1973, Natural selection of mutants of vesicular stomatitis virus by cultured cells of *Drosophila melanogaster*, *J. Gen. Virol.* **20**:341.

Nagata, I., Kimura, Y., Ito, Y., and Tanaka, T., 1972, Temperature-sensitive phenomenon of viral maturation observed in BHK cells persistently infected with HVJ, *Virology* **49**:453.

Narayan, O., Griffin, D. E., and Chase, J., 1977a, Antigenic shift of visna virus in persistently infected sheep, *Science* **197**:376.

Narayan, O., Griffin, D. E., and Silverstein, A. M., 1977b, Slow virus infection: Replication and mechanisms of persistence of visna virus in sheep, *J. Infect. Dis.* **135**:800.

Narayan, O., Griffin, D. E., and Clements, J. E., 1978, Virus mutation during "slow infection": Temporal development and characterization of mutants of visna virus recovered from sheep, *J. Gen. Virol.* **41**:343.

Nishiyama, Y., 1977, Studies of L cells persistently infected with VSV: Factors involved in the regulation of persistent infection, *J. Gen. Virol.* **35**:265.

Nishiyama, Y., Ito, Y., Shimokata, K., Kimura, Y., and Nagata, I., 1976, Relationship between establishment of persistent infection of haemagglutinating virus of Japan and properties of the virus, *J. Gen. Virol.* **32**:73.

Nishiyama, Y., Ito, Y., and Shimokata, K., 1978, Properties of viruses selected during persistent infection of L cells with VSV, *J. Gen. Virol.* **40**:481.

Norrby, E., 1967, A carrier cell line of measles virus in Lu106 cells, *Arch. Gesamte Virusforsch.* **20**:215.

Norrby, E., and Kristensson, K., 1978, Subacute encephalitis and hydrocephalus in hamsters caused by measles virus from persistently infected cell cultures, *J. Med. Virol.* **2**:305.

Norval, M., 1979, Mechanism of persistence of rubella virus in LLC MK₂ cells, *J. Gen. Virol.* **43**:289.

Ohuchi, M., and Homma, M., 1976, Trypsin action on the growth of Sendai virus in tissue culture cells. IV. Evidence for activation of Sendai virus by cleavage of a glycoprotein, *J. Virol.* **18**:1147.

Payne, F. E., and Baublis, J. V., 1973, Decreased reactivity of SSPE strains with measles virus antibody, *J. Infect. Dis.* **127**:505.

Peleg, J., and Stollar, V., 1974, Homologous interference in *Aedes aegypti* cell cultures infected with Sindbis virus, *Arch. Gesamte Virusforsch.* **45**:309.

Perekrest, V. V., Gavrilov, V. I., Demidova, S. A., and Borisova, S. M., 1974, A new model of persistent influenza infection in a continuous line of pig embryo kidney cells, *Acta Virol.* **18**:391.

Perrault, J., 1976, Cross-linked double-stranded RNA from a defective vesicular stomatitis virus particle, *Virology* **70**:360.

Perrault, J., and Leavitt, R. W., 1978, Characterization of snap-back RNAs in vesicular stomatitis defective interfering virus particles, *J. Gen. Virol.* **38**:21.

Pfau, C. J., 1978, The immunological basis of persistent infection and disease in lymphocytic choriomeningitis virus-infected mice, in: *Animal Models of Comparative and Developmental Aspects of Immunity and Disease* (M. E. Gershwin, ed.), pp. 298–309, Pergamon Press, Oxford.

Popescu, M., and Lehmann-Grube, F., 1976, Diversity of lymphocytic choriomeningitis virus: Variation due to replication of the virus in the mouse, *J. Gen. Virol.* **30**:113.

Popescu, M., and Lehmann-Grube, F., 1977, Defective interfering particles in mice infected with lymphocytic choriomeningitis virus, *Virology* **77**:78.

Porter, D. D., Larsen, A. E., and Porter, H. G., 1969, The pathogenesis of Aleutian disease of mink. I. *In vivo* viral replication and the host antibody response to viral antigen, *J. Exp. Med.* **130**:575.

Porter, D. D., Larsen, A. E., and Porter, H. G., 1973, The pathogenesis of Aleutian disease of mink. III. Immune complex arteritis, *Am. J. Pathol.* **71**:331.

Porter, D. D., Larsen, A. E., Cox, N. A., Porter, H. G., and Suffin, S. C., 1977, Isolation of Aleutian disease virus of mink in cell culture, *Intervirology* **8**:129.

Preble, O. T., and Youngner, J. S., 1972, Temperature-sensitive mutants isolated from L cells persistently infected with Newcastle disease virus, *J. Virol.* **9**:200.

Preble, O. T., and Youngner, J. S., 1973*a*, Temperature-sensitive defect of mutants isolated from L cells persistently infected with Newcastle disease virus, *J. Virol.* **12**:472.

Preble, O. T., and Youngner, J. S., 1973*b*, Selection of temperature-sensitive mutants during persistent infection: Role in maintenance of persistent Newcastle disease virus infections of L cells, *J. Virol.* **12**:481.

Pringle, C. R., 1977, Genetics of rhabdoviruses, in: *Comprehensive Virology*, Vol. 9 (H. Fraenkel-Conrat and R. R. Wagner, eds.), pp. 239–289, Plenum Press, New York.

Pringle, C. R., Shirodaria, P. V., Cash, P., Chiswell, D. J., and Malloy, P., 1978, Initiation and maintenance of persistent infections by respiratory syncytial virus, *J. Virol.* **28**:199.

Printz, P., 1970, Adaption du virus de la stomatite vésiculaire à *Drosophila melanogaster*, *Ann. Inst. Pasteur Paris* **119**:520.

Ramig, R. F., and Fields, B. N., 1977, Method for rapidly screening revertants of reovirus temperature-sensitive mutants for extragenic suppression, *Virology* **81**:170.

Ramig, R. F., and Fields, B. N., 1979, Revertants of temperature-sensitive mutants of reovirus: Evidence for frequent extragenic suppression, *Virology* **92**:155.

Ramig, R. F., White, R. M., and Fields, B. N., 1977, Suppression of the temperature-sensitive phenotype of a mutant of reovirus type 3, *Science* **195**:406.

Ramseur, J. M., and Friedman, R. M., 1977, Prolonged infection of interferon-treated cells by vesicular stomatitis virus: Possible role of temperature-sensitive mutants and interferon, *J. Gen. Virol.* **37**:523.

Ramseur, J. M., and Friedman, R. M., 1978, Prolonged infection of L cells with vesicular stomatitis virus: Defective interfering forms and temperature-sensitive mutants as factors in the infection, *Virology* **85**:253.

Rapp, F., 1964, Plaque differentiation and replication of virulent and attenuated strains of measles virus, *J. Bacteriol.* **88**:1448.

Rapp, F., and Jerkofsky, M. A., 1973, Persistent and latent infections, in: *The Herpesviruses* (A. S. Kaplan, ed.), pp. 271–289, Academic Press, New York.

Reeve, P., and Poste, G., 1971, Studies on the cytopathogenicity of Newcastle disease virus: Relation between virulence, polykaryocytosis and plaque size, *J. Gen. Virol.* **11**:17.

Rima, B. K., Martin, S. J., and Gould, E. A., 1979, A comparison of polypeptides in measles and SSPE virus strains, *J. Gen. Virol.* **42**:603.

Rodriguez, J. E., ter Meulen, V., and Henle, W., 1967, Studies on persistent infections of tissue cultures. VI. Reversible changes in Newcastle disease virus populations as a result of passage in L cells or chick embryos, J. Virol. **1**:1.

Roux, L., and Holland, J. J., 1979, Role of defective interfering particles of Sendai virus in persistent infections, *Virology* **93**:91.

Rustigian, R., 1962, A carrier state in HeLa cells with measles virus (Edmonston strain) apparently associated with non-infectious virus, *Virology* **16**:101.

Rustigian, R., 1966a, Persistent infection of cells in culture by measles virus. I. Development and characteristics of HeLa sublines persistently infected with complete virus, *J. Bacteriol.* **92**:1792.

Rustigian, R., 1966b, Persistent infection of cells in culture by measles virus. II. Effect of measles antibody on persistently infected HeLa sublines and recovery of a HeLa clonal line persistently infected with incomplete virus, *J. Bacteriol.* **92**:1805.

Sabin, A. B., 1961, Reproductive capacity of polioviruses of diverse origins at various temperatures: Concepts of role of temperature in infection by polioviruses, *Perspect. Virol.* **2**:90.

Sato, M., Yamada, T., Yamamoto, K., and Yamamoto, N., 1976, Evidence for hybrid formation between rubella virus and a latent virus of BHK-21/WI-2 cells, *Virology* **69**:691.

Sato, M., Tanaka, H., Yamada, T., and Yamamoto, N., 1977, Persistent infection of BHK-21/WI-2 cells with rubella virus and characterization of rubella variants, *Arch. Virol.* **54**:333.

Sato, M., Urade, M., Maeda, N., Miyazaki, T., Watanabe, M., Shibata, T., and Yamamoto, N., 1978a, Isolation and characterization of a new rubella variant with DNA polymerase activity, *Arch. Virol.* **56**:89.

Sato, M., Urade, M., Yoshida, H., Maeda, N., Yura, Y., Shirasuna, K., and Miyazaki, T., 1978b, Evidence for phenotypic mixing between NDV and a latent virus of BHK-21/WI-2 cells in the early passaged BHK 21/WI 2 cells persistently infected with NDV, *Arch. Virol.* **56**:157.

Scheid, A., and Choppin, P., 1976, Protease activation mutants of Sendai virus. Activation of biologic properties by specific proteases, *Virology* **69**:265.

Schloer, G. M., and Hanson, R. P., 1968, Relationship of plaque size and virulence for chickens of 14 representative Newcastle disease virus strains, *J. Virol.* **2**:40.

Sekellick, M. J., and Marcus, P. I., 1978, Persistent infection. I. Interferon-inducing defective-interfering particles as mediators of cell sparing: Possible role in persistent infection by vesicular stomatitis virus, *Virology* **85**:175.

Sekellick, M. J., and Marcus, P. I., 1979, Persistent infection. II. Interferon-inducing temperature-sensitive mutants as mediators of cell sparing: Possible role in persistent infection by vesicular stomatitis virus, *Virology* **95**:36.

Shenk, T. E., Koshelnyk, K. A., and Stollar, V., 1974, Temperature-sensitive virus from *Aedes albopictus* cells chronically infected with Sindbis virus, *J. Virol.* **13**.439.

Shipman, C., Vander Weide, G. C., and Ilma, B., 1971, Prevalence of type R virus-like particles in clones of BHK-21 cells, *Virology* **38**:707.

Simizu, B., and Takayama, N., 1969, Isolation of two plaque mutants of Western equine encephalitis virus differing in virulence for mice, *J. Virol.* **4**:799.

Simizu, B., and Takayama, N., 1971, Relationship betwen neurovirulence and temperature sensitivity of an attenuated Western equine encephalitis virus, *Arch. Gesamte Virusforsch.* **34**:242.

Simpson, R. W., and Iinuma, M., 1975, Recovery of infectious proviral DNA from mammalian cells infected with RS virus, *Proc. Natl. Acad. Sci. USA* **72**:3230.

Spandidos, D. A., and Graham, A. F., 1976, Generation of defective virus after infection of newborn rats with reovirus, *J. Virol.* **20**:234.

Stanners, C. P., Francoeur, A. M., and Lam, T., 1977, Analysis of vesicular stomatitis virus mutant with attenuated cytopathogenicity: Mutation in viral function, P, for inhibition of protein synthesis, *Cell* **11**:273.

Stanwick, T. L., and Hallum, J. V., 1976, Comparison of RNA polymerase associated with Newcastle disease virus and a temperature-sensitive mutant of Newcastle disease virus isolated from persistently infected L cells, *J. Virol.* **17**:68.

Stohlman, S. A., and Weiner, L. P., 1978, Stability of neurotropic mouse hepatitis virus (JHM strain) during chronic infection of neuroblastoma cells, *Arch. Virol.* **57**:53.

Stollar, V., Peleg, J., and Shenk, T. E., 1974, Temperature sensitivity of a Sindbis virus mutant isolated from persistently infected *Aedes aegypti* cell culture, *Intervirology* **2**:337.

Stowring, L., Haase, A. T., and Charman, H. P., 1979, Serologic definition of the lentivirus group of retroviruses, *J. Virol.* **29**:523.

Straver, P. J., and van Bekkum, J. G., 1972, Plaque production by carrier strains of foot-and-mouth disease virus in BHK-monolayers incubated at different temperatures, *Arch. Gesamte Virusforsch.* **37**:12.

Straver, P. J., Bool, P. H., Claessens, A. M., and van Bekkum, J. G., 1970, Some properties of carrier strains of foot-and-mouth disease virus, *Arch. Gesamte Virusforsch.* **29**:113.

Sutmoller, P., and Gaggero, A., 1965, Foot-and-mouth disease carriers, *Vet. Rec.* **77**:968.

Takemoto, K. K., and Habel, K., 1959, Virus-cell relationship in a carrier culture of HeLa cells and Coxsackie A9 virus, *Virology* **7**:28.

Taylor-Papadimitriou, J., and Stoker, M., 1971, Effect of interferon on some aspects of transformation by polyoma virus, *Nature (London) New Biol.* **230**:114.

ter Meulen, V., Koprowski, H., Iwasaki, Y., Käckell, Y. M., and Müller, D., 1972, Fusion of cultured multiple sclerosis brain cells with indicator cells: Presence of nucleocapsids and virions and isolation of parainfluenza type virus, *Lancet* **2**:1.

Thacore, H. R., and Youngner, J. S., 1969, Cells persistently infected with Newcastle disease virus. I. Properties of mutants isolated from persistently infected L cells, *J. Virol.* **4**:244.

Thacore, H. R., and Youngner, J. S., 1970, Cells persistently infected with Newcastle disease virus. II. Ribonucleic acid and protein synthesis in cells infected with mutants isolated from persistently infected L cells, *J. Virol.* **6**:42.

Thacore, H. R., and Youngner, J. S., 1971, Cells persistently infected with Newcastle disease virus. III. Thermal stability of hemagglutinin and neuraminidase of a mutant isolated from persistently infected L cells, *J. Virol.* **7**:53.

Thormar, H., and Palsson, P. A., 1967, Visna and Maedi—Two slow infections of sheep and their etiological agents, *Perspect. Virol.* **5**:291.

Thormar, H., Mehta, P. D., and Brown, H. R., 1978, Comparison of wild-type and subacute sclerosing panencephalitis strains of measles virus, *J. Exp. Med.* **148**:674.

Truant, A. L., and Hallum, J. V., 1977*a*, A persistent infection of baby hamster kidney-21 cells with mumps virus and the role of temperature-sensitive variants, *J. Med. Virol.* **1**:49.

Truant, A. L., and Hallum, J. V., 1977*b*, A latent infection of baby hamster kidney 21 cells with mumps virus, *Proc. Soc. Exp. Biol. Med.* **156**:470.

Tsai, K.-S., 1977, Replication of parainfluenza type 3 virus in alveolar macrophages: Evidence of *in vivo* infection and of *in vitro* temperature sensitivity in virus maturation, *Infect. Immun.* **18**:780.

Urade, M., Sato, M., Yoshida, H., Shirasuna, K., Miyazaki, T., and Yamamoto, N., 1978, Effect of concanavalin A on the infectivity of rubella virus and its variants, *Arch. Virol.* **56**:359.

van Bekkum, J. G., Fraenkel, H. S., Frederiks, H. H. J., and Fraenkel, S., 1959, Observations on the carrier state of cattle exposed to foot-and-mouth disease virus, T, *Diergeneeskd. Mem.* **84**:1159.

Vickerman, K., 1974, Antigenic variation in African trypanosomes, in: *Symposium on Parasites in the Immunized Host: Mechanisms of Survival, Ciba Foundation Symposium*, Vol. 25, pp. 53–80, Associated Scientific Publishers, Amsterdam.

Villarreal, L. P., and Holland, J. J., 1976, RNA synthesis in BHK 21 cells persistently infected with vesicular stomatitis virus and rabies virus, *J. Gen. Virol.* **33**:213.

Wagner, R. R., Levy, A., Snyder, R., Ratcliff, G., and Hyatt, D., 1963, Biologic properties of two plaque variants of vesicular stomatitis virus (Indiana serotype), *J. Immunol.* **91**:112.

Walker, D. L., and Hinze, H. C., 1962, A carrier state of mumps virus in human conjunctiva cells. I. General considerations, *J. Exp. Med.* **116**:739.

Webster, R. G., and Laver, W. G., 1975, Antigenic variation of influenza viruses, in: *The Influenza Viruses and Influenza* (E. D. Kilbourne, ed.), pp. 269–314, Academic Press, New York.

Wechsler, S. L., and Fields, B. N., 1978, Differences between the intracellular polypeptides of measles and subacute sclerosing panencephalitis virus, *Nature (London)* **272**:458.

Wechsler, S. L., Weiner, H. L., and Fields, B. N., 1979, Immune response in subacute sclerosing panencephalitis: Reduced antibody response to the matrix protein of measles virus, *J. Immunol.* **123**:884.

Wertz, G. W., and Youngner, J. S., 1970, Interferon production and inhibition of host synthesis in cells infected with vesicular stomatitis virus, *J. Virol.* **6**:476.

Wiktor, T. J., and Clark, H. F., 1972, Chronic rabies virus infection of cell cultures, *Infect. Immun.* **6**:988.

Wild, T. F., and Dugre, R., 1978, Establishment and characterization of a subacute sclerosing panencephalitis (measles) virus persistent infection in BGM cells, *J. Gen. Virol.* **39**:113.

Youngner, J. S., and Quagliana, D. O., 1975, Temperature-sensitive mutants isolated from hamster and canine cell lines persistently infected with Newcastle disease virus, *J. Virol.* **16**:1332.

Youngner, J. S., and Quagliana, D. O., 1976, Temperature-sensitive mutants of vesicular stomatitis virus are conditionally defective particles that interfere with and are rescued by wild-type virus, *J. Virol.* **19**:102.

Youngner, J. S., Dubovi, E. J., Quagliana, D. O., Kelly, M., and Preble, O. T., 1976, Role of temperature-sensitive mutants in persistent infections initiated with vesicular stomatitis virus, *J. Virol.* **19**:90.

Youngner, J. S., Preble, O. T., and Jones, E. V., 1978*a*, Persistent infection of L cells with vesicular stomatitis virus: Evolution of virus populations, *J. Virol.* **28**:6.

Youngner, J. S., Preble, O. T., Jones, E. V., and Creager, R. S., 1978*b*, Evolution of virus populations in persistent infections of L cells with vesicular stomatitis virus, in: *Persistent Infections* (J. G. Stevens, G. J. Todaro, and C. F. Fox, eds.), *ICN-UCLA Symp. Mol. Cell. Biol.*, Vol. 11, pp. 417–429, Academic Press, New York.

CHAPTER 3

Defective Interfering RNA Viruses and the Host-Cell Response

John J. Holland, S. Ian T. Kennedy, Bert L. Semler, Charlotte L. Jones, Laurent Roux, and Elizabeth A. Grabau

Department of Biology
University of California, San Diego
La Jolla, California 92093

1. INTRODUCTION

This chapter will emphasize recently derived knowledge concerning the nature of defective interfering (DI) particles of RNA animal viruses, their biological origins and functions, and their involvement in long-term persistent infections. We will not attempt to review all of the DI literature, and we will confine ourselves to DI particles of RNA viruses. The previous review by Huang and Baltimore (1977) amply documents the occurrence and behavior of DI particles in a wide variety of DNA and RNA viruses and discusses their biological effects, and a very thorough recent review of rhabdovirus DI particles by Reichmann and Schnitzlein (1978) provides excellent in-depth coverage of many areas not covered by the present chapter as well as some alternate viewpoints of areas which are considered here. We will omit DNA virus DI particles from extensive consideration because of space limitations and because they are generally less well characterized at present.

However, at the end of the chapter we will briefly cite recent studies implicating DI particles in some persistent infections by DNA viruses.

DI particles were first recognized in preparations of influenza virus propagated *in vivo*. The first clear definition of DI particles was that of von Magnus (1954) who showed that homologous interference exerted by the yields from serial undiluted passages of influenza virus in eggs was due to replication of "incomplete particles" which showed hemagglutinating and interfering ability but not infectivity. In fact, Henle and Henle (1943) first reported a "paradoxical behavior" in which late-harvest virus from eggs showed lower infectivity in mice when undiluted than when diluted one thousandfold. Because of the resistance of the interfering agent to UV light and heat, they concluded that interference was due to "inactivated" infectious virus, but their results were almost certainly due to the presence of DI particles. Cooper and Bellett (1959) and Bellett and Cooper (1959) showed that a similar phenomenon occurred with vesicular stomatitis virus (VSV) on undiluted passage in cell culture. They demonstrated that the interfering component was transmissible and that it sedimented more slowly than infectious virus. However, they were unable to rule out interferon and for some reason were unable to neutralize these DI particles with immune serum. Hackett (1964) demonstrated by electron microscopy that VSV DI particles were shorter than standard infectious virus, and several years later it was shown that discrete VSV DI particles could be separated from standard virus on sucrose gradients (Huang *et al.*, 1966; Crick *et al.*, 1966; Hackett *et al.*, 1967). This allowed purification and study of the effects of DI particles (Huang and Wagner, 1966a). It is even possible to achieve greater than a billionfold purification of VSV DI particles by repeated cycles of velocity sedimentation in sucrose gradients and to obtain milligram quantities of DI particles totally freed of infectious virus for biological studies (Doyle and Holland, 1973). The converse, however, is not true—it is not possible to remove all DI particles from standard virus by velocity sedimentation because a percentage of the smaller DI particles will always aggregate and cosediment along with standard virus. However, VSV DI particles can be biologically eliminated or reduced in number by serial cloning (Stampfer *et al.*, 1971). Small amounts of infectious virus picked directly from a plaque may be and usually are free of DI particles, but high-titer pools prepared directly from a plaque isolate are always contaminated by DI particles (Holland *et al.*, 1976a). Since VSV generates DI particles at a rate of 10^{-7}–10^{-8} for each infectious standard virus particle replicated (Holland *et al.*, 1976b), these DI particles are present in such low amounts that they cannot be visualized directly. They can be observed only after several further serial undiluted passages during which they undergo 10^4-fold amplification during each passage (Holland et al., 1976a,b) with support of the helper standard virus. Thus the need for serial undiluted passages in the "von Magnus phenomenon" is probably a requirement for amplification of DI particles and not for their generation. Removal of DI particles from standard virus is a particular problem for the paramyxoviruses since cloning alone does not work (Rima et al., 1977). To overcome this difficulty these authors suggest "an intermediate dilution of $1:1000$ be used so that the virus growth period is relatively short."

Huang and Baltimore (1970) were the first to call attention to the widespread occurrence of DI particles among nearly all groups of animal viruses, and they proposed the name DI for virus particles which (1) lack a portion of the genome; (2) contain normal virus structural proteins; (3) can replicate only with the aid of helper standard infectious virus; and (4) interfere specifically with replication of homologous standard helper virus. Another important characteristic of DI particles is the fact that their generation and their interfering capacity may show enormous variability in different cell types (Choppin, 1969; Huang and Baltimore, 1970; Perrault and Holland, 1972a; Holland et al., 1976a). In the case of the positive-strand viruses, even the final size and structure of the DI genome is strictly controlled by the cell type which generates the DI particles (Stark and Kennedy, 1978). This is discussed in detail below.

Members of each group of the negative-strand viruses have been found to produce DI particles or DI-like particles. These include the orthomyxoviruses (e.g., influenza A), paramyxoviruses (e.g., Sendai, measles viruses), rhabdoviruses (e.g., VSV, rabies virus), arenaviruses (e.g., LCM and parana viruses), and probably bunyaviruses (e.g., La Crosse and Uukuniemi) (references are given below). Among the positive-strand RNA viruses of class IV (Baltimore, 1971), DI particles have been identified in stocks of picornaviruses (Cole et al., 1971; McClure et al., 1980) and togaviruses (Schlesinger et al., 1972). As yet, there has been no report of DI particles of any member of the coronavirus group, but this probably reflects the present paucity of information regarding the properties of the coronaviruses. Among the double-stranded RNA viruses, reovirus has clearly been shown to generate DI particles (Nonoyama et al., 1970), and there is suggestive evidence for DI particles of infectious pancreatic necrosis virus of trout (Nicholson and Dunn, 1972).

The history of picornavirus, reovirus, and togavirus DI particles dates back to the early years of this decade. In 1970 Nonoyama *et al.* reported the presence of DI particles in reovirus stocks. The elegant studies of Cole *et al.* (1971) established the existence of poliovirus DI particles, and the following year two groups independently reported the existence of DI particles of the togavirus, Sindbis virus (SV) (Inglot and Chudzio, 1972; Schlesinger *et al.*, 1972). For poliovirus, 16–18 serial passages in HeLa cells were required before DI particles became detectable. Fewer passages—six to eight—were required for SV DI particles to become apparent in virus stocks propagated in either chicken or hamster cells. With the exception of some recent work on mengovirus DI particles (McClure *et al.*, 1980), poliovirus remains the only picornavirus system for which DI particles have been formally identified. Reovirus DI particles (Nonoyama and Graham, 1970) were detected after seven high-multiplicity passages of several different clones of type 3 reovirus. Almost all work concerning DI particles of togaviruses has been done with either SV or Semliki Forest virus (SFV), both alphaviruses. Very little has been reported about DI particles of flaviviruses.

In summary, DI particles are deletion mutants (usually genome recombinants) which cannot replicate by themselves and which interfere specifically with replication of the homologous infectious helper virus that they require for their own generation and replication. Below, we review their structural, biological, and biochemical properties and the evidence for their role in persistence. Because of their rather significant distinguishing characteristics, we will deal with the DI particles of negative-strand viruses separately from those of the positive-strand viruses.

2. STRUCTURE AND GENOME ARRANGEMENT OF DI PARTICLES

2.1. DI Particles of Negative-Strand Viruses

The structure of VSV and its DI particles with respect to overall morphology and protein composition has been reviewed (Huang, 1973; Wagner, 1975; Huang and Baltimore, 1977) and will not be reiterated here. For most of the negative-strand RNA viruses, the DI particles appear to be identical to the standard virus in both their protein composition and overall morphological characteristics. In some cases DI are smaller in size, however.

The genome RNA of DI particles from negative-strand viruses has been characterized in a number of different ways. However, since most of the data on DI RNA structure comes from studies on VSV and Sendai virus, this section will focus almost entirely on these two viruses. Using velocity sedimentation and hybridization, it was originally shown for VSV (Huang and Wagner, 1966*b*; Brown *et al.*, 1967; Schaffer *et al.*, 1968) and Sendai virus (Kingsbury *et al.*, 1970) that DI RNA is a deleted form of the standard virus RNA. In addition, it was shown by RNA-RNA annealing that any given DI particle contains a specific portion of the standard virus genome and not random pieces encapsidated into mature DI particles (Schincariol and Howatson, 1972; Stamminger and Lazzarini, 1974).

Identification of those virion genes represented within various VSV DI-particle isolates has been achieved by hybridization of purified DI RNAs to the purified mRNA fractions obtained from VSV-infected cell extracts (Leamnson and Reichmann, 1974; Stamminger and Lazzarini, 1974; Schnitzlein and Reichmann, 1976; Adler and Banerjee, 1976) and to the total mRNA synthesized *in vitro* by purified virions treated with detergent (Roy and Bishop, 1972). It was found that most of the DI RNAs originated from the 5' end of the standard virus genome and that these DI particles exhibited homotypic interference. However, a single DI-particle isolate (HR DI) was unique in that it arose from the 3' end of the standard virus RNA (Leamnson and Reichmann, 1974; Stamminger and Lazzarini, 1974; Schnitzlein and Reichmann, 1976). This isolate of Indiana DI particles was also unique in that it exhibited heterotypic interference with New Jersey VSV (Prevec and Kang, 1970; Schnitzlein and Reichmann, 1976). Its difference from nearly all other DI particles was further demonstrated when it was shown to be the only known DI particle to transcribe some functional mRNA both *in vivo* (Chow *et al.*, 1977; Johnson and Lazzarini, 1977) and *in vitro* (Colonno *et al.*, 1977), presumably because it has the transcriptional initiation site contained at the 3' terminus of standard virus RNA. In addition, recent evidence has shown that the HR DI particle isolate contains RNAs with internal genome deletions that retain the standard VSV 3' and 5' terminus (Perrault and Semler, 1979; Lazzarini, personal communication).

DI particles from VSV may contain minus strands (Roy and Bishop, 1972; Stamminger and Lazzarini, 1974) or unlinked plus and minus strands of RNA (Roy *et al.*, 1973; Leamnson and Reichmann, 1974; Reichmann *et al.*, 1974; Schnitzlein and Reichmann, 1976; Perrault and Leavitt, 1977*a*). Sendai RNA isolated from DI nucleocapsids obtained from the infected cell also appears to have considerable plus and minus strand polarity (Kolakofsky, 1976). In addition, a rather unique structural feature of the RNA of some isolates of VSV DI particles results from packaging of covalently linked plus and minus strands. These are referred to as "snap-back" RNA (Lazzarini *et al.*, 1975; Perrault, 1976; Perrault and Leavitt, 1977*a*). It was suggested that this RNAse-resistant, snap-back structure may be a modified version of a normal VSV RNA replicating intermediate which becomes packaged into some types of DI particle (Perrault, 1976). It may have biological significance, since it has been detected at varying levels in quite a few different DI particle isolates (Perrault and Leavitt, 1977*a*).

The RNA from influenza virus DI particles was first shown to differ from standard virus RNA in that it completely or partially lacked the largest segment of viral RNA (Duesberg, 1968; Choppin and Pons, 1970). Other data (Bean and Simpson, 1976; Nayak *et al.*, 1978) indicate that influenza DI particles do not always selectively lose a particular RNA segment. Instead, there appears to be a relative reduction of one or more of the four largest viral RNA segments packaged by DI particles concomitant with packaging of subviral-size RNAs. This rather nonspecific loss of viral RNA segments has been suggested as the basis for the loss of infectivity in influenza DI particles (Nayak *et al.*, 1978). The apparent discrepancies in DI genome composition may be explained by a rather considerable variability in the reduction of viral RNA segments in DI RNA preparations obtained from different clones of influenza virus (Janda *et al.*, 1979).

In addition to cistron representation and RNA packaging, recent work suggests that the RNA termini of DI particles may be important in DI particle generation and interference. Inverted complementary sequences have been found in Sendai virus (Kolakofsky, 1976; Leppert *et al.*, 1977) and VSV DI RNAs (Perrault and Leavitt, 1977*b*; Perrault *et al.*, 1978). These terminal "stem" sequences of RNA in Sendai virus vary in length from 110 to 150 nucleotide pairs, depending on which DI particle isolate they are derived from (Leppert *et al.*, 1977). In VSV DI RNAs the terminal complementary regions span approximately 60 nucleotide pairs in those DI particles so far analyzed (Perrault and Leavitt, 1977*b*; Perrault *et al.*, 1978). Hybridization studies with the isolated DI stems and standard virus genome indicate that only the 5' and not the 3' terminus of the standard virus RNA is conserved in the DI RNAs. This is true for both Sendai virus (Leppert *et al.*, 1977; Kolakofsky *et al.*, 1978) and VSV (Perrault and Leavitt, 1977*b*; Perrault *et al.*, 1978). Additionally, the 3' termini of most DI RNAs are complementary copies of the 5' end of standard virus RNA. To date, the HR DI particle of VSV has the only DI RNA known to contain both the 3' and 5' termini of the standard virus and hence cannot form the terminally base-paired stems found in other DI RNAs (Perrault *et al.*, 1978; Perrault and Semler, 1979). On the basis of these and other data, two similar models for DI particle generation employing a replicase-switching and copy-back mechanism have been proposed (Leppert *et al.*, 1977; Huang, 1977). A possible role in DI-particle autointerference has been suggested for the inverted complementary terminal sequences (Perrault *et al.*, 1978), as discussed below. Neither interference nor the proposed models for DI-particle generation can be based solely on RNA structure since other factors like protein type within the DI nucleocapsid also have an influence on the interference phenomenon (Schnitzlein and Reichmann, 1977). It is also likely that the generation of the HR DI particle and its interference with standard VSV occur by different mechanisms than the ones proposed since the structure of its RNA termini is different from that of other DI particles (Perrault and Semler, 1979).

Although most of the data concerning the 3' and 5' termini of standard and DI RNAs were obtained from electron microscopy and hybridization studies, the following studies employing nucleotide sequencing of VSV (Indiana serotype) RNAs have lent further support to the polarity assignments given to the various RNA termini:

1. The first 17 nucleotides at the 3' end of the DI RNA are similar (but not identical) to those at the 3' end of the standard virus RNA, and this similarity then diverges to a complete lack of homology for the next 50 or so nucleotides past the first 17 (Keene *et al.*, 1978).
2. The sequence of the 46 nucleotide *in vitro* RNA transcript templated by the 3' end of the DI RNA (Semler *et al.*, 1978; Holland *et al.*, 1978; Schubert *et al.*, 1978) is significantly different from the sequence of the leader RNA (Colonno and Banerjee, 1978), which is known to be synthesized directly from the 3' end of standard virus RNA (Colonno and Banerjee, 1976).
3. The sequence of the 5' end of standard virus RNA is identical to the 5' end of DI particle RNAs for at least 46 nucleotides in from the terminus (Perrault *et al.*, 1978; Semler *et al.*, 1979).

Our knowledge to date of the sequences at the 5' and 3' ends of VSV (Indiana serotype) and DI RNAs is presented in Fig. 1A and

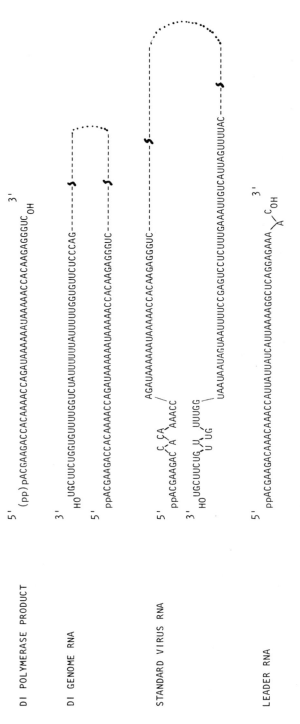

Fig. 1A. Nucleotide sequences of RNA species from VSV (Indiana serotype). These data reflect direct sequencing as well as inferred sequences taken from the following: DI polymerase product (Semler *et al.*, 1978; Holland *et al.*, 1978; Schubert *et al.*, 1978); DI genome RNA—direct sequencing of the first 17 nucleotides of the 3′ end (Keene *et al.*, 1978); DI genome RNA—inferred sequences of both the 5′ and 3′ termini by hybridization and duplex sizing (Perrault *et al.*, 1978; Semler *et al.*, 1978); standard virus RNA—direct sequencing of the 3′ terminus (Keene *et al.*, 1978; Rowlands, 1979; McGeoch and Dolan, 1979); standard virus RNA—inferred sequence of the 3′ terminus by hybridization (Colonno and Banerjee, 1978); standard virus RNA—direct sequencing of the 5′ terminus (Semler *et al.*, 1979); standard virus RNA—inferred sequence of the 5′ terminus by hybridization and duplex sizing (Perrrault *et al.*, 1978; Semler *et al.*, 1978); and the leader RNA (Colonno and Banerjee, 1978). Note that the proposed recombination point that generates the DI genome RNA must be just a few nucleotides internal to that region on the DI RNA which is protected by the DI polymerase product (see text).

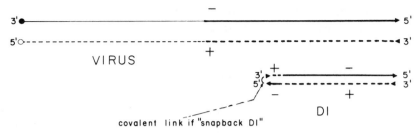

Fig. 1B. Schematic representation of VSV standard virus RNA and the DI RNA which is derived from it. The DI RNA has the same nucleotide sequence at the 3' end (and the 5' end) of both the plus and the minus strands, but the standard virus RNA has a different sequence at the 3' end of its plus and minus strands despite some partial identity. Note that the 5' terminus of the minus strand's virion RNA is conserved in the DI RNA, while the 3' end is not. "Snap-back RNA" DI particles are a special type containing covalently linked plus- and minus-strand RNA. Thick lines indicate the 5' half of the genome (encoding the L protein).

schematized in Fig. 1B. Since the stem structures are only slightly longer than the region coding for the DI polymerase product RNA, it is clear that the recombination point which generates most VSV DI particles is at the internal end of the stem sequence, and this is only slightly beyond (internal to) the end of the 46-nucleotide region coding for DI product RNA. Intriguingly, RNA sequence analysis has revealed a common hexamer oligonucleotide found in just this region for four different VSV DI-particle RNAs (Schubert et al., 1979), and it was proposed that this hexamer may represent a specific internal replicase recognition site that is a necessary aspect of the strand-switching and copy-back models for DI-particle generation. Further sequencing of other DI-particle RNAs and replicase binding experiments will determine the importance of such sequences in DI-particle generation.

Whether these structures are a general feature in other negative-strand DI particles must await further investigation. Evidence from electron microscopy of other negative-strand virus groups has shown circular nucleocapsid structures as well as linear molecules of greater than normal length. These have been reported for measles-infected cells (Thorne and Dermott, 1976), and from virions of LaCrosse virus (Obijeski et al., 1976) and Lumbo virus (Samso et al., 1975) (two serologically related bunyaviruses). Circular nucleocapsids as well as circular RNAs have been observed in Uukuniemi virus which is an unrelated bunyavirus (Petterson and von Bonsdorff 1975; Petterson and Hewlett, 1976; Hewlett et al., 1977). The status of any of these structures as DI-particle components is unclear. All of these could be indicative of inverted complementary terminal sequences, but proof awaits further biochemical and nucleotide sequence analysis of RNAs from these and other negative-strand virus groups.

2.2. DI Particles of Positive-Strand Viruses

Because the genome of DI particles is a truncated form of the standard virus genome, the size of DI particles is often smaller than that of the standard virus (e.g., VSV, see above). This difference is commonly employed as an experimental basis for the physical separation of DI particles from their standard virus. The physical difference, in turn, facilitates the characterization of the DI-particle genome. For the positive-strand RNA viruses this difference, although greater for the picornaviruses than for the alphaviruses, is considerably less than for rhabdoviruses. Thus for poliovirus several cycles of density-gradient centrifugation are required to effect essentially complete purification of its DI particles. The modest difference between the buoyant density of poliovirus and its DI particles is reflected in the relatively small difference between the size of the DI genome and that of the standard virion. Figure 2 shows an RNA-RNA duplex between poliovirus DI RNA and negative-strand RNA from replicative form (Nomoto *et al.*, 1978). This technique, together with other techniques which probe the sequence relationship between standard and DI poliovirus RNA, clearly established that about 13–16% of the nucleotide sequence of standard virus RNA is deleted in the DI RNA and that this deletion is located about 20% inward from the 5' end of the standard virus genome. This latter observation is in agreement with the earlier finding that the deletion in poliovirus DI RNA maps in the N1 region which from biochemical and genetic analysis was shown to be in the 5' terminal half of the genome (Cole and Baltimore, 1973*a*). In a recent study Lunquist *et al.* (1979) showed that at least five distinct types of polio DI particles can be generated and that single, double, and possibly triple deletions can occur in the viral genome. All of these mutations occur in the capsid gene region. In addition, despite their heterogeneity, the DI genomes are quite similar in physical size.

For SV and SFV there is even less difference between the buoyant density of the standard virion and its DI particles than for the poliovirus counterparts. Two reports (Shenk and Stollar, 1973; Bruton and Kennedy, 1976) suggested that alphavirus DI particles can be slightly more dense than the standard virus. Other workers (Weiss and Schlesinger, 1973) failed to resolve standard and DI SV particles on

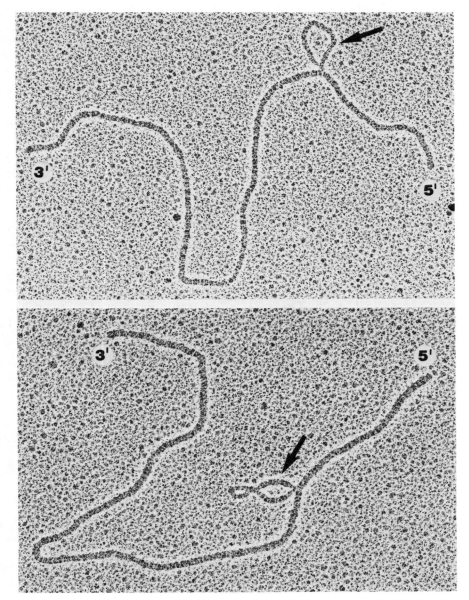

Fig. 2. Electron micrograph of an RNA-RNA duplex formed between poliovirus DI RNA and negative strand from RF isolated from cells infected with standard virus. From Nomoto *et al*. (1978) with permission.

density gradients. The reason for the similarity in the density of standard and DI alphaviruses is, however, unrelated to that of the poliovirus system. From ribonuclease T_1 oligonucleotide fingerprinting (Kennedy, 1976; Kennedy *et al.*, 1976) it was clearly established that the nucleotide sequence of alphavirus DI RNA is only a very small fraction of that of the standard virus genome. Therefore, in order to reconcile this marked sequence difference between standard and DI particle RNA with the close similarity between the buoyant density of standard and DI particles, it was suggested that each alphavirus DI particle contains several copies of DI RNA (Kennedy *et al.*, 1976). Indeed, there may be intracellular packaging "rules" which put into each nucleocapsid one standard virus RNA (molecular weight 4.4×10^6) or the almost exact mass equivalent of DI RNA. This mass equivalent may be two molecules of half-length DI RNA, three molecules of about one-third-length RNA, and so on up to six molecules of about one-sixth-length RNA. (We shall consider this point again later.) How these several copies of DI RNA are arranged in the DI particle is not known, but the observation that they can exist as circles with short panhandle tails (Fig. 3a) suggests that they may form concatameric structures of the type shown in Fig. 3b. These structures would be formed by hydrogen bonding between a short nucleotide sequence at the 5′ end of the DI RNA and its inverted complement at the 3′ end either within the same strand (to form a circle) or between strands (to form a concatamer). Inverted complementary nucleotide sequences have been shown to exist

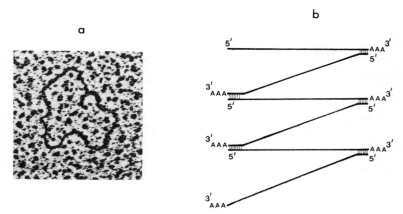

Fig. 3.   Conformation of SFV DI RNA. (a) Electron micrograph of DIssD RNA (see Fig. 4) from purified DI particles of SFV. The RNA was spread under partially denaturing conditions (Simons and Kennedy, unpublished). (b) Schematic representation of six molecules of alphavirus DI RNA arranged in a concatamer.

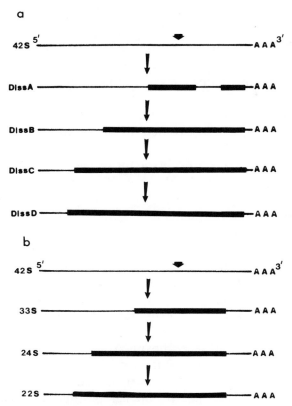

Fig. 4. Sequence organization of alphavirus DI RNAs. For SFV (a) the DI RNAs are denoted DIssA, DIssB, DIssC, and DIssD (Stark and Kennedy, 1978); for SV (B) the DI RNAs are denoted 33 S, 24 S and 22 S according to their sedimentation coefficient (Guild and Stollar, 1977). The ▬▬▬ denotes deleted sequences which are approximately to scale. The heavy arrows indicate the junction between the nonstructural (polymerase) genes (to the left) and the structural genes in standard virus 42 S RNA.

at the ends of both standard and DI SFV RNA (Kennedy, unpublished observations).

Using oligonucleotide fingerprinting (Kennedy, 1976; Stark and Kennedy, 1978) and RNA-RNA hybridization (Guild and Stollar, 1977), the sequence arrangements shown in Fig. 4 have been established for standard RNA and the RNA of several DI particles generated during the course of high-multiplicity serial passaging of SV and SFV. Several points emerge from these studies. First, during the serial passaging, several species of DI RNA appear. Second, in all cases the 5' and 3' extremities of standard virus RNA are retained in DI RNA.

Thus all species of alphavirus RNA are internally deleted forms of the standard genome. Third, with the exception of minor deletion differences, the deletions which generate SFV DI RNA (Fig. 4a) are very similar to those generating SV DI RNA (Fig. 4b). In addition to these sequence relationship findings several groups have observed that during the course of serial passaging the size of alphavirus DI RNA progressively decreases (Johnston et al., 1975; Guild et al., 1977; Stark and Kennedy, 1978). These two sets of observations strongly suggest that during serial passaging a series of sequential internal deletions occurs whereby each DI RNA acts as progenitor for the next smallest in the series until the smallest DI RNA of all (e.g., DIssD for SFV) is generated. For both SV and SFV this is an RNA with a molecular weight one-sixth that of the genome.

Reovirus DI particles have essentially the same buoyant density as standard virus. However, DI-particle cores can be resolved from those of standard virus. The density difference is consistent with the observation that the largest (L_1) segment of the ten-segment double-stranded RNA genome is missing in DI particles (Nonoyama and Graham, 1970). Interestingly, however, no smaller, deleted version of the L_1 segment is apparent, which by analogy with DI particles of influenza virus might have been expected (see above). A second study of reovirus DI particles has shown that temperature-sensitive mutants of groups C and F more rapidly generate DI particles than wild-type virus. In this case the L_1 segment is missing but on further passage another segment is deleted (Schuerch et al., 1974).

3. MECHANISMS OF DI-PARTICLE GENERATION, REPLICATION, AND INTERFERENCE

3.1. DI Particles of Negative-Strand Viruses

This section must involve some speculation on the biochemical mechanisms of DI-particle generation, replication, and interference. These can only be inferred but cannot be proved from data presently available.

3.1.1. DI-Particle Generation

Mechanisms of DI-particle generation remain undefined since some complex recombination mechanism must occur to shorten the virus genome internally and to add a new 3' terminus which is a copy of the standard virus 5' terminus (see above). The "strand-switching, copyback" model proposed by Leppert *et al.* (1977) and Huang (1977) (in which the viral replicase falls off its template RNA, reattaches to the nascent RNA, and "reads back" on the nascent RNA) is a very plausible one, but experimental support is lacking since DI-particle generation takes place within the confines of an infected cell. Obviously, any inter- or intramolecular recombination event, whether legitimate (involving regions of sequence homology) or illegitimate, would be compatible with the data presently available. Indeed, it is not clear whether the recombination event occurs during replication at the positive- or negative-strand level or, alternatively, whether a splicing event occurs. Simple-minded *in vitro* attempts to generate DI particles or modify their size (by mutagenesis or by shear breakage of standard virus or DI nucleocapsid) do not succeed (Holland *et al.*, 1976a). Furthermore, future attempts to achieve DI-particle generation *in vitro* by enzymatic or other means of RNA genome rearrangement will be hampered by the fact that naked virion RNA from negative-strand DI particles is biologically inactive (Holland *et al.*, 1976a). The minimal infectious structure is the membrane-free nucleocapsid (Brown *et al.*, 1967; Holland *et al.*, 1976a), and *in vitro* reassembly has yet to be achieved with any negative-strand virus or DI nucleocapsid.

It can be demonstrated using low-titer clonal isolates that VSV DI-particle generation is a rather random event, and any DI-particle-free clone can generate a wide array of different-size DI particles in different passage series from the clone (Holland *et al.*, 1976a). Others have reported that single clones seem to have a genetic capacity to regularly generate the same DI particles in a given cell type (Reichmann *et al.*, 1971; Kang *et al.*, 1978). However, this result is inevitable whenever the starting clone of virus is contaminated with DI particles which amplify during subsequent passage series, and both of these investigations started with high-titer virus pools prepared from clonal isolates. Since the rate of DI particle generation is about 10^{-7}–10^{-8} per infectious particle replication (Holland *et al.*, 1976b), any VSV pool containing more than about 10^7–10^8 pfu must be suspect with regard to the possibility that DI particles are already present. Ideally, a very early small plaque should be picked and used for such studies if the isolate contains 10^6 or less total infectious virus pfu. The multiple-plaque harvest technique of Stampfer *et al.* (1971) is a good method to obtain low-titer virus pools free or nearly free of DI (Holland *et al.*, 1976b). Kolakofsky (1979) has also found random generation of different DI particles of Sendai virus on independent serial passages of a multiply cloned plaque isolate, and Janda *et al.* (1979) have obtained similar results with some clones of influenza virus. Recently, a major technical advance for the preparation of VSV pools free of DI particles has been reported (Kang and Allen, 1978). Pretreatment of host cells with actinomycin D before virus growth was reported to deplete a host-cell factor required for DI particle generation. This technique has not been repeated by others, so its general applicability is not yet known.

3.1.2. DI-Particle Replication and Interference

The most notable fact regarding negative-strand virus DI-particle replication is their complete inability to replicate RNA without helper infectious virus. This is in contrast to DI particles from some positive-strand viruses such as poliovirus, which can carry out viral RNA synthesis but lack genetic information encoding capsid proteins (see below). The vast majority of VSV DI particles are nontranscribing and therefore genetically inert (Huang and Manders, 1972; Perrault and Holland, 1972*b*). The one known transcribing VSV DI particle (HR DI) does not code for the L protein, a major transcriptase and replicase polypeptide (Colonno *et al.*, 1977), but it has been reported to be capable of killing cells (Marcus *et al.*, 1977).

DI-particle interference was suggested independently by Huang and Manders (1972) and by Perrault and Holland (1972*b*) to be due to competition between DI particles and infectious virus RNA templates for viral replicase molecules. This replicative competition model was based on the following observations: (1) DI particles are genetically inert but replicate well in the presence of helper virus; (2) DI particles contain all the proteins of the helper virus; (3) DI particles do not inhibit primary transcription of standard virus added to cells in large amounts in the presence of cycloheximide; (4) DI particles strongly inhibit the replication of full-size viral genome RNA following primary transcription in the absence of cycloheximide, and there is a parallel inhibition of synthesis of the large amounts of viral messenger RNA normally transcribed from these secondary (newly replicated) viral RNA templates; (5) concomitant with this suppression of standard virus RNA replication and secondary messenger RNA transcription there is a striking synthesis of DI genome-size RNA (i.e., DI particle RNA replication). All these results strongly suggest but do not prove that DI particles compete at the replicative level. An even stronger indication for replicative interference is given by the fact that in pig kidney cells in which VSV DI particles do not interfere (Perrault and Holland, 1972a) there is no strong inhibition of viral RNA or viral messenger RNA synthesis despite high levels of replication of DI genome-size RNA in the same cells (Perrault and Holland, 1972b). Khan and Lazzarini (1977) have repeated and extended these replicative competition studies and conclude also that replicase competition could explain interference. However, it should be recognized that DI-particle interference could involve a number of mechanisms, including perhaps effects on viral protein synthesis or turnover rates. Rima and Martin (1979) report that measles virus DI particles cause a selective inhibition of synthesis of all other measles virus proteins except the N protein. However, Little and Huang (1977) found that DI interference caused no selective inhibition of synthesis of VSV proteins.

Khan and Lazzarini (1977) and Schnitzlein and Reichmann (1977) observed that there is much less interference by Indiana serotype DI particles when coinfecting cells with VSV New Jersey serotype helper virus even though the VSV Indiana DI particles replicate well with the heterotypic helper virus. Thus DI-particle replication can be dissociated from virus replication in heterotypic interference just as it can be from homologous interference in "low-interference" cell lines such as pig kidney cells (Perrault and Holland, 1972a). This ability to obtain DI-particle replication with little or no interference under certain conditions does not eliminate replicase competition as the site of interference (wherever interference does occur). In fact, Schnitzlein and Reichmann (1977) obtained strong heterotypic interference if the VSV Indiana DI genome RNA was encapsidated within VSV New Jersey proteins by one prior cycle of replication in the presence of VSV New Jersey helper virus. Clearly, the interaction of viral proteins with each other is important in determining the replicative and interfering efficiency of DI nucleocapsid templates. Furthermore, the reduced availability of viral proteins (resulting from reduced viral mRNA synthesis) may render replicative and interference phenomena more complex if limited availability of viral matrix and glycoprotein membrane proteins results in a buildup of DI and viral nucleocapsids within the cytoplasm. Also, the existence of low-interference cell lines (Choppin, 1969; Huang and Baltimore, 1970; Kingsbury and Portner, 1970; Perrault and Holland, 1972a; Holland et al., 1976a) suggests a major role of cellular factors in determining DI-particle interference. These factors may act as replicase components or in other ways. Obviously, interference mechanisms remain largely unexplored at the biochemical level, and definitive studies may require development of cell-free replication systems. Even if the replicase competition model proves to be substantially correct, quantitative regulatory aspects may prove to be more important than qualitative mechanisms. DI genome size could well be a factor in interference among the positive-strand RNA viruses (see below), but it appears to play little if any role in interference by negative-strand RNA viruses since large, medium, and small DI particles replicate and interfere with about equal efficiency. In growth competition experiments the smallest DI particles do not seem to replicate faster and hence outcompete larger DI particles; on the contrary, DI particles of various sizes outcompete other DI particles of various sizes in a random manner depending to a considerable extent on the cells in which they are replicating (Holland *et al.*, 1976*a*).

Finally, it is clear that the structure of the DI RNA genome is important in interference since Prevec and Kang (1970) observed heterotypic interference with New Jersey serotype VSV by VSV DI particles of the HR (transcribing DI) class. Further sequencing and interference studies are needed to compare this unique class of DI particles to the major class of DI particles. This may be difficult at present because all stocks of HR DI which we have examined are contaminated with other DI particles of the nontranscribing class (Holland, unpublished), Adachi and Lazzarini (1978) and Reichmann and Schnitzlein (1978) have reported that their preparations of HR DI do interfere normally. The differences in the 3' end sequences in this DI class as compared to the majority class predict that it should behave quite differently in interference (at least if the altered 3' ends of the majority class of VSV DI particle are critical determinants of DI replicative and interfering ability as has been suggested (Perrault *et al.*, 1978). Most VSV DI particles contain the same RNA sequence at the 3' end of both their minus-strand and plus-strand RNA homologues (Perrault *et al.*, 1978). Since this sequence is found only at the 3' end of the plus (but not the minus) strand RNA of the standard infectious virus, any selective affinity for this sequence by the viral replicase should favor DI-particle replication over standard virus replication. This model would also predict that a completely pure preparation of the unique HR DI particle with RNA whose 3' end is identical to that of standard virus RNA would not exhibit homologous interference as effectively as that of the major class of VSV DI particles. If the HR DI preparation of Reichmann and Schnitzlein (1978) and Adachi and Lazzarini (1978) (which exhibited strong interfering ability) was free of significant levels of the major class DI, then the new RNA 3' end possessed by the major class DI must not be a critical requirement for interference. Another possible explanation for the replicative advantage and interfering ability of DI particles lies in the fact that the recombination point which generates the inverted "stems" is about 60 nucleotides or less from the 3' end of each DI RNA molecule (Perrault et al., 1978). This nearby recombination point might greatly alter the secondary and tertiary structure of DI RNA 3' ends and greatly increase their affinity for replicase as compared to standard virus RNA 3' ends. Since DI particles arise at a rather high frequency, only those 3' end recombinants with a favorable replicase affinity would replicate preferentially and be selected. Clearly, our knowledge of the mechanisms of interference is still fragmentary.

3.2. DI Particles of Positive-Strand Viruses

3.2.1. DI-Particle Replication and Interference

Interference with standard virus multiplication by DI particles of poliovirus and alphaviruses occurs at the level of standard virus RNA synthesis and proviral assembly. For reovirus neither the mechanism of interference nor of enrichment is known. Two distinct functional classes of viral RNA are found in cells infected with either standard poliovirus or standard alphaviruses. These are single-stranded positive-polarity RNA and replicative intermediate (RI) RNA. For poliovirus a single size of positive-strand RNA (35 S) exists which acts as mRNA for both the viral structural proteins and polymerase polypeptides. In contrast, cells infected with standard alphaviruses contain two size classes of positive-strand RNA. The first of these (42 S RNA) is the viral genome and acts in the infected cell as mRNA for the polymerase polypeptides. The mRNA for the alphavirus structural proteins is a subgenomic fragment (26 S RNA) whose nucleotide sequence is the 3' terminal one-third of 42 S RNA. For both poliovirus and the alphaviruses, RI RNA consists of genome-length template RNA to which is hydrogen bonded several nascent RNA strands. This class of RNA is probably derived from cytoplasmic replication complexes active in the synthesis of both positive- and negative-strand viral RNA.

Cells infected with alphavirus DI particles alone or with DI particle RNA do not synthesize any virus-specified components (Bruton et al., 1976). Thus alphavirus DI particles, although adsorbed, appear totally unable to initiate any virus-specific synthetic event. The reason for this inertness lies in the sequence relationship between standard virus RNA and DI RNA (see previous section). All alphavirus DI RNAs have a deletion across the junction region between the polymerase and structural protein genes in 42 S RNA. Since the polymerase genes are translated to form a polyprotein whose C-terminal coding region is absent in all the DI RNAs, these RNAs, even if potentially capable of translation (i.e., are capped, polyadenylated, and have a ribosome binding site; Kennedy, unpublished; Bruton *et al.*, 1976; Clegg and Kennedy, unpublished), would seem *a priori* to be unable to direct the synthesis of functional polymerase and therefore unable to initiate the first step in multiplication. That this is a reasonable hypothesis to account for the metabolic inactivity of alphavirus DI particles is supported by the finding that neither SV DI RNA nor SFV DI RNA can serve as mRNA either *in vitro* or *in vivo* (Weiss *et al.*, 1974; Bruton *et al.*, 1976).

Cells coinfected with alphavirus stocks which contain DI particles synthesize several species of virus-specific RNA distinct from those which characterize multiplication of standard particles alone. These new species comprise not only single-stranded (ss) DI RNAs but also RI RNAs whose template strands are involved in replicating these ss DI RNAs (Weiss *et al.*, 1974; Bruton *et al.*, 1976; Kennedy *et al.*, 1976; Guild *et al.*, 1977). In addition, the total amount of viral RNA synthesis in cells coinfected with DI particles plus a given amount of standard virus is less than that in cells infected with the same amount of standard virus alone (Guild and Stollar, 1975). This reduction in total viral RNA synthesis depends on the ratio of DI particles to standard virus in the inoculum. The recognition of intracellular DI RI RNA, the lack of mRNA function of the ssDI RNA, and their sequence relationship to the standard genome, together with the dependence of total virus-specified RNA on the input ratio of DI particles to standard virus, all have led to the following model for alphavirus interference and selective propagation. Since all species of positive-strand DI RNA have the same 3' nucleotide sequence as standard viral RNA, it seems likely that DI RNA and standard viral RNA can compete with one another for available viral polymerase. Since DI RNA is shorter than 42 S RNA, in a given period of time more DI negative-strand RNA than 42 S negative-strand RNA will be made. Since the DI and standard negative-strand RNAs also have common 3' termini, competition for polymerase will again occur and, using the same length-difference argument, more DI positive-strand RNA than 42 S (or 26 S) positive-strand RNA will be synthesized. These two "competition" processes, when operating sequentially, result not only in a marked reduction in the synthesis of all standard virus RNAs compared to their DI counterparts but also in a selective propagation of DI particles over standard virions. Although it may merely be the marked difference in length between DI and standard RNA which results in the synthesis of the former at the expense of the latter, other factors such as a greater affinity of DI RNA standard virus RNA for polymerase may also play a role. For example, the secondary and/or tertiary structure of the RNAs may determine their relative rates of replication at the intiation and/or elongation stage. In any event the model not only affords an explanation for interference by and selective propagation of alphavirus DI particles but also predicts that as soon as a short DI RNA is generated it will compete for polymerase not only with standard virus RNAs but also with any longer DI RNAs present in the same cell. This prediction has recently been confirmed for SV DI RNA (Guild et al., 1977) and SFV DI RNA (Stark and Kennedy, 1978). In addition, it now seems clear that foreshortening of alphavirus DI RNA occurs by a process of sequential internal deletions (see preceding sections). A second level at which interference may occur in the alphavirus system is in nucleocapsid assembly. Since the extent of structural protein synthesis is determined by the level of 26 S RNA, interference with the synthesis of this RNA by mechanisms discussed above will reduce synthesis of structural proteins. Consequently, newly synthesized genomic 42 S RNA and positive-strand DI RNA will compete for available structural proteins, specifically, available nucleocapsid protein. To what extent this level of competition plays a role in determining the overall decrease in standard virus multiplication is not known, but if it does play a role it is likely to be a minor one.

One notable feature of the alphavirus DI system is the marked effect exerted by the host cell on the generation and replication of DI particles. This effect was first recognized by Levin et al. (1973). In a more detailed study Stark and Kennedy (1978) showed that certain types of cell—for example, the mouse 3T3 cell and the rat NRK cell—generate and enrich SFV DI particles extremely rapidly such that within three or four passages the yield of standard virus has dropped by two to three orders of magnitude, and DI particles constitute over 95% of the final progeny. By contrast, 12 passages are required to generate detectable DI particles in pig PK15 cells, and 20 passages are necessary in one line of HeLa cells. However, the deletion pathway of DI RNA is the same in all the cell types, and in almost every cell type the size and nucleotide sequence of the final DI RNA (DIssD; Fig. 4) which is generated are the same. Pig PK15 (Stark and Kennedy, 1978) cells are, however, an interesting and to date a unique exception in that they appear unable to support the final two deletion events, and the "terminal" DI particles contain DIssB (FIg. 4). The host cell, then, determines the timing of generation and even the kinetics of enrichment, i.e., the differential rate of multiplication of DI particles compared to standard virus and even the competitive ability of a larger DI RNA when a shorter one appears. However, it (the cell) plays little if any direct role in determining the primary nucleotide sequence of the DI RNAs, this property being the exclusive domain of the virus.

Alphavirus multiplication occurs not only in vertebrate but also in invertebrate cells (e.g., Stevens, 1970; Davey and Dalgarno, 1974). Early attempts to generate SV DI particles in invertebrate (mosquito) cells by high-multiplicity serial passaging failed (Igarashi and Stollar, 1976), as did attempts in those cells to replicate DI particles generated in a vertebrate cell system (Eaton, 1975; Igarashi and Stollar, 1976). Recently, we have been examining the generation of SFV DI particles in several clones derived from the original *Aedes albopictus* mosquito cell line of Singh (1967). In contrast to earlier findings both we and Logan (1979) have observed that several cell clones, all of which support the multiplication of standard SFV to levels greatly exceeding that obtained with uncloned cells, generate DI particles in the very first cycle of multiplication. furthermore, the DI RNA of these particles is indistinguishable by oligonucleotide mapping from that of particles generated in the vertebrate cells (Tooker and Kennedy, submitted). In addition, these several clones permit the multiplication of DI particles generated in vertebrate cells. Thus it now appears that at least a proportion of the cells in uncloned stocks of *A albopictus* cells are indeed capable of generating and replicating SFV DI particles and that these particles are identical to those produced in the vertebrate cell. We shall return to the question of DI particles in invertebrate cells when we consider alphavirus persistence (see next section).

In marked contrast to alphavirus DI RNA, poliovirus DI RNA is capable of acting as mRNA (Cole and Baltimore, 1973a,b). However, although coding for polymerase, poliovirus DI RNA does not contain a functional set of capsid genes, and consequently no progeny particles are produced in cells infected with DI particles alone. In coinfected cells standard RNA and DI RNA appear to be replicated independently of one another, each with its own RI RNAs. Moreover, and again unlike the alphavirus system, the total level of viral RNA synthesis in cells coinfected with standard and DI poliovirus is essentially the same as in cells infected with standard virus alone. Since infected cells are limited to the extent of total viral RNA synthesis which they can support, the replication of standard virus RNA in coinfected cells in decreased by a percentage which is close to the percentage of DI particles in the inoculum. Synthesis of procapsid is reduced by a similar amount. Furthermore, DI and standard RNA compete for available procapsid in the assembly of progeny particles. These two levels of interference are independent of one another and multiply together so that the percentage of standard virus produced in co-infected cells is the square of the percentage of standard virus in the inoculum. The enrichment of poliovirus DI particles is about 6% per multiplication cycle (Cole and Baltimore, 1973c). This value is small compared to that of the alphaviruses, where, depending to an extent on the host cell, enrichment is between 20% and 80% per multiplication cycle. Presently, it is unclear at the molecular level how poliovirus DI enrichment occurs, but pulses of inhibition of protein synthesis during virus multiplication in coinfected cells have suggested that enrichment occurs early—perhaps during the first cycles of RNA synthesis (Baltimore *et al.*, 1974).

3.2.2. DI-Particle Generation

The molecular mechanism of genesis of poliovirus and alphavirus DI particles, like that of all other DI systems, is obscure. One of the simplest hypotheses is that, having initiated RNA synthesis, the polymerase detaches from its template and rejoins it downstream near the 5' end. Alternatively, if splicing occurs at either the nascent or post-transcriptive level, then a mistake in this process could generate a DI RNA. At this time, however, there is no evidence that splicing occurs in the normal fashioning of either picornavirus or alphavirus RNAs. It is also unclear whether deletion occurs during the synthesis of positive-strand RNA or negative-strand RNA. However, it is clear that the host cell can greatly influence the genesis of DI RNA. For example, in 3T3 cells, SFV particles are generated within two passages. Yet with one line of HeLa cells DI particles were not apparent even after 200 passages (Stark and Kennedy, 1978). This phenomenon is not due to differences in the ability of the two cell lines to support the multiplication of DI particles (or standard virus). Perhaps some feature of the cytoplasmic architecture of the RNA-synthesizing apparatus or some host-coded component of the polymerase plays a role in determining DI-particle genesis.

Two other aspects of DI-particle genesis are worthy of consideration. First, it is not clear if the several discrete sizes of DI RNA seen
during serial passaging of the alphaviruses constitute the only species of
DI RNA capable of being generated. It is possible that a larger
spectrum of DI RNAs can be generated but because of size and/or
sequence constraints (for example, during packaging) only a few
discrete sizes survive to be extensively amplified during successive
cycles of virus multiplication. Second, one can ask if in DI RNA any
microsequence heterogeneity exists around the junction region between
conserved parts of the progenitor. Recently an answer to this question
has been obtained for poliovirus DI RNA. Using RNA-RNA duplex
mapping, a number of hybrid molecules formed between poliovirus DI
RNA and standard negative-strand RNA were examined. These studies
showed that both the extent and position of the deletion in DI RNA
was somewhat variable (Nomoto *et al.*, 1978). This in turn indicates
that deletion may not involve recognition of a specific sequence of only
a few nucleotides but rather a region delimiting some feature of secondary structure, for example, a hairpin loop.

4. ROLE OF DI PARTICLES IN LONG-TERM VIRAL PERSISTENCE

4.1. Negative-Strand Viruses

4.1.1. Persistent Infections by Enveloped RNA Viruses Other Than Rhabdoviruses

Persistent infections have been established with many different
virus groups (Walker, 1964; Rima and Martin, 1977), and several
hypotheses have been advanced to account for this persistence. These
include reverse transcription and integration of the viral genome into
the host-cell DNA (Zhdanov, 1975; Simpson and Iinuma, 1975),
temperature sensitivity of the virus (Preble and Youngner, 1975), and
the presence of DI particles (Huang and Baltimore, 1970). This chapter
will limit itself to the involvement of DI particles in persistent infection.
(See Chapter 2 for a review of the role of temperature sensitive mutants.)
Relatively few persistent infections have been closely examined for
the presence of DI particles. However, there are a number of cases
where the investigators have not studied DI particles directly, but
report evidence that may suggest their presence. Several criteria for
their possible involvement are (1) all or at least a large majority of the

cells in the carrier culture contain viral antigen; (2) carrier cultures are resistant to challenge by homologous virus but support normal replication of heterologous virus; and (3) the virus shed by the carrier culture shows highly reduced infectivity to particle ratio and shows strong interference with infectious virus. Studies which suggest the possible presence of DI particles by more than one of the above criteria include persistent infections by lymphocytic choriomeningitis (LCM) virus (Trowbridge and Pfau, 1970; Lehmann-Grube *et al.*, 1969; Staneck *et al.*, 1972), measles virus (Wild and Dugre, 1978), and Sendai virus (Kimura *et al.*, 1975; Nishiyama *et al.*, 1976). Stronger evidence for the involvement of DI particles in persistent infection is provided by the following studies where the investigators have characterized the persistently infected cultures with regard to the presence of DI particles.

4.1.1a.   Arenaviruses

Persistent infection of L cells by LCM virus has been established (Welsh and Pfau, 1972) and has been shown to produce little if any infectious virus after 50–60 cell divisions, although virtually all the cells contain viral antigen by immunofluorescence. These persistently infected cultures contain a component that specifically interferes with LCM virus plaque formation. The interfering component further characterized by Welsh *et al.* (1972) closely resembles DI particles. This component does not replicate in the absence of standard virus, and it appears to contain the same viral proteins since LCM immune serum reduces the interfering activity. It is also more resistant to UV inactivation than standard virus, suggesting that it may contain a subgenomic portion of the standard virus RNA.

Persistent infection of BHK cells by LCM virus was examined by Stanwick and Kirk (1976). After 21 passages of the persistently infected cells, infectious virus could no longer be detected by inoculation into mice. However, 90% of the cells showed presence of viral antigen, and the cultures continued to produce LCM virus particles which protected mice from subsequent intracranial challenge by infectious LCM virus. These interfering particles have not been further characterized but may well be defective. Staneck and Pfau (1974) have reported that a persistent infection established in BHK cells by another arenavirus, Parana virus, also shares many of the properties of other DI-particle-mediated systems, including resistance to homologus but not heterologous superinfection and the shedding of an interfering component which has a smaller target to UV inactivation than the infectious virus.

Recently, Welsh and Oldstone (1977) have characterized L cells persistently infected with LCM virus and showed that early after acute infection LCM antigens were expressed at the cell surface; these cells were efficiently lysed by complement plus antibody and by LCM-immune T cells. After several days, however, strongly interfering DI arose and cell surface expression of viral antigens greatly decreased so that immune T cells were less effective in causing lysis and antibody plus complement was ineffective. However, nearly all cells showed high intracellular levels of virus antigen and continued to do so throughout ensuing weeks of persistent infection despite a continuing suppression of viral surface antigen expression. The authors concluded that DI particles caused reduced surface antigen expression which may allow cells to escape immune surveillance during persistent infection. They found no evidence for *ts* mutants in LCM persistence.

4.1.1b. Paramyxoviruses

Rima *et al.* (1977) established persistent infections of Vero cells by the Edmonston strain of measles virus. Persistent infection was readily obtained only with inocula which has been passaged serially without dilution. They showed that the infectivity-to-hemagglutinin ratio decreases in the undiluted passage stocks and that the interfering ability increases. The interfering activity was sensitive to UV inactivation and was sedimentable by ultracentrifugation. No accumulation of *ts* mutations could be demonstrated in undiluted passage stocks. When a sixth undiluted passage capable of establishing persistent infection was passed twice at limiting dilution or plaque purified, it lost the ability to establish persistent infection. Such undiluted passages of measles virus have been shown to cause an accumulation of defective interfering particles containing an encapsidated RNA smaller than the 52 S RNA contained in the infectious particle (Hall *et al.*, 1974). Similarly, after infection of Vero cells with undiluted-passage measles virus, Kiley *et al.* (1974) have demonstrated the presence of intracellular viral nucleocapsids of small size (110 S) along with the full size nucleocapsid (200 S). 200 S nucleocapsids alone were detected in cells infected with the original plaque-purified virus.

Holland *et al.* (1976c) have also reported establishing a persistent infection of HeLa cells with undiluted passages of measles virus. In the same way they have established persistent infections of BHK cells with mumps and influenza virus. In contrast, the original viral stocks were highly cytopathic and led to the destruction of the infected monolayers.

However, infection by the virus from fifth undiluted passages led to survival of these cultures, and these became carrier cultures which survived for months. In view of the recent characterization of influenza DI particles by Nayak *et al.* (1978), it seems likely that the DI particles of influenza virus play a role in persistent infection similar to that which has been described for other systems. Nayak *et al.* (1978) and Nakajima *et al.* (1978) observed very small RNA species in influenza DI-particle preparations. These apparently represent genome deletion mutants for various genome segments.

Persistent infection of BHK cells by Sendai virus has recently been established by mixed infection of standard and DI virus stocks (Roux and Holland, 1979). As in all the persistent infections discussed so far, the majority of the cells contained viral antigen and were resistant to superinfection by homologous but not heterologous virus. Characterization of intracellular nucleocapsids showed the continual synthesis of two size classes of viral nucleocapsid RNA: a genome-size 50 S RNA and a smaller size class. When persistent infection was established by infecting the cells with a stock of standard virus alone and selecting for the few surviving cells, both standard virus and DI-article-size classes of intracellular viral nucleocapsid RNA were observed. This appears to be a result of amplification of a DI particle known to be present in this standard virus stock (Kolakofsky, 1979). The contaminating DI particles were probably responsible for the survival of a few cells after standard virus infection. In both cultures Roux and Holland consistently observed a ten- to hundredfold greater amount of the smaller size class RNA compared to 50 S RNA after 24-hr labeling. On day-to-day analysis no overall change in the ratio of DI to standard RNA synthesis could be observed (Roux and Holland, 1980). However, the composition of the DI size class of RNA varied constantly: some species of DI RNA disappeared and others appeared with continued passage of the persistently infected cells. No selection toward a particular size class RNA was observed during the 12-month period of analysis. Interestingly, challenge infection of these carriers with standard virus either caused no change in nucleocapsid RNA ratios or stimulated synthesis of more molecules of DI RNA than of standard virus RNA.

4.1.2. Persistent Infection by Rhabdoviruses

Wagner *et al.* (1963) were the first to establish persistent rhabdovirus infections with VSV in cultured L cells, and they showed clearly that small-plaque mutants were greatly favored in their ability to establish persistence. Holland and Villarreal (1974) showed the DI particles were essential for establishment of persistent infection, along with *ts* mutant infectious virus of VSV. These persistently infected carrier cells continuously shed low levels of infectious virus and DI particles. DI particles recovered from these carrier cells were able to reestablish persistent infection of BHK21 cells when coinfected with either wild-type or *ts* mutant infectious virus, whereas the "wild-type DI particle" originally employed could help establish persistence only with the group III (matrix protein) mutant *ts* G31. This original BHK21-VSV Indiana carrier (abbreviated herafter as CAR4) has now been maintained for over 6 years as a persistently infected carrier culture and has been extensively characterized. It has shed only low levels of mature virus and DI particles even though all or nearly all cells are continuously infected, grow at near-normal rates, and exhibit large amounts of virus antigen in the cytoplasm. Large amounts of biologically active DI RNP can be recovered from the cytoplasm of disrupted cells, and these will reinitiate persistent infection when coinfecting with infectious virus. Shed virus is temperature sensitive, and all isolates are very slow growing small-plaque mutants at any temperature. However, these cannot reinitiate persistent infection of BHK21 cells at any multiplicity without addition of DI particles to attenuate cytopathic effects. It appears that intracellular DI nucleocapsids suppress viral RNA synthesis to such low levels at any temperature that cells maintain nearly normal cell synthesis and growth (Villarreal and Holland, 1976). No evidence for a role of interferon or for integrated DNA copies of viral RNA could be obtained.

Another rhabdovirus, rabies virus, is notably different from VSV in causing generally less cytopathology in cultured cells and in the relative ease with which it establishes persistent infections *in vitro* (Fernandes *et al.*, 1964). Wiktor and Clark (1972) characterized hamster cells and other cells chronically infected with rabies virus and observed cyclic variations in titers of infectious virus shed by carrier cultures. They concluded that interferon might be regulating these fluctuations in yield. Kawai *et al.* (1975) established BHK21 rabies virus carrier cultures and showed that the cyclic variations in virus yield correlated with cyclic patterns of rising and falling levels of rabies virus DI particles. These cyclical patterns of virus and DI-particle production were strikingly similar to the cyclic rising and falling of VSV virus and DI particle production which occurs when fresh uninfected cells are added regularly to cultures infected with VSV (Palma and Huang, 1974). Furthermore, no interferon could be detected or induced in the persistently infected BHK21 cells of Kawai *et al.* (1975), and these carrier cells were resistant to homologous rabies virus challenge but fully susceptible to heterologous challenge by VSV. Small-plaque, slightly *ts* mutants arose in these carrier cultures and eventually displaced wild-type infectious virus. These cloned small-plaque mutant viruses caused greater cytopathology than wild-type virus and could not by themselves induce persistent infection. These small-plaque mutants generate both interfering and noninterfering defective particles (Kawai and Matsumoto, 1977). Strangely, the rabies small-plaque mutants were resistant to homologous interference caused by the DI particles generated by large-plaque, wild-type HEP rabies virus. However, the DI particles which they generated interfered with both large-plaque wild-type HEP Flury rabies virus and with the small-plaque mutant virus which generated them. Obviously, this specificity of DI interference could play a role in selection of virus mutants surviving during persistence. In much less thorough studies of rabies persistence, Holland *et al.* (1976c) have also implicated DI-particle involvement, and greatly reduced levels of rabies virus directed RNA synthesis (Villarreal and Holland, 1976).

The most extensively studied carrier system is that of VSV in BHK21 cells (Holland and Villarreal, 1974; Holland *et al.*, 1976c, 1978). Studies of this persistently infected culture over a period of 5 years have shown that DI particles and their nucleocapsids play a critical role in the establishment and the maintenance of long-term persistence. In sharp contrast to this system where the role of DI particles is clear, a variety of L-cell–VSV carriers have been described where other factors (including or excluding the presence of DI particles) are implicated. The L-cell–VSV carrier cells of Youngner *et al.* (1976) appear not to involve DI particles but strongly involve viral mutation to temperature sensitivity (see also the chapter by Youngner and Preble in this volume). Ramseur and Friedman (1977) also implicated *ts* mutants and showed a role of interferon in establishing persistence in L cells and perhaps in maintaining it. They also showed that high levels of anti-IF could terminate this chronic infection. Nishiyama (1977) implicated *ts* small-plaque mutants, DI particles, and interferon as being involved in his L cells persistently infected with VSV. He also found that only 5–30% of cells showed viral antigens, and he showed that treatment with antiviral antibody led to curing of the carrier cells. As with the carrier cells of Ramseur and Friedman (1977), the involvement of interferon was reflected in the ability of these cells to resist heterologous challenge by Mengo virus or EMC virus (as well as resistance to homologous VSV challenge). Stanners *et al.* (1977) have reported that a *ts* mutant (T1026) of VSV able to establish persistence in cells is a double mutant affecting RNA polymerase activity and shutoff of protein synthesis. Finally, Nishiyama *et al.* (1978) have characterized *ts* small-plaque mutants recovered from persistently infected L cells and showed that these were better inducers of interferon than wild-type VSV, and they are also more sensitive to the action of exogenous interferon and can initiate persistence without added interferon when infecting L cells at low multiplicity of infection. Holland *et al.* (1976*b,c*) observed high levels of DI particles produced by L cells persistently infected by VSV plus DI particles, but these never gave long-term persistence and despite numerous attempts these carriers spontaneously cured within several weeks or several months as was observed by Ramseur and Friedman (1977).

Clearly, L-cell VSV carriers can involve a number of factors; DI particles may be involved in some of these persistent infections and not in others. This is in sharp contrast to the BHK21-VSV and BHK21-rabies carriers described above in which DI particles play an essential and continuing role. Recently, we reported a HeLa cell line which replicates VSV DI particles very poorly at times or not at all at other times (Holland *et al.*, 1976*a*). We have utilized this HeLa cell line in an attempt to analyze VSV persistence in the absence of DI particles. One persistently infected VSV carrier culture established with these HeLa cells shed DI particles (apparently due to selection of DI-particle-producing cells) (Holland *et al.*, 1976*a*). Another VSV-HeLa cell carrier designated CAR49 (Holland *et al.*, 1978) shed VSV for nearly 1 year until it cured spontaneously. At no time did this carrier shed detectable DI particles. This allowed critical comparison of this type of culture with the DI-particle-producing type. Table 1 compares and contrasts what is known about the DI-particle-producing rhabdovirus-persistent infections (e.g., BHK21-VSV or BHK21-rabies) with those which do not (or need not) involve DI particles (e.g., HeLa-VSV-CAR49 and L-Cell–VSV carriers).

It can be seen in Table 1 that there are many distinguishing characteristics between the type of persistent infection involving DI particles and those not involving DI particles. The most striking difference lies in the fact that all or nearly all cells are infected at all times in the DI-particle-producing carrier cells, whereas only a small percentage of cells are usually infected and exhibiting virus antigen in the DI-particle-negative carrier cells. The ease with which these latter carriers are cured by antibody treatment suggests that these carrier cultures lacking DI particles are persistently infected only at the popula-

TABLE 1

General Characteristics of Persistently Infected Vertebrate Cells in Which DI Particles Are Involved as Compared to Those Lacking (Or Not Requiring) DI Involvement[a]

Characteristic examined	Carriers with DI involvement (VSV-BHK and rabies-BHK)	Carriers lacking or not requiring DI (L-cell-VSV or HeLa-VSV-Car49)
Percentage of cells showing virus antigen	Always ~100%	Low (<0.1% to 20–30%)
Duration of persistence	Indefinite [many years] (very stable persistence at the individual cell level)	Usually short term—tend to "cure"[b] or to be destroyed by severe crises (unstable persistent state maintained at the population level)
Effect of antiviral antibody	No effect on confluent cell monolayers; antibody "cures" only very light monolayer with well isolated cells[b]	Antibody "cures" confluent cell monolayers as well as isolated cells[b]
Response to virus challenge	Resistant to homologous challenge; fully sensitive to heterologous challenge virus	Not resistant to homologous or heterologous challenge (HeLa-VSV-CAR49) or resistant to both because of interferon presence
Interferon involvement	Never detected	Often present
DI nucleocapsid accumulation in cytoplasm	Large amounts	Not present or not required
Frequency and severity of crises of cytopathology	Infrequent, usually not pronounced	Frequent and often involve large percentage of cells
Selection and replacement of input virus by ts and small-plaque mutants during persistence	Yes	Yes
Cloned ts, small-plaque mutants able to induce persistent infection without DI or interferon	No	Yes

[a] This table is based on data presented in Holland et al (1976c, 1978, Youngner et al. (1976), Ramseur and Friedman (1977), Nishiyama (1977), Nishiyama et al. (1978), Kawai et al. (1975), and Kawai and Matsumoto (1977).

[b] The term "cure" refers to carrier cultures which no longer shed infectious virus even after cocultivation, which are no longer expressing virus antigen detectably, which show no resistance to challenge infection, and which lack viral nucleic acid by annealing.

tion level so that immune isolation of cells from each other leads to rapid curing. In contrast, the buildup of interfering DI nucleocapsids in the cytoplasm of cells of the DI-particle-mediated carrier state (Holland *et al.*, 1976c; Roux and Holland, 1979) can allow slow noncytocidal replication of virus within cells for months or years in the presence of antiviral antibody (Holland *et al.*, 1976c) and even within carrier cells transplanted into nude mice for months or years (Reid *et al.*, 1979, and see below).

In vivo cell surface antigenic modulation by antibody as well as by DI particles may be required to prevent lysis of persistently infected cells by antibody plus complement or by immunocytes (Joseph and Oldstone, 1975). Whether persistent infections of the non-DI-particle-producing type can survive for months or years *in vivo* in intact animals remains to be established. Perhaps this type might be maintained better in cases where there is extreme immunological deficit (whether virus antigen specific or nonspecific). However, it is well established that persistent RNA virus disease can occur in the absence of general or virus antigen-specific immunodeficiency (Welsh and Oldstone, 1977; Perrin *et al.*, 1977).

The distinguishing characteristics delineating DI-particle-positive and DI-particle-negative persistent infections (listed in Table 1) may prove generally useful as an indicator of the factors involved in any particular *in vitro* persistent infection by enveloped RNA viruses. Determination of such parameters *in vivo* will be much more difficult. Note in Table 1 that both types of carrier culture share one very important common characteristic: in both types of persistence there is strong selection of *ts* and small-plaque mutants. Slow-growing small-plaque mutants nearly always appear even when the mutant virus is not *ts* (or is only slightly *ts*). These mutants are often lower in polymerase activity and more sensitive to interferon and induce interferon more efficiently (see above). All of these phenotypic characteristics of mutant virus from persistent infection could be explained by a single unifying hypothesis: namely, that multiple mutations occur in the genome of viruses during persistence. This hypothesis has been confirmed by T_1 ribonuclease oligonucleotide mapping of VSV infectious virus recovered from BHK21-CAR4 carrier cells persistently infected for more than 5 years (Holland *et al.*, 1978, 1979). Beginning within 1 year and continuing thereafter beyond 5 years, the original cloned input virus has undergone massive and continuing genome rearrangement which probably represents dozens or even hundreds of mutations. Figure 5 shows the T_1 RNAse oligonucleotide differences between the original

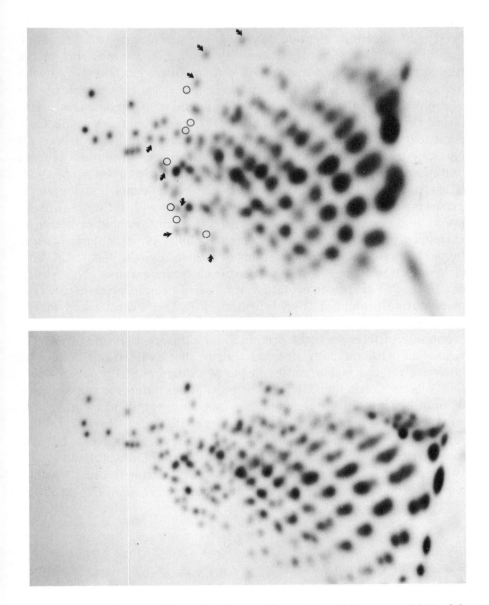

Fig. 5. Ribonuclease T1 oligonucleotide map. Comparison of the genome RNA of the original clone of vesicular stomatitis virus used to establish persistent infection of BHK21 cells (bottom panel) with the genome RNA of a clone of small-plaque *ts* mutant recovered from the BHK21-VSV-Ind-CAR4 carrier cells after 5 years of persistent infection at 37°C (top panel). The arrows indicate new oligonucleotides which have appeared and the circles indicate where oligonucleotide spots have disappeared during 5 years of persistent infection.

virus and the small-plaque *ts* mutants recovered after 5 years of persistent infection. Peptide mapping studies in progress (Holland, unpublished) also show significant alterations in the proteins of the recovered small-plaque mutants. These small-plaque, slowly growing mutants do not readily undergo reversion either phenotypically or genotypically (Holland *et al.*, 1979). While the virus genome is accumulating these massive mutations, the DI population recoverable from persistently infected cells is constantly changing, with newly arising DI particles replacing previous DI particles. Since numerous genome mutations do not accumulate on repeated lytic passage of VSV (Clewley *et al.*, 1977; Holland *et al.*, 1979), it appears that long-term persistent infection selects for massive mutation within the virus population, and persistence may well be important in the rapid evolution of enveloped RNA virus genomes. This possibility is particularly intriguing with regard to antigenic variants of influenza virus. Persistent Visna virus infection is known to give rise to antigenic variants (Narayan *et al.*, 1977). A less drastic evolution of measles virus M protein may take place during prolonged CNS infection in SSPE (Wechsler and Fields, 1978; Hall *et al.*, 1978). However, Hall *et al.* (1979) found electrophoretic differences in M protein among different strains of measles virus, but with no pattern characteristic of SSPE strains. They did observe a relative lack of antibodies to M protein in SSPE patients.

Whether changing DI particle populations influence the selection of multiply mutant virus genomes is not clear (Holland *et al.*, 1979), but the DI specificity observed for rabies mutants by Kawai and Matsumoto (1977) is suggestive in this regard. However, in HeLa-cell DI-free carriers of VSV, multiple mutations accumulate (Holland *et al.*, 1979), and at least some mutations must be occurring in other non-DI-particle-producing carrier states (e.g., Youngner *et al.*, 1976; Mudd *et al.*, 1973).

4.2. Positive-Strand Viruses

Togaviruses, picornaviruses, and reoviruses are usually cytocidal for vertebrate cells in tissue culture. Persistently infected cultures are therefore often difficult to establish; we are aware of only a single report of a picornavirus persistent infection in cell culture (Crowell and Syverton, 1961). In contrast, there is accumulating evidence of picornavirus persistent infection in human patients suffering from agammaglobulinemia (Wilfert *et al.*, 1977); the picornavirus system is therefore worthy of further study. For the alphaviruses, both Western encephalitis virus and SV have been established in a persistent state in L cells (Chambers, 1957; Inglot *et al.*, 1973). Persistent infection of BHK cells with SV (Weiss, *et al.*, 1980) and SFV has also been initiated. Persistent infection of rabbit kidney cells with Japanese encephalitis virus has been reported (Schmaljohn and Blair, 1977). Alphaviruses (and flaviviruses) readily establish persistent infections in cultured invertebrate cells (Rahacek, 1968; Peleg, 1969; Stollar and Shenk, 1973). These systems are of considerable interest because of the natural transmission cycle of togaviruses from vertebrates through insects and back to vertebrates. L cells, CHO cells, and Vero cells have been employed to study reovirus persistence in culture (Taber *et al.*, 1976; Ahmed and Graham, 1977). Reovirus has also been employed to study persistence in small rodents (Graham, 1977).

At the present time the evidence for the involvement of DI particles in togavirus persistent infection in vertebrate cells in cultures is accumulating. Inglot *et al.* (1973) suggested that DI particles of SV may play a role in persistent L-cell infection. These authors also pointed to the involvement of interferon in this system. Recent data also indicate that, for SFV, interferon plays a major role in maintaining the persistent state in L cells and that DI particles are not involved in maintenance, although they do greatly facilitate the establishment of the carrier state (Meinkoth and Kennedy, 1979). In BHK cells on the other hand, DI particles are indispensible in establishing persistence, and at all times examined (over 3 years) the carrier culture contains substantial amounts of DI particles. Interferon appears to play little or no role in this system. Persistence in cultures of rabbit kidney cells and Vero cells could readily be established by the flavivirus Japanese encephalitis virus (Schmaljohn and Blair, 1977). In this study only serial undiluted passage fluid could establish the persistent infection in the rabbit cells, and culture fluid from these cells was used to establish the carrier state in Vero cells. The virus produced from the rabbit cells was tentatively identified as containing DI particles. Although these observations are indicative of a role for DI particles in both the establishment and the maintenance of the carrier state, final proof awaits additional experimentation.

Considerable effort has been invested in evaluating the role of DI particles in alphavirus persistence in invertebrate cells, notably in the *Aedes albopictus* cell line. In contrast to the vertebrate cell, persistent infection in the mosquito cell can readily be established with standard virus alone (Stollar and Shenk, 1973; Davey and Dalgarno, 1974; Igarashi *et al.*, 1977; Eaton, 1977). In these studies infection resulted in rapid multiplication of virus followed after about 4–6 days by a decline in virus yield which lasted several weeks and which culminated in a plateau level of virus production. This level remained constant for as long as the cultures were maintained. Although suggested by earlier studies (Stollar and Shenk, 1973), it has only recently become clear that persistently infected mosquito cells produce DI particles. Igarashi *et al.* (1977) presented evidence that double-stranded RNA characteristic of replicative form derived from DI RI RNA (see preceding section) was formed in SV persistently infected mosquito cells by 10 weeks after infection. Eaton (1977) showed that the pattern of RNA synthesis in BHK cells infected with culture fluid from SV persistently infected mosquito cells was characteristic of infection with stocks containing DI particles and concluded that the persistently infected cells were releasing DI particles into the extracellular medium. Thus there is now evidence that cultured mosquito cells can produce DI particles. It is premature at this time, however, to implicate DI particles in any essential role in maintaining the carrier state.

The studies of Ahmed and Graham (1977) have pointed to the importance of DI particles in persistent reovirus infection in L cells and Vero cells. Passages of reovirus rich in DI particles which were extensively deleted in the L_1, L_3, and M_1 segments of the genome (see earlier) could readily initiiate persistence. The greater the proportion of DI particles in the inoculum, the greater was the capacity of the virus stock to initiate persistence. By contrast, DI-particle-free stocks were unable to initate persistence, and the infected cultures perished. About 80% of the cells in the persistent state continuously produced virus, and in this system frequent crises were observed. Analysis of the carrier cultures during the first 18 passages showed that defective particles were always present. However, the status of these particles as true interfering DI particles was not demonstrated; therefore, the role of DI interference in maintaining the carrier state was and indeed remains unclear. One additional feature of these studies was that, although persistence was established using a *ts* mutant of the standard virus, the phenotype of the standard virus isolated from the carrier culture was that of wild type. This situation is in contrast to many other virus-carrier states where evolution of *ts* mutants occurs (e.g., Preble and Youngner, 1975; Younger *et al.*, 1976; Youngner and Quagliana, 1975). Thus for reovirus there is compelling evidence for a role for DI-like particles in establishing persistence *in vitro* (and also *in vivo*—see below). The role of DI virus in maintaining the carrier state is less clear.

4.3. *In Vivo* Evidence for DI-Particle Protection

Since DI particles are able to interfere with the growth of standard virus in cell culture, their ability to affect the outcome of infection in animals is of particular interest. DI particles clearly can be generated and replicated *in vivo*. The first characterization of DI particles was carried out "*in vivo*" with influenza in eggs (von Magnus, 1951). Sendai virus (Kingsbury *et al.*, 1970) also was shown to generate large quantities of DI particles in eggs. However, the chorioallantoic membrane of embryonated eggs, where most virus replicates, in many respects more closely resembles a cell culture monolayer than a whole animal. However, recent studies demonstrate that DI particles can also be generated *in vivo* in animals. VSV generates DI particles more readily in baby mice than in adults (Holland and Villarreal, 1975). DI particles have also been found to be generated intracerebrally by rabies virus in baby mice (Holland and Villarreal, 1975), by Rift Valley fever virus in mice (Mims, 1956), and by LCM virus in mice (Popescu and Lehmann-Grube, 1977).

To determine whether interference by DI particles could prevent viral disease, von Magnus (1954) attempted to protect mice against challenge with influenza virus by use of a high-passage virus stock containing large numbers of DI particles; he obtained fewer deaths and reduced virus multiplication compared to controls. Similar experiments by Holland and Doyle (1973) with influenza virus and VSV showed an inhibition of virus multiplication but no significant protection. However, subsequent work with VSV indicated that these early failures were probably due to contaminating infectious virions in the DI particle preparation and probably also to DI particles in the standard virus preparation. In more careful studies in which large numbers of highly purified VSV DI particles (completely freed of infectious virus) were injected into mice along with a low but otherwise lethal challenge dose of standard virus, the purified DI particles provided complete prophylaxis (Doyle and Holland, 1973). As the dosage of challenge virus was increased, fewer mice survived. However, those that died succumbed after a lengthened course of disease and exhibited a different syndrome as compared to control animals. Crick and Brown (1977) in a follow-up study concluded that the protective effect of DI might be due to the immunizing capacity of inactivated DI since chemically inactivated infectious virus provides good immunization when given 2 days before the challenge. Also, they observed some homologous and heterologous prophylactic effect when inactivated DI particles were injected simultaneously with challenge virus. These effects were quantitated as shifts in LD_{50} (i.e., by summing results at different challenge doses and averaging results).

Recently, Jones and Holland (1980) have examined this approach using UV-inactivated DI particles (and UV-inactivated standard virus as control). In these experiments they employed low challenge virus dosages given simultaneously with, or 3 days subsequent to, DI-particle administration. No prophylactic protection from death was obtained with any UV-inactivated standard virus or UV-inactivated DI particle, whereas noninactivated DI particles gave strong prophylactic protection. However, in agreement with the data of Crick and Brown (1977) on nonspecific protection, it was observed that UV-inactivated snap-back DI particles (i.e., those containing covalently linked plus and minus RNA) did prolong the life of animals challenged simultaneously with standard virus (but failed to protect them from death). However, UV-inactivated non-snap-back DI particles gave no effect when administered simultaneously with challenge. These effects may be attributable to interferon induction. A similar induction of interferon by the DI particles employed by Crick and Brown could explain the slight nonspecific protection they observed since "snap-back DI particles" are rather common (Perrault and Leavitt, 1977a) and since they are known to be powerful inducers of interferon (Marcus and Sekellick, 1977). We conclude that prophylactic protection of mice by VSV DI particles requires replicating and interfering ability and is due to true homologous interference. Additional factors such as interferon induction and antigenic immunization may also play a role in protection. Dimmock and Kennedy (1978) reached similar conclusions for DI protection against SFV. They observed that the DI particles must be inoculated into mice slightly before or concurrently with the challenge virus to obtain prophylactic protection. As with VSV, DI particles provided protection from a normally fatal dosage of SFV; however, in this system there was no alteration of the disease syndrome in the presence of DI particles. Another system in which DI particles were shown to provide protection is the infection of 2-day-old rats with reovirus (Spandidos and Graham, 1976). Additionally, in this system a very high percentage of the surviving animals was affected by a severe runting syndrome; these animals chronically shed virus and DI particles. In addition to their ability to prevent disease or to alter its course, DI particles may be involved in altering virus–cell interactions with the immune system as cited above. Welsh and Oldstone (1977) and Huang et al. (1978) have also shown reduced virus antigen expression on the surface of infected cells coinfected with DI; this results in reduced susceptibility to immune attack.

Rabies DI particles were shown by Wiktor *et al.* (1977) to have some protective effect against intracerebrally inoculated (but not against peripherally inoculated) challenge virus. However, Wunner and Clark (1978) were unable to ascribe a protective role to rabies DI particles in comparisons of virus stocks containing DI particles when these were titrated intracerebrally in mice. Obviously, more work is needed to determine whether DI particles are protective in rabies virus infections.

As one would expect, the large dosages of DI particles necessary to give protection are immunogenic (Doyle and Holland, 1973), and a protective immune response was seen after 3 or more days even with inactivated DI particles which are capable of protection against concomitant challenge. Large numbers of DI particles were necessary for prophylaxis with VSV, SFV, and reovirus. Minimum effective numbers of VSV DI particles were at least 10^8 per mouse, while 10^7 generally were necessary for SFV and reovirus. Since the lethal dose of standard virus in these systems can probably be produced by the yield from one infected cell, effective prophylaxis requires that DI particles must coinfect every cell initially infected by standard virus. This could explain the dependence on large numbers of DI particles.

Finally, Faulkner *et al.* (1979) have employed dissociated neuron cultures from mice to study the neuronal role of VSV DI particles. Standard virus alone replicated to high levels selectively in neuronal (as compared to nonneuronal CNS cells) and caused cell death within 1–2 days. Coinfection with large amounts of DI particles completely suppressed virus replication and greatly delayed neuronal cell death. This is strong evidence that true DI-particle interference can take place in CNS neurons.

4.4. *In Vivo* Evidence for DI-Particle Persistence

When LCM virus was studied *in vivo* in mice using a sensitive interference focus assay for DI particles, DI particles were found in the organs of both acutely infected adults and in carrier mice which were infected neonatally (Popescu and Lehmann-Grube, 1977). The ratio of DI particles to infectious virions differed in various organs; these ratios declined with time in the carrier mice. These observations *in vivo* appear to correlate with the variation in the ability of different cell culture lines to support DI particle replication and with the relative ease of generating VSV DI particles in baby mice vs. adult mice. Welsh and Oldstone (1977) have recently provided evidence that peritoneal macrophages of LCM carrier mice contain DI particles, and Welsh *et al.* (1977) have recently demonstrated that DI particles of LCM virus can provide strong protection against cerebellar LCM disease and LCM virus antigen expression in baby rats coinfected with LCM virus homologous DI particles. Coupled with the finding of LCM virus DI particles in many tissues of persistenty infected mice (Popescu and Lehmann-Grube, 1977), these results suggest a likely involvement of DI particles in acute and persistent LCM virus infections *in vivo*.

DI particles also play an important role in persistent infections of newborn rats with reovirus (Spandidos and Graham, 1976; Graham, 1977). When infected intracerebrally with DI-particle-free stocks, all the rats died within 12–14 days. However, when the inoculum contained DI particles, over 60% of the rats survived and developed the usual runting syndrome of a chronic infection. Defective virus (not shown to be interfering) was detected in the brain of a runted rat 24–30 days after infection. It has also been shown *in vivo* that the tumorigenicity of established cultured tumor cell lines is strikingly abrogated by persistent infection with enveloped RNA viruses (Yamada and Hatano, 1972; Reid *et al.* 1979). This suppression of tumorigenicity of BHK 21 cells by DI-particle-mediated persistent VSV infection in nude mice is due to natural killer lymphocytes (Minato *et al.*, 1979). These natural killer cells are not only capable of killing the persistently infected cells with greater efficiency than they kill uninfected cells but also appear to be more efficiently induced by infected cells. These natural killer cells are strongly activated by interferon. This induction of interferon could in turn be due to the snap-back class of DI particles (Marcus and Sekellick, 1977). Moreover, Ito *et al.* (1975) have shown that Sendai persistently infected cells can induce interferon.

This ability to maintain persistently infected tumor cells *in vitro* offers an ideal tool for *in vivo* study of persistence. We have found that DI and virus function *in vivo* in these cells in a manner similar to *in vitro* VSV persistence (Reid *et al.*, 1979) and biologically altered virus mutants can be selected when persistently infected cells able to escape the natural killer cell response are selected (Reid *et al.*, 1979; Minato *et al.*, 1979). These nude mouse persistence models should lead to significant insight into *in vivo* parameters of persistence. Little is known about long-term *in vivo* persistence at present, although Wagner (1974) and Stanners and Goldberg (1975) showed that *ts* mutants injected into animals give an altered disease process with reduced death rate and prolonged time until death. Rabinowitz *et al.* (1976) showed that different *ts* mutants of VSV cause quite different histopathological changes and quite different degrees of virulence. Whether such infections ever lead to long-term persistence and whether DI appear during their course is not yet known.

Similarly, work with class B and C mutants of reovirus type 3 in newborn rats showed that more rats survived inoculation with either mutant type than with the wild-type virus. Also, following inoculation with the class B mutant virus, more of the surviving rats developed the runting syndrome indicative of chronic infection (Fields, 1972). It is of interest that these mutants appear to generate DI particles more readily than the wild-type virus in cell culture (Spandidos *et al.*, 1976).

5. RECENT PRELIMINARY EVIDENCE FOR DI-PARTICLE INVOLVEMENT IN PERSISTENCE OF DNA VIRUSES

In contrast to the situation with RNA viruses there has, until very recently, been almost no serious investigation of the possible role of DI particles in persistent infections by DNA viruses. This is understandable since there might appear to be no need for DI particle involvement in persistence of DNA viruses. Viral DNA integration into cell chromosomal DNA offers a simpler, more straightforward, and well-established mechanism for DNA virus persistence. Nevertheless, some DNA virus–cell systems may involve a role of DI particles in persistence if some very recent preliminary studies are confirmed and extended.

Norkin (1979) has clearly demonstrated the involvement of DI particles in one type of SV40 virus persistence in monkey cells, with considerable levels of DI particle DNA being present throughout the course of persistent infection. Henry *et al.* (1979) described conditions for efficient production of DI particles of equine herpesvirus type 1 and alluded to as yet unpublished evidence that they can play a role in establishing persistent infection by this herpesvirus. Likewise, Stinski *et al.* (1979) and Mocarski and Stinski (1979) have described the production of DI particle DNA by serial high-multiplicity passages of cytomegalovirus and cite very preliminary evidence for their involvement in establishing persistent infection and their production by persistently infected cells.

It is difficult to see why DI particles and DI genome DNA would be necessary or important in persistent infection by herpesviruses, papovaviruses, or other DNA viruses able to integrate their genomes. If they do prove to be important in some types of DNA virus persistence *in vitro*, it will be interesting to look for their presence and possible involvement in latent and recurrent herpesvirus infections of humans. Stevens (1978) has already shown that replication-defective *ts* mutants of Herpes simplex virus establish central nervous system persistent infections with high efficiency. Whether DI particles or their subgenomic DNAs also can play a role in natural infections must await sensitive quantitative assays for DI particles of these and other DNA viruses.

It may ultimately be found that integration of complete genomes suffices for persistence in some DNA virus–cell systems, whereas a constantly mutating plasmid state with DI particle interference may prove necessary for others. A smoldering plasmid state with DI cycling and selection of viable multiple mutants of standard virus might offer the same advantages for persistence of DNA viruses that it offers for RNA viruses (more frequent release of infectious virus, selection of viable mutants with ability to break through the immune response occasionally, etc.).

6. CONCLUSION

DI particles are clearly able to affect standard virus replication *in vitro* and *in vivo* in animals and are clearly involved (along with massive mutational change of the infectious virus) in at least some types of enveloped RNA virus persistence. In at least these complex types of persistence, single point mutations to temperature sensitivity cannot alone explain long-term persistence. Details of the altered interactions between the constantly changing infectious virus population with selection of massive mutational change and the constantly changing DI population remain to be clarified.

The reasons for DI particle presence in some types of vertebrate cell–virus persistence and not in other types are not clear as yet. There are some obvious correlations: (1) The most highly susceptible cells which produce the highest yields of infectious virus generally tend to generate and replicate DI particles more efficiently than do less susceptible cell types; (2) these high-virus-producing, high-DI-particle-producing cell types generally tend to produce more stable persistent infections (Holland *et al.*, 1976c, 1978) in which nearly 100% of the cells are usually involved and in which DI particles are present. In contrast, less susceptible lines which are poor DI-particle producers more often tend to initiate less stable, non-DI-particle-producing carrier states at the cell population level. In this case a low percentage of cells are infected at any given time and total destruction of the population is avoided through the antiviral effect of interferon and/or by attenuation of the virus. Spontaneous cell curing by unknown mechanisms may affect the balance between infected and uninfected cells.

Insect cells such as *Drosophila* cells in culture represent a unique case in which only very low levels of VSV can be produced (Mudd *et al.*, 1973) and in which we have consistently failed to detect even traces of DI particles. Nevertheless, every VSV infection of these cells invariably leads to long-term persistent infection. The same is true of *Aedes albopictus* cells infected with VSV (Holland, unpublished data). However, Kennedy (unpublished data) has cloned these *A. albopictus* cells and categorized clonal populations into those which are highly susceptible to SFV, those which are moderately susceptible, and those which replicate virus only to very low levels. The cloned populations producing large amounts of virus also generate and replicate large numbers of DI particles and show continuing production of virus and DI particles during long-term persistence. In contrast, uncloned *A. albopictus* cells and low-producer cloned cell populations produce no DI particles either on initial infection or during prolonged persistence. Perhaps there is a threshold level of virus production below which DI particle production cannot be initiated or maintained and below which DI-particle production is not useful for cell and tissue survival after virus infection. Indeed, it is possible to envisage a class of persistent infection in which the host cell and the infectious virus establish a symbiotic relationship without recourse to either DI-particle modulation of cellular defense. Persistent infection of invertebrates which are devoid of immunosurveillance or possibly even persistent infection of vertebrates for which immunodefense is not available may be examples of such a virus–cell relationship.

Clearly, there is a dearth of knowledge regarding biological mechanisms of DI-particle generation, DI-particle interference, and DI-particle protective effects in tissues and organs of intact animals. Although structural studies of DI RNA and viral RNA allow formulation of some reasonable hypotheses regarding DI-particle generation, replication ,and interference, these studies remain unsupported by hard experimental evidence and probably shall remain so until cell-free viral and DI-particle replication systems are developed.

Studies of the influences by DI particles on the course of virus infections in intact animals are difficult to assess for a variety of reasons. Among these are (1) the presence of at least low levels of DI particles in most standard virus stocks prior to *in vivo* inoculation, (2) difficulties in quantitating the presence of small numbers of DI particles *in vivo*, especially when a vigorous immune response limits replication of infectious virus to low levels, and (3) the need for large numbers of purified DI for *in vivo* prophylaxis (over 10^8 particles per mouse in the case of VSV). This last problem is particularly troublesome since even this rather small mass of viral antigen might stimulate the immune system and interferon, and complicate interpretation of protective effects. Smaller numbers of DI particles are probably ineffective because they would have a vanishingly low probability of coinfecting one of the few brain cells initially infected by the infectious particles of the low-input inoculum, thereby leading to foci of massive infectious virus production prior to any DI-particle involvement. Obviously, more refined experimental approaches are needed to answer most biological questions regarding DI-particle involvement in natural disease and in virus persistence, but it is already clear that they are ubiquitous and can be involved *in vivo* both in acute and in persistent infections of certain kinds.

The advent of rapid RNA sequencing, the continuing elucidation of viral defense mechanisms in the whole animal, and the prospect of cell-free viral and DI RNA replication all promise to make the next few years of research into the biology of DI particles and persistence extremely exciting.

NOTE ADDED IN PROOF

Since this review was written, a number of relevant studies have appeared, and these are briefly cited below.

DI Particle Genome Structure.   Perrault and Semler (1979, *Proc. Natl. Acad. Sci. USA* **76**:6191), Clerx-van Haaster *et al.* (1980, *J. Virol.* **33**:807), and Epstein *et al.* (1980, *J. Virol.* **33**:818) have now shown that internal deletion is involved in generation of the rare transcribing class of VSV DI particle. Perrault and Semler also confirmed that purified preparations of this transcribing class of DI particle compete very poorly with the standard class DI particles. Also, Schubert *et al.* (1979) have shown that three different DI particles of the standard class have complementary stems. One of these was 45 and the other two were 48 base pairs in length (see page 142, third paragraph, and page 154, second paragraph, for related discussion.)

Obijeski *et al.* (1980, *Nucleic Acids Res.* **8**:2431) have now shown that the two smallest RNA segments from LaCrosse virus have termini with extensive complementarity.

McClure *et al.* (1980, *Virology* **100**:408) reported a new type of DI particle of poliovirus and mengovirus with only 4–6% of the genome deleted, and no detectable density change from that of standard virus.

Rao and Huang (1979, *Proc. Natl. Acad. Sci. USA* **76**:3742) and Leppert *et al.* (1979, *Cell* **18**:735) have shown synthesis of small RNA copies of DI particle RNA 3′ termini in infected cells.

Virus and DI Particles in Persistence. Rowlands *et al.* (1980, *Cell* **19**:871) showed that all VSV proteins have altered peptide maps after 5 years of persistent infection, and the multiply mutated virus is so slow growing that it can now establish persistent infection without DI particle coinfection, although DI particles are quickly generated. Ahmed *et al.* (1980, *J. Virol.* **34**:285 and **34**:383) have shown genetic evidence for multiple mutations and the presence of extragenically suppressed *ts* lesions resulting from reovirus persistence and in high passage stocks of wild-type virus. Henry *et al.* (1980, *J. Gen. Virol.* **47**:343) have shown alterations in equine herpesvirus protein synthesis due to DI particles. Yogo *et al.* (1980, *Virology* **103**:241) have shown the presence of free BK virus defective virus DNA in a hamster tumor induced by this human papovirus. Jones *et al.* (1980, *Virology* **103**:158) have shown that the natural-killer (NK) cell response to cells persistently infected with VSV can be escaped by a number of different *viral* mutations. Horodyski and Holland (1980, *J. Virol.*, in press) have found evidence for selection of standard virus mutants by DI particles during persistent VSV infection. Finally, Reid *et al.* (1980, *Proc. Natl. Acad. Sci. USA*, submitted for publication) showed that treatment of nude mice with anti-mouse-interferon antibody prevents rejection of persistently-infected tumor cells, and these rapidly form large tumors.

ACKNOWLEDGMENTS

We thank Deborah Spector, Jacques Perrault, and David Rowlands for helpful comments and careful reading of the manuscript. The research was supported by Grants USPHS AI15087 (IK) and A114627 (JH) and NSF PCM 77-19383 (IK).

7. REFERENCES

Adachi, T., and Lazzarini, R. A., 1978, Elementary aspects of autointerference and the replication of defective interfering virus particles, *Virology* **87**:152.

Adler, R., and Banerjee, A. K., 1976, Analysis of the RNA species isolated from defective particles of vesicular stomatitis virus, *J. Gen. Virol.* **33**:51.

Ahmed, R., and Graham, A. F., 1977, Persistent infections in L cells with temperature sensitive mutants of reovirus, *J. Virol.* **23**:250.

Baltimore, D., 1971, Expression of animal virus genomes, *Bacteriol. Rev.* **35**:235.

Baltimore, D., Cole, C. N., Villa-Komaroff, L., and Spector, D., 1974, Poliovirus defective interfering particles, in: *Mechanisms of Virus Disease: ICN-UCLA Symposia on Molecular and Cellular Biology*, Vol. 1 (W. S. Robinson and C. F. Fox, eds), pp. 117–130, Academic Press, New York.

Bean, W. J., Jr., and Simpson, R. W., 1976, Transcriptase activity and genome composition of defective influenza virus, *J. Virol.* **18**:365.

Bellett, A. J. D., and Cooper, P. D., 1959, Some properties of the transmissible interfering component of vesicular stomatitis virus preparations, *J. Gen. Microbiol.* **21**:498.

Brown, F., Martin, S. J., Cartwright, B., and Crick, J., 1967, The ribonucleic acids of the infective and interfering components of vesicular stomatitis virus, *J. Gen. Virol.* **1**:479.

Bruton, C. J., and Kennedy, S. I. T., 1976, Defective interfering particles of Semliki Forest virus: Structural differences between standard virus and defective interfering particles, *J. Gen. Virol.* **31**:383.

Bruton, C. J., Porter, A., and Kennedy, S. I. T., 1976, Defective interfering particles of Semliki Forest virus: Intracellular events during interference, *J. Gen. Virol.* **31**:397.

Chambers, V. C., 1957, The prolonged persistence of western equine encephalitis in cultures of strain L cells, *Virology* **3**:62.

Choppin, P. W., 1969, Replication of influenza virus in a continuous cell line: High yield of infective virus from cells inoculated at high multiplicity, *Virology* **39**:130.

Choppin, P. W., and Pons, M. W., 1970, The RNAs of infective and incomplete influenza virus grown in MDBK and HeLa cells, *Virology* **42**:603.

Chow, J. M., Schnitzlein, W. M., and Reichmann, M. E., 1977, Expression of genetic information contained in the RNA of a defective interfering particle of vesicular stomatitis virus, *Virology* **77**:579.

Clewley, J. P., Bishop, D. H. L., Kang, C. Y., Coffin, J., Schnitzlein, W. M., Reichmann, M. E., and Shope, R. E., 1977, Oligonucleotide fingerprints of RNA species obtained from rhabdoviruses belonging to the vesicular stomatitis virus subgroup, *J. Virol.* **23**:152.

Cole, C. N., and Baltimore, D., 1973a, Defective interfering particles of poliovirus. 2. Nature of the defect, *J. Mol. Biol.* **76**:325.

Cole, C. N., and Baltimore, D., 1973b, Defective interfering particles of poliovirus. 3. Interference and enrichment, *J. Mol. Biol.* **76**:345.

Cole, C. N., and Baltimore, D., 1973c, Defective interfering particles of poliovirus. 4. Mechanisms of enrichment, *J. Virol.* **12**:1414.

Cole, C. N., Smoler, D., Wimmer, E., and Baltimore, D., 1971, Defective interfering particles of poliovirus. 1. Isolation and physical properties, *J. Virol.* **7**:478.

Colonno, R. J., and Banerjee, A. K., 1976, A unique RNA species involved in initiation of vesicular stomatitis virus RNA transcription *in vitro*, *Cell* **8**:197.

Colonno, R. J., and Banerjee, A. K., 1978, Complete nucleotide sequence of the leader RNA synthesized *in vitro* by vesicular stomatitis virus, *Cell* **15**:93.

Colonno, R. J., Lazzarini, R. A., Keene, J. D., and Banerjee, A. K., 1977, *In vitro* synthesis of messenger RNA by a defective interfering particle of vesicular stomatitis virus, *Proc. Natl. Acad. Sci. USA* **74**:1884.

Cooper, P. D., and Bellett, A. J. D., 1959, A transmissible interfering component of vesicular stomatitis virus preparations, *J. Gen. Microbiol.* **21**:485.

Crick, J., and Brown, F., 1977, *In vivo* interference in vesicular stomatitis virus infection, *Infect. Immun.* **15**:354.

Crick, J., Cartwright, B., and Brown, F., 1966, Interfering components of vesicular stomatitis virus, *Nature (London)* **211**:1204.

Crowell, R. L., and Syverton, J. T., 1961, Poliovirus persistent infection in cell culture, *J. Exp. Med.* **113**:419.

Davey, M. W., and Dalgarno, L., 1974, Semliki Forest virus replication in cultured *Aedes albopictus* cells: Studies on the establishment of persistence, *J. Gen. Virol.* **24**:453.

Dimmock, N. J., and Kennedy, S. I. T., 1978, Protection of lethally infected mice with low doses of defective-interfering Semliki Forest virus, *J. Gen. Virol.* **39**:231.

Doyle, M., and Holland, J. J., 1973, Prophylaxis and immunization in mice by use of virus-free defective T particles to protect against intracerebral infection by vesicular stomatitis virus, *Proc. Natl. Acad. Sci. USA* **70**:2105.

Duesberg, P. H., 1968, The RNAs of influence virus, *Proc. Natl. Acad. Sci. USA* **59**:930.

Eaton, B. T., 1975, Defective interfering particles of Semliki Forest virus do not interfere with viral RNA synthesis in *Aedes albopictus* cells, *Virology* **68**:534.

Eaton, B. T., 1977, Evidence for the synthesis of defective interfering particles by *Aedes albopictus* cells persistently infected with Sindbis virus, *Virology* **77**:843.

Faulkner, G., Dubois-Dalcq, M., Hoogke-Peters, E., McFarland, H. F., and Lazzarini, R. A., 1979, Defective interfering particles modulate VSV infection of dissociated neuron cultures, *Cell* **17**:979.

Fernandes, M. V., Wiktor, T. J., and Koprowski, H., 1964, Endosymbiotic relationship between animal viruses and their host cells, *J. Exp. Med.* **120**:1099.

Fields, B. N., 1972, Genetic manipulation of reovirus—A model for modification of disease? *N. Engl. J. Med.* **287**:1026.

Graham, A. F., 1977, Possible role of defective virus in persistent infection, in: *Microbiology 1977* (D. Schlessinger ed.). pp. 445–450, American Society for Microbiology, Washington, D.C.

Guild, G. M., and Stollar, V., 1975, Defective interfering particles of Sindbis virus. 3. Intracellular viral RNA species in chick embryo cell cultures, *Virology* **67**:24.

Guild, G. M., and Stollar, V., 1977, Defective interfering particles of Sindbis virus. 5. Sequence relationships between SV_{STD} 42 S RNA and intracellular defective viral RNAs, *Virology* **77**:175.

Guild, G. M., Flores, L., and Stollar, V., 1977, Defective interfering particles of Sindbis virus. 4. Virion RNA species and molecular weight determination of defective double-stranded RNA, *Virology* **77**:158.

Hackett, A. J., 1964, A possible morphological basis for the autointerference phenomenon in vesicular stomatitis virus, *Virology* **24**:51.

Hackett, A. J., Schaffer, F. L., and Madin, S. H., 1967, The separation of infectious and autointerfering particles in vesicular stomatitis virus preparations, *Virology* **31**:114.

Hall, W. W., Martin, S. J., and Gould, E., 1974, Defective interfering particles produced during the replication of measles virus, *Med. Microbiol. Immunol.* **160**:155.

Hall, W. W., Kiessling, W., and ter Meulen, V., 1978, Membrane proteins of subacute sclerosing panencephalitis and measles viruses, *Nature (London)* **272**:460.

Hall, W. W., Lamb, R. A., and Choppin, P. W., 1979, Measles and subacute sclerosing panencephalitis virus proteins: Lack of antibodies to the M protein in patients with subacute sclerosing panencephalitis, *Proc. Natl. Acad. Sci. USA* **76**:2047.

Henle, W., and Henle, G., 1943, Interference of inactive virus with the propagation of virus of influenza, *Science* **98**:87.

Henry, B. E., Newcomb, W. W., and O'Callaghan, D. J., 1979, Biological and biochemical properties of defective interfering particles of equine herpesvirus type 1, *Virology* **92**:495.

Hewlett, M. J., Petterson, R. F., and Baltimore, D., 1977, Circular forms of Uukuniemi virion RNA: An electron microscopic study, *J. Virol.* **21**:1085.

Holland, J. J., and Doyle, M., 1973, Attempts to detect homologous autointerference *in vivo* with influenza virus and vesicular stomatitis virus, *Infect. Immun.* **7**:526.

Holland, J. J., and Villarreal, L. P., 1974, Persistent noncytocidal vesicular stomatitis virus infections mediated by defective T particles that suppress virion transcriptase, *Proc. Natl. Acad. Sci. USA* **71**:2956.

Holland, J. J., and Villarreal, L. P., 1975, Purification of defective interfering T particles of vesicular stomatitis and rabies viruses generated *in vivo* in brains of newborn mice, *Virology* **67**:438.

Holland, J. J., Villarreal, L. P., and Breindl, M., 1976*a*, Factors involved in the generation and replication of Rhabdovirus defective T particles, *J. Virol.* **17**:805.

Holland, J. J., Villarreal, L. P., Breindl, M., Semler, B. L., and Kohne, D., 1976*b*, Defective interfering virus particles attenuate virus lethality *in vivo* and *in vitro*, in: *Animal Virology* (D. Baltimore, A. S. Huang, and C. F. Cox, eds.), pp. 773–786, Academic Press, New York.

Holland, J. J., Villarreal, L. P., Welsh, R. M., Oldstone, M. B. A., Kohne, D., Lazzarini, R., and Scolnick, E., 1976*c*, Long-term persistent vesicular stomatitis virus and rabies virus infection of cells *in vitro*, *J. Gen. Virol.* **33**:193.

Holland, J. J., Semler, B. L., Jones, C., Perrault, J., Reid, L., and Roux, L., 1978, Role of DI, virus mutation, and host response in persistent infections by envelope RNA viruses, in: *Persistent Viruses* (J. Stevens, G. Todaro, and C. F. Fox, eds.), pp. 57–73 Academic Press, New York.

Holland, J. J., Grabau, E., Jones, C. L., and Semler, B. L., 1979, Evolution of multiple genome mutations during long term persistent infection by vesicular stomatitis virus, *Cell* **16**:495.

Huang, A. S., 1973, Defective interfering virus, *Annu. Rev. Microbiol.* **27**:101.

Huang, A. S., 1977, Viral pathogenesis and molecular biology, *Bacteriol. Rev.* **41**:811.

Huang, A. S., and Baltimore, D., 1970, Defective viral particles and viral disease processes, *Nature (London)* **226**:325.

Huang, A. S., and Baltimore, D., 1977, Defective interfering animal viruses, in: *Comprehensive Virology*, Vol. 10 (H. Fraenkel-Conrat and R. R. Wagner, eds.), pp. 73–116, Plenum Press, New York.

Huang, A. S., and Manders, E. K., 1972, Ribonucleic acid synthesis of vesicular stomatitis virus. 4. Transcription by standard virus in the presence of defective intefering virus particles, *J. Virol.* **9**:909.

Huang, A. S., and Wagner, R. R., 1966a, Defective T particles of vesicular stomatitis virus. 2. Biologic role in homologous interference, *Virology* **30**:173.

Huang, A. S., and Wagner, R. R., 1966b, Comparative sedimentation coefficients of RNA extracted from plaque-forming and defective particles of vesicular stomatitis virus, *J. Mol. Biol.* **22**:381.

Huang, A. S., Greenwalt, J. W., and Wagner, R. R., 1966, Defective T particles of vesicular stomatitis virus. 1. Preparation, morphology, and some biologic properties, *Virology* **30**:161.

Huang, A. S. Little, S. P., Oldstone, M. B. A., and Rao, D., 1978, Defective interfering particles: Their effect on gene expression and replication of vesicular stomatitis virus, in: *Persistent Viruses* (J. Stevens, G. Todaro, and C. F. Fox, eds.), pp. 399–408, Academic Press, New York.

Igarashi, A., and Stollar, V., 1976, Failure of defective interfering particles of Sindbis virus produced in BHK or chicken cells to affect viral replication in *Aedes albopictus* cells, *J. Virol.* **19**:398.

Igarashi, A., Koo, R., and Stollar, V., 1977, Evolution and properties of *Aedes albopictus* cell cultures persistently infected with Sindbis virus, *Virology* **82**:69.

Inglot, A. D., and Chudzio, T., 1972, Incomplete Sindbis virus, in: *Proceedings of the Second International Congress for Virology* (J. L. Melnick, ed.), pp. 158–162, Karger, New York.

Inglot, A. D., Albin, M., and Chudzio, T., 1973, Persistent infection of mouse cells with Sindbis virus: Role of virulence of strains, auto-interfering particles and interferon, *J. Gen. Virol.* **20**:105.

Ito, Y., Nishiyama, Y., Shimokata, K., Kimura, Y., Nagata, I., Shimizu, K., and Kunii, A., 1975, Interferon induction in mice by BHK cells persistently infected with HVJ, *J. Gen. Virol.* **27**:93.

Janda, J. M., David, A. R., Nayak, D. P., and De, B. K., 1979, Diversity and generation of defective interfering influenza virus particles, *Virology* **95**:48.

Johnson, L. D., and Lazzarini, R. A., 1977, Replication in viral RNA by a defective interfering vesicular stomatitis virus particle in the absence of helper virus, *Proc. Natl. Acad. Sci. USA* **74**:4387.

Johnston, R. E., Jovell, D. R. Brown, D. T., and Falkner, P., 1975, Interfering passages of Sindbis virus: Concomitant appearance of interference, morphological variants and truncated viral RNA, *J. Virol.* **16**:951.

Jones, C. L., and Holland, J. J., 1980, Requirements for DI particle prophylaxis against VSV infection *in vivo*, *J. Gen. Virol.* (in press).

Joseph, B. S., and Oldstone, M. B. A., 1975, Immunologic injury in measles infection. II. Suppression of immune injury through antigenic modulation, *J. Expl. Med.* **142**:864.

Kang, C. Y., and Allen, R., 1978, Host function—dependent induction of defective interfering particles of vesicular stomatitis virus, *J. Virol.* **25**:202.

Kang, C. Y., Glimp, T., Clewley, J. P., and Bishop, D. H. L., 1978, Studies on the generation of vesicular stomatitis virus (Indiana serotype) defective interfering particles, *Virology* **84**:142.

Kawai, A., and Matsumoto, S., 1977, Interfering and noninterfering defective particles generated by a rabies small plaque variant virus, *Virology* **76**:60.

Kawai, A., Matsumoto, S., and Tanabe, K., 1975, Characterization of rabies viruses recovered from persistently infected BHK cells, *Virology* **67**:520.

Keene, J. D., Schubert, M., Lazzarini, R. A., and Rosenberg, M., 1978, Nucleotide sequence homology at the 3' termini of RNA from vesicular stomatitis virus and its defective interfering particles, *Proc. Natl. Acad. Sci. USA* **75**:3225.

Kennedy, S. I. T., 1976, Sequence relationships between the genome and the intracellular RNA species of standard and defective interfering Semliki Forest virus, *J. Mol. Biol.* **108**:491.

Kennedy, S. I. T., Bruton, C. J., Weiss, B., and Schlesinger, S., 1976, Defective interfering passages of Sindbis virus: Nature of the defective virion RNA, *J. Virol.* **19**:1034.

Khan, S. R., and Lazzarini, R. A., 1977, The relationship between autointerference and the replication of a defective interfering particle, *Virology* **77**:189.

Kiley, M. P., Gray, R. H., and Payne, F. E., 1974, Replication of measles virus: Distinct species of short nucleocapsids in cytoplasmic extracts of infected cells, *J. Virol* **13**:721.

Kimura, Y., Ito, Y., Shimokata, K., Nishiyama, Y., Nagata, I., and Kitoh, J., 1975, Temperature sensitive virus derived from BHK cells persistently infected with HVJ, *J. Virol.* **15**:55.

Kingsbury, D. W., and Portner, A., 1970, On the genesis of incomplete Sendai virions, *Virology* **42**:872.

Kingsbury, D. W., Portner, A., and Darlington, R. W., 1970, Properties of incomplete Sendai virions and subgenomic viral RNAs, *Virology* **42**:857.

Kolakofsky, D., 1976, Isolation and characterization of Sendai virus DI RNAs, *Cell* **8**:547.

Kolakofsky, D., 1979, Studies on the generation and amplification of Sendai virus DI genomes, *Virology* **93**:589.

Kolakofsky, D., Leppert, M., and Kort, L., 1978, A genetic map of Sendai virus DI RNAs, in: *Negative Strand Viruses and the Host Cell* (B. W. J. Mahy and R. D. Barry, eds.), pp. 539–553, Academic Press, New York.

Lazzarini, R. A., Weber G. H., Johnson, L. D., and Stamminger, G. M., 1975, Covalently linked message and anti-message (genomic) RNA from a defective vesicular stomatitis virus particle, *J. Mol. Biol.* **97**:289.

Leamnson, R. N., and Reichmann, M. E., 1974, The RNA of defective vesicular stomatitis virus in relation to viral cistrons, *J. Mol. Biol.* **85**:551.

Lehmann-Grubbe, F., Slenzka, W., and Reef Tees, 1969, A persistent and inapparent infection of L cells with the virus of lymphocytic choriomeningitis, *J. Gen. Virol.* **5**:63.

Leppert, M., Kort, L., and Kolakofsky, D., 1977, Further characterization of Sendai virus DI RNAs: A model for their generation, *Cell* **12**:539.

Levin, J. G., Ramseur, J. M., and Grimley, P. M., 1973, Host effect on arbovirus replication: Appearance of defective interfering particles in murine cells, *J. Virol.* **12**:1401.

Lunquist, R. E., Sullivan, M., and Maizel, J. V., 1979, Characterization of a new isolate of poliovirus defective interfering particles, *Cell* **18**:79.

Little, S. P., and Huang, A. S., 1977, Synthesis and distribution of VSV specific polypeptides in the absence of progeny production, *Virology* **81**:37.

Logan, K. B., 1979, Generation of defective interfering particles of Semliki Forest virus in a clone of *Aedes aldopictus* (mosquito) cells, *J. Virol.* **30**:38.

Marcus, P. I., and Sekellick, M. J., 1977, Defective interfering particles with covalently linked [±] RNA induce interferon, *Nature (London)* **266**:815.

Marcus, P. I., Sekellick, M. J., Johnson, L. D., and Lazzarini, R. A., 1977, Cell killing by viruses. V. Transcribing defective interfering particles of VSV function as cell killing particles, *Virology* **82**:242.

McClure, M. A., Holland, J. J., and Perrault, J., 1980, Generation of defective interfering particles in picornaviruses, *Virology* **100**:408.

McGeoch, D. J., and Dolan, A., 1979, Sequence of 200 nucleotides at the 3′ terminus of the genome RNA of vesicular stomatitis virus, *Cell* **6**:3199.

Meinkoth, J., and Kennedy, S. I. T., 1979, Semliki Forest virus persistence in mouse L929 cells, *Virology* **100**:141.

Mims, C. A. C., 1956, Rift Valley fever in mice. 4. Incomplete virus: Its production and properties, *Br. J. Exp. Pathol.* **37**:129.

Minato, N., Bloom, B. R., Jones, C., Holland, J. J., and Reid, L. M., 1979, Mechanism of rejection of virus persistently infected tumor cells by athymic nude mice, *J. Exp. Med.* **149**:1117.

Mocarski, E. S., and Stinski, M. F., 1979, Persistence of the cytomegalovirus genome in human cells, *J. Virol.* **31**:761.

Mudd, J. A., Leavitt, R. W., Kingsbury, D. T., and Holland, J. J., 1973, Natural selection of mutants of vesicular stomatitis virus by cultured cells of *Drosophila melanogaster*, *J. Gen. Virol.* **20**:341.

Narayan, O., Griffin, D. E., Chase, J., 1977, Antigenic shift of Visna virus in persistently infected sheep, *Science* **197**:376.

Nayak, D. P., Tobita, K., Janda, J. M., Davis, A. R., and De, B. K., 1978, Homologous interference mediated by defective interfering influence virus derived from a temperature-sensitive mutant of influenza virus, *J. Virol.* **28**:375.

Nicholson, B. L., and Dunn, J., 1972, Autointerference in the replication of the infectious pancreatic necrosis (IPN) virus of trout, *Bacteriol. Proc.* **72**:196.

Nishiyama, Y., 1977, Studies of L cells persistently infected with VSV: Factors involved in the regulation of persistent infection, *J. Gen. Virol.* **35**:265.

Nishiyama, Y., Ito, Y., Shimokata, K., Kimura, Y., and Nagata, J., 1976, Relationship between establishment of persistent infection of heamagglutinating virus of Japan and the properties of the virus, *J. Gen. Virol.* **32**:73.

Nishiyama, Y., Ito, Y., and Shimokata, K., 1978, Properties of viruses selected during persistent infection of L cells with VSV, *J. Gen. Virol.* **40**:481.

Nomoto, A., Jacobson, A., Lee, Y. F., Dunn, J., and Wimmer, E., 1978, Defective interfering particles of poliovirus: Mapping of the deletion and evidence that the deletion in the genome of DI (1), (2) and (3) is located in the same region. *J. Mol. Biol.* **128**:179.

Nonoyama, M., and Graham, A. F., 1970, Appearance of defective virions in clones of reovirus, *J. Virol.* **6**:693.

Nonoyama, M., Watanabe, Y., and Graham, A. F., 1970, Defective virions of reovirus, *J. Virol.* **6**:693.

Norkin, L. C., 1979, The emergence of simian virus 40 variants in a persistent infection of Rhesus monkey kidney cells, and their interaction with standard simian virus 40, *Virology* **95**:598.

Obijeski, J. F., Bishop, D. H. L., Palmer, E. L., and Murphy, F. A., 1976, Segmented genome and nucleocapsid of La Crosse virus, *J. Virol.* **20**:664.

Palma, E. L., and Huang, A. S., 1974, Cyclic production of vesicular stomatitis virus caused by defective interfering particles, *J. Infect. Dis.* **126**:402.

Peleg, J., 1969, Inapparent persistent virus infection in continuously grown *Aedes aegypti* mosquito cells, *J. Gen. Virol.* **5**:463.

Perrault, J., 1976, Cross-linked double-stranded RNA from a defective vesicular stomatitis virus particle, *Virology* **70**:360.

Perrault, J., and Holland, J. J., 1972*a*, Variability of vesicular stomatitis virus autointerference with different host cells and virus serotypes, *Virology* **50**:148.

Perrault, J., and Holland, J. J., 1972*b*, Absence of transcriptase activity or transcription-inhibiting activity in defective interfering particles of vesicular stomatitis virus, *Virology* **50**:159.

Perrault, J., and Leavitt, R. W., 1977*a*, Characterization of snap-back RNAs in vesicular stomatitis defective interfering virus particles, *J. Gen. Virol.* **38**:21.

Perrault, J., and Leavitt, R. W., 1977*b*, Inverted complementary terminal sequences in single-stranded RNAs and snap-back RNAs from vesicular stomatitis defective interfering particles, *J. Gen. Virol.* **38**:35.

Perrault, J., and Semler, B. L., 1979, Internal genome deletions in two distinct classes of defective interfering particles of vesicular stomatitis virus, *Proc. Natl. Acad. Sci. USA* **76**:6191.

Perrault, J., Semler, B. L., Leavitt, R. W., and Holland, J. J., 1978, Inverted complementary sequences in defective interfering particle RNAs of vesicular stomatitis virus and their possible role in autointerference, in: *Negative Strand Viruses and the Host Cell* (B. W. J. Mahy and R. D. Barry, eds.), pp. 527–538, Academic Press, New York.

Perrin, L., Tishon, A., and Oldstone, M. B. A., 1977, Immuniologic injury in measles virus infection. 3. Presence and characterization of human cytotoxic lymphocytes, *J. Immunol.* **118**:282.

Petterson, R. F., and Hewlett, M. J., 1976, The structure of the RNA of Uukuniemi virus, a proposed Bunyavirus, in: *Animal Virology* (D. Baltimore, A. S. Huang, and C. F. Fox, eds.), pp. 515–527, Academic Press, New York.

Petterson, R. F., and Von Bonsdorff, C. H., 1975, Ribonucleoproteins of Uukuniemi virus are circular, *J. Virol.* **15**:386.

Popescu, M., and Lehmann-Grube, F., 1977, Defective interfering particles in mice infected with lymphocytic choriomeningitis virus, *Virology* **77**:78.

Preble, O. T., and Youngner, J. S., 1975, Temperature sensitive mutant viruses and the etiology of chronic and inapparent infections, *J. Infect. Dis.* **131**:467.

Prevec, L., and Kang, C. Y., 1970, Homotypic and heterotypic interference by defective particles of vesicular stomatitis virus, *Nature (London)* **228**:25.

Rabinowitz, S. G., Dal Canto, M. C., and Johnson, T. C., 1976, Comparison of central nervous system disease produced by wild type and temperature-sensitive mutants of vesicular stomatitis virus, *Infect. Immun.* **13**:1242.

Rahacek, J., 1968, Persistent infection of mosquito cells grown *in vitro* with Murray Valley encephalitis and Japanese encephalitis viruses, *Acta Virol.* **12**:340.

Ramseur, J. M., and Friedman, R. M., 1977, Prolonged infection of interferon-treated cells by VSV: Possible role of temperature sensitive mutants and interferon, *J. Gen. Virol.* **37**:523.

Reichmann, M. E., and Schnitzlein, W. M., 1978, Defective interfering particles of rhabdoviruses, *Curr. Top. Microbiol. Immunol.* **86**:124.

Reichmann, M. E., Pringle, C. R., and Follett, E. A. C., 1971, Defective particles in BHK cells infected with temperature sensitive mutants of vesicular stomatitis virus, *J. Virol.* **8**:154.

Reichmann, M. E., Villarreal, L. P., Kohne, D., Lesnaw, J., and Holland, J. J., 1974, RNA polymerase activity and poly(A) synthesizing activity in defective T particles of vesicular stomatitis virus, *Virology* **58**:240.

Reid, L. M., Jones, C. L., and Holland, J., 1979, Virus carrier state suppresses tumorigenicity of tumor cells in athymic (nude) mice, *J. Gen. Virol.* **42**:609.

Rima, B. K., and Martin, S. J., 1977, Persistent infection of tissue culture cells by RNA viruses, *Med. Microbiol. Immunol.* **162**:89.

Rima, B. K., and Martin, S. J., 1979, Effect of undiluted passage on the polypeptides of measles virus, *J. Gen. Virol.* **44**:135.

Rima, B. K., Davidson, W. B., and Martin, S. J., 1977, The role of defective interfering particles in persistent infection of vero cells by measles, *J. Gen. Virol.* **35**:89.

Roux, L., and Holland, J. J., 1979, Role of defective interfering particles of Sendai virus in persistent infections, *Virology* **93**:91.

Roux, L., and Holland, J. J., 1980, Viral genome synthesis in BHK21 cells persistently infected with Sendai virus, *Virology* **100**:53.

Rowlands, D. J., 1979, Sequences of VSV RNA in the region coding for leader RNA, N mRNA and their function, *Proc. Natl. Acad. Sci. USA* **76**:4793.

Roy, P., and Bishop, D. H. L., 1972, Genome homology of vesicular stomatitis virus and defective T particles and evidence for the sequential transcription of the virion ribonucleic acid, *J. Virol.* **9**:946.

Roy, P., Repik, P., Hefti, E., and Bishop, D. H. L., 1973, Complementary RNA species isolated from vesicular stomatitis (HR) strain defective virions, *J. Virol.* **11**:915.

Samso, A., Bouloy, M., and Hannoun, C., 1975, Présence de ribonucléoproteines circulaires dans le virus Lumbo (Bunyavirus), *C. R. Acad. Sci. Ser. D* **280**:213.

Schaffer, F. L., Hackett, A. J., and Soergel, M. E., 1968, Vesicular stomatitis virus RNA: Complementarity between infected cell RNA and RNAs from infectious and autointerfering viral fractions, *Biochem. Biophys. Res. Commun.* **31**:685.

Schincariol, A. L., and Howatson, A. F., 1972, Replication of vesicular stomatitis virus. 2. Separation and characterization of virus-specific RNA species, *Virology* **49**:766.

Schlesinger, S., Schlesinger, M., and Burge, B. W., 1972, Defective virus particles from Sindbis virus, *Virology* **48**:615.

Schmaljohn, C., and Blair, C. D., 1977, Persistent infection of cultured mammalian cells by Japanese encephalitis virus, *J. Virol.* **24**:580.

Schnitzlein, W. M., and Reichmann, M. E., 1976, the size and cistronic origin of defective vesicular stomatitis virus particle RNAs in relation to homotypic and heterotypic interference, *J. Mol. Biol.* **101**:307.

Schnitzlein, W. M., and Reichmann, M. E., 1977, A possible effect of viral proteins on the specificity of interference by defective vesicular stomatitis virus particles, *Virology* **80**:275.

Schubert, M., Keene, J. D., Lazzarini, R. A., and Emerson, S. U., 1978, The complete sequence of a unique RNA species synthesized by a DI particle of VSV, *Cell* **15**:103.

Schubert, M., Keene, J. D., and Lazzarini, R. A., 1979, A specific internal RNA polymerase recognition site of VSV RNA is involved in the generation of DI particles, *Cell* **18**:749.

Schuerch, A. R., Matsuhisa, T., and Joklik, W. K., 1974, Temperature-sensitive mutants of reovirus. 6. Mutant ts447 and ts556 particles that lack either one or two genome segments, *Intervirology* **3**:36.

Semler, B. L., Perrault, J., Abelson, J., and Holland, J. J., 1978, Sequence of a RNA templated by the 3'-OH RNA terminus of defective interfering particles of vesicular stomatitis virus, *Proc. Natl. Acad. Sci. USA* **75**:4704.

Semler, B. L., Perrault, J., and Holland, J. J., 1979, The nucleotide sequence of the 5' terminus of vesicular stomatitis virus RNA, *Nucl. Acids Res.* **6**:3923.

Shenk, T. E., and Stollar, V., 1973, Defective interfering particles of Sindbis virus. 1. Isolation and some chemical and biological properties, *Virology* **53**:162.

Simpson, R. W., and Iinuma, M., 1975, Recovery of infectious proviral DNA from mammalian cells infected with respiratory syncitial virus, *Proc. Natl. Acad. Sci. USA* **72**:3230.

Singh, K. R. P., 1967, Cell cultures derived from larvae of *Aedes albopictus* (SRuse) and *Aedes aegypti* (L), *Curr. Sci.* **36**:506.

Spandidos, D. A., and Graham, A. F., 1976, Generation of defective virus after infection of newborn rats with reovirus, *J. Virol.* **20**:234.

Spandidos, D. A., Krystal, G., and Graham, A. F., 1976, Regulated transcription of the genomes of defective virions and temperature-sensitive mutants of reovirus, *J. Virol.* **18**:7.

Stamminger, G., and Lazzarini, R. A., 1974, Analysis of the RNA of defective VSV particles, *Cell* **3**:85.

Stamminger, G. M., and Lazzarini, R. A., 1977, RNA synthesis in standard and autointerfered vesicular stomatitis infections, *Virology* **77**:202.

Stampfer, M., Baltimore, D., and Huang, A. S., 1971, Absence of interference during high multiplicity infection by clonally purified vesicular stomatitis virus, *J. Virol.* **7**:409.

Staneck, L. D., and Pfau, C. J., 1974, Interfering particles from a culture persistently infected with parana virus, *J. Gen. Virol.* **22**:437.

Staneck, L. D., Trowbridge, R. S., Welsh, R. M., Wright, E. A., and Pfau, C. J., 1972, Arenaviruses: Cellular response to long-term *in vitro* infection with parana and lymphocytic choriomeningitis viruses, *Infect. Immun.* **6**:444.

Stanners, C. P., and Goldberg, V. J., 1975, On the mechanism of neurotropism of VSV in newborn hamsters. Studies with temperature-sensitive mutants, *J. Gen. Virol.* **29**:281.

Stanners, C. P., Francoeur, A. M., and Larn, T., 1977, Analysis of VSV mutant with attenuated cytopathogenicity: Mutation in viral function P for inhibition of protein synthesis, *Cell* **11**:273.

Stanwick, T. L., and Kirk, B. F., 1976, Analysis of baby hamster kidney cells persistently infected with lymphocytic choriomeningitis virus, *J. Gen. Virol.* **32**:361.

Stark, C., and Kennedy, S. I. T., 1978, The generation and propagation of defective interfering particles of Semliki Forest virus in different cell types, *Virology* **89**:285.

Stevens, J., 1978, Latent herpetic infections in the central nervous system of experimental animals, in: *Persistent Viruses* (J. Stevens, G. J. Todaro, and C. F. Fox, eds.), p. 701, Academic Press, New York.

Stevens, T. M., 1970, Arbovirus replication in mosquito cell lines (Singh) grown in monolayer or suspension culture, *Proc. Soc. Exp. Biol. Med.* **134**:356.

Stinski, M. F., Mocarski, E. S., and Thomsen, D. R., 1979, DNA of human cytomegalovirus: Size heterogeneity and defectiveness resulting from serial undiluted passages, *J. Virol.* **31**.231.

Stollar, V., and Shenk, T. E., 1973, Homologous viral interference in *Aedes albopictus* cultures chronically infected with Sindbis virus, *J. Virol.* **11**:592.

Taber, R., Alexander, V., and Whitford, W., 1976, Persistent reovirus infection of CHO cells resulting in virus resistance, *J. Virol.* **17**:513.

Thorne, H. V., and Dermott, E., 1976, Circular and elongated forms of measles virus nucleocapsid, *Nature (London)* **264**:473.

Trowbridge, R. S., and Pfau, C. J., 1970, Persistent infection of cultured $BHK_{21}/13C$ cells by lymphocytic choriomeningitis virus, *Bacteriol. Proc.*, p. 199.

Villarreal, L. P., and Holland, J. J., 1976, RNA synthesis in BHK_{21} cells persistently infected with vesicular stomatitis virus and rabies virus, *J. Gen. Virol.* **33**:213.

Von Magnus, P., 1951, Propagation of the PR 8 strain of influenza virus in chick embryos. 3. Properties of the incomplete virus produced in serial passages of undiluted virus, *Acta Pathol. Microbiol. Scand.* **29**:156.

von Magnus, P., 1954, Incomplete forms of influenza virus, *Adv. Virus Res.* **2**:59.

Wagner, R. R., 1974, Pathogenicity and immunogenicity for mice of temperature sensitive mutants of vesicular stomatitis virus, *Infect. Immun.* **10**:309.

Wagner, R. R., 1975, Reproduction of rhabdoviruses, in: *Comprehensive Virology*, Vol. 4 (H. Fraenkel-Conrat and R. R. Wagner, eds.), pp. 1–93, Plenum Press, New York.

Wagner, R. R., Levy, A., Snyder, R., Ratcliff, G., and Hyatt, D., 1963, Biologic properties of two plaque variants of vesicular stomatitis virus (Indiana serotype), *J. Immunol.* **91**:112.

Walker, D. L., 1964, The viral carrier state in animal cultures, *Progr. Med. Virol.* **6**:111.

Wechsler, S. L., and Fields, B. N., 1978, Differences between the intracellular polypeptides of measles and subacute sclerosing panencephalitis virus, *Nature (London)* **272**:458.

Weiss, B., and Schlesinger, S., 1973, Defective interfering passages of Sindbis virus: Chemical composition, biological activity and mode of interference, *J. Virol.* **12**:862.

Weiss, B., Goran, D., Cancedda, R., and Schlesinger, S., 1974, Defective interfering passages of Sindbis virus: Nature of the intracellular defective viral RNA, *J. Virol.* **14**:1189.

Weiss, B., Rosenthal, R., and Schlesinger, S., 1980, Establishment and maintenance of persistent infection by Sindbis virus in BHK cells, *J. Virol.* **33**:463.

Welsh, R. M., and Oldstone, M. B. A., 1977, Inhibition of immunologic injury of cultured cells infected with lymphocytic choriomeningitis virus: Role of defective interfering virus in regulating viral antigenic expression, *J. Exp. Med.* **145**:1449.

Welsh, R. M., and Pfau, C. J., 1972, Determinants of lymphocytic choriomeningitis interference, *J. Gen. Virol.* **14**:177.

Welsh, R. M., O'Connell, C. M., and Pfau, C. J., 1972, Properties of defective lymphocytic choriomeningitis virus, *J. Gen. Virol.* **17**:355.

Welsh, R. M., Lampert, P. W., and Oldstone, M. B. A., 1977, Prevention of virus-induced cerebral disease by defective interfering lymphocytic choriomeningitis virus, *J. Infect. Dis.* **136**:391.

Wiktor, T. J., and Clark, H. F., 1972, Chronic rabies virus infection of cell cultures, *Infect. Immun.* **6**:988.

Wiktor, T. J., Dietyzsehold, B., Leamnson, R. N., and Koprowski, H., 1977, Induction and biological properties of defective interfering particles of rabies virus, *J. Virol.* **21**:626.

Wild, T. F., and Dugre, R., 1978, Establishment and characterization of a subacute sclerosing panencephalitis (measles) virus persistent infection in BGM cells, *J. Gen. Virol* **39**:113.

Wilfert, C. M., Buckley, R., Rosen, F. S., Whismant, J., Oxman, M. N., Griffith, J. F., Katz, S. L., and Moure, M., 1977, Persistent enterovirus infections in agammaglobulinemia, in: *Microbiology 1977* (D. Schlesinger, ed.), pp. 488–493, American Society for Microbiology, Washington, D.C.

Wunner, W. H., and Clark, H. F., 1978, Study of virulent and avirulent rabies viruses and their defective RNA-containing particles, in: *Negative Strand Viruses and the Host Cell* (B. Mahy and R. Barry, eds.), pp. 599–606, Academic Press, London.

Yamada, T., and Hatano, M., 1972, Lowered transplantability of cultured tumor cells by persistent infection with paramyxovirus (HVJ), *Gann* **63**:647.

Youngner, J. S., and Quagliana, D. O., 1975, Temperature-sensitive mutants isolated from hamster and canine cell lines persistently infected with Newcastle disease virus, *J. Virol.* **16**:1332.

Youngner, J., Dubovi, E. J., Quagliana, D. O., Kelly, M., and Preble, O. T., 1976, Role of temperature sensitive mutants in persistent infections initiated with vesicular stomatitis virus, *J. Virol.* **19**:90.

Zhdanov, V. M., 1975, Integration of viral genomes, *Nature (London)* **256**:471.

CHAPTER 4

Persistence and Transmission of Cytomegalovirus

Fred Rapp

Department of Microbiology
and
Specialized Cancer Research Center
The Pennsylvania State University
College of Medicine
Hershey, Pennsylvania 17033

1. INTRODUCTION

The herpesviruses comprise a diverse group of double-stranded DNA-containing viruses. As a virus group they are unpredictable in that individual group members exhibit different basic characteristics, including host specificity and genome complexity. Cytomegalovirus (CMV) is a herpesvirus that is particularly interesting from an academic as well as a clinical viewpoint (Table 1). Also known as salivary gland virus (Weller, 1970), it was originally named for the enlarged cells containing intranuclear and cytoplasmic inclusions produced by infection with the virus. Cytomegalovirus was first isolated by three investigators working independently in their laboratories. Smith (1956) in St. Louis isolated the virus from submaxillary salivary gland tissue of a dead infant; Rowe *et al.* (1956) in Bethesda discovered the virus in cultures of adenoidal tissues from three children; and Weller and his associates (1957) in Boston isolated a CMV from an infant with cytomegalic inclusion disease (CID). From this time on,

TABLE 1

Biological Properties of Human Cytomegalovirus

Site of latency unknown
Epithelial target cell *in vivo*
Replication cycle in cell culture (diploid fibroblasts) of 36–48 hr
Low to intermediate virus yield (10^4–10^7) in cell culture
Highly species specific

many investigations have focused on CMV and its role in diseases of man.

2. PHYSICAL, MORPHOLOGICAL, AND MOLECULAR CHARACTERISTICS

In 1963, Smith and Rasmussen demonstrated that the structure of CMV is that of a herpesvirus and that CMV nucleic acid stains as DNA. They also observed other properties of CMV that were similar to herpes simplex virus (HSV), including the presence of an envelope and well-defined capsomeres. Of particular interest was their observation that the particle-to-infectivity ratio is extremely high, with only about one infectious unit forming per 1000 infected cells. Using 5-fluorodeoxyuridine (FUdR), Goodheart *et al.* (1963) found evidence that CMV is a DNA-containing virus and that FUdR separates the processes of development of cytopathology and virus synthesis in CMV-infected cells. Another study in 1963 (McAllister *et al.*) followed the development of virus cytopathology over a 96-hr period and demonstrated cell rounding 24 hr after infection. By 48 hr after infection, virus antigen was detectable in cytoplasmic lesions and the nucleus. The most significant events occurred approximately 72 hr after infection. At this time infectious virus was detectable in cells and supernatant, and DNA was present in the cytoplasmic lesion. By 96 hr after infection, the begining of cell degeneration was evident. McGavran and Smith (1965) extended the studies of McAllister *et al.* (1963) and observed that the cytoplasmic body is composed of aggregates of lysosomes and is formed as virus enters the cytoplasm from the nucleus. In addition, they determined that the second cytoplasmic coat of CMV is actually derived from the inner nuclear membrane as the virus leaves the nucleus, a property similar to that observed in other herpesviruses.

Thermal inactivation studies (Krugman and Goodheart, 1964) revealed that CMV is a relatively heat-labile virus and that the half-life at 37°C is less that 1 hr. Plummer and Lewis (1965) also studied thermoinactivation of CMV and, in contrast to Krugman and Goodheart (1964), observed a plateau in all inactivation curves of CMV at 36°C and 22°C. CMV was also found to be less stable at 4°C and 10°C than at 22°C.

A concise review on the replication of herpesviruses has been presented by Roizman and Furlong (1974). In addition St. Jeor and Rapp (1973), Vonka *et al.* (1976), Figueroa *et al.* (1978), and Furukawa *et al.* (1978) have studied the replication of viruses in CMV-infected and CMV-transformed cells. Ihara and associates (1978) studied the replication of CMV using temperature-sensitive mutants and observed that human CMV may induce two distinct species of DNA polymerase. Furukawa *et al.* (1973) described cytopathology within 6–24 hr after infection of human cells and suggested that a protein is synthesized in infected cells approximately 2 hr after infection since inhibitors of pro-

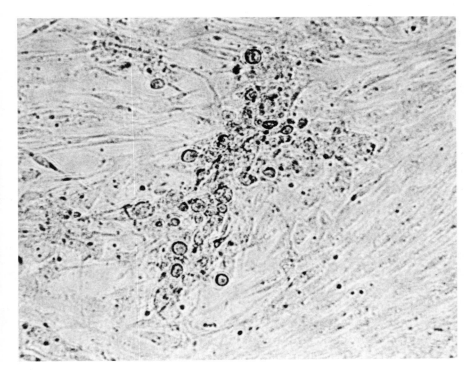

Fig. 1.   Focus of cytomegalovirus cytopathology in human embryo lung cells.

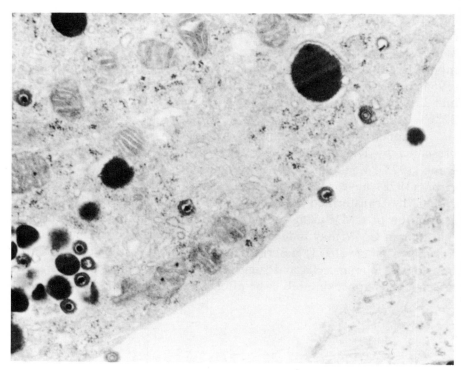

Fig. 2.   Electron micrograph of intracytoplasmic and "budding" cytomegalovirions in human cells (kindly supplied by Dr. M. Webber). Note the bar-shaped nucleoid within the virions.

tein synthesis prevented the cytopathic effect. It is obvious that CMV is less cytopathic (Fig. 1) than HSV. Smith and deHarven (1973) studied the sequence of HSV and CMV replication in WI38 cells. They found the following differences between the two viruses: cytoplasmic CMV capsids were coated, whereas those of HSV were not, and there was a variation in the structure of the HSV and CMV cores (Fig. 2). Other observations paralleled those of earlier reports in that CMV required 4 days for replication and release of progeny. Smith and deHarven do not concur with an earlier report (McGavran and Smith, 1965) that cytoplasmic dense bodies in CMV-infected cells represent lysosomes; however, they do suggest (Smith and deHarven, 1978) that dense bodies bud into lysosomes and acquire an envelope in the process. The longer time cycle for CMV replication is probably not due to an adsorption or penetration mechanism, since timing for these events is the same for HSV and CMV.

In 1974, St. Jeor *et al.* reported the stimulation of cellular DNA synthesis by human CMV (Fig. 3). This was followed by Tanaka *et al.* (1975), who reported the stimulation of host cell RNA synthesis during early stages of infection with human CMV. A recent study (Tanaka *et al.*, 1978) has demonstrated that an increase in activity of the three major classes of RNA polymerases is involved in the stimulation of cell RNA synthesis and that a CMV-induced early protein(s) is responsible for the induction of the RNA polymerase. A study by Albrecht *et al.* (1976) in which hamster cells were abortively infected with CMV demonstrated that CMV-infected cells had increased rates of cell DNA replication and mitotic activity. DeMarchi and Kaplan (1977) reported that defective CMV particles are very important in the stimulation of cellular DNA synthesis in permissive cultures and that detection of stimulation of cellular DNA synthesis is possible mainly in cells infected with virus incapable of producing a productive infection. In

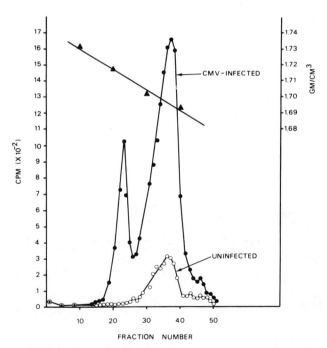

Fig. 3. Induction of DNA synthesis in human embryo lung cells infected with cytomegalovirus. Infected (●) and uninfected (○) cells were extracted for DNA following exposure to [³H]thymidine for 24–48 hr. (▲) indicates density. The DNA was centrifuged to equilibrium in a gradient of cesium chloride. Infected cells demonstrate synthesis of CMV DNA and increase in synthesis of cellular DNA as measured by uptake of the labeled thymidine. From St. Jeor *et al.* (1974).

addition, studies from this laboratory (Miller *et al.*, 1977) demonstrated that CMV induces high levels of cellular thymidine kinase and does not code for a virus thymidine kinase. These observations have been confirmed by the work of Estes and Huang (1977) and Závada *et al.* (1976).

Cytomegalovirus nuclear antigens have been detected from 1 hr to 4 days after infection as reported by Rapp *et al.* (1963), Jack and Wark (1972), Laing (1974), Smith and deHarven (1974), Geder (1976), and, most recently, Michelson-Fiske *et al.* (1977).

Cytomegalovirus-specific early antigens (Fig. 4) were detected when fibroblasts were infected in the presence of cytosine arabinoside (The *et al.*, 1974). The presence of these early antigens was used to study the antibody response in acutely infected and healthy individuals. It was observed that acutely infected patients had antibodies to early and late antigens, whereas healthy individuals produced antibodies to late antigens only. When serum was taken from patients prior to onset of illness, antibodies to either early or late antigens could not be detected. Early antigens of CMV, HSV, and Epstein-Barr virus (EBV) do not cross-react (Giraldo *et al.*, 1977).

The proteins of CMV have been studied by several investigators (Sarov and Abady, 1975; Edwards, 1976; Fiala *et al.*, 1976; Stinski, 1976, 1977; Gupta *et al.*, 1977; Gupta and Rapp, 1978). Reports present variable data, with numbers of proteins ranging from 20 to 32 and molecular weights ranging from 13,500 to greater than 235,000. Of the proteins identified by Fiala *et al.* (1976), six polypeptides were present in virions, four were present in dense bodies, and the remainder

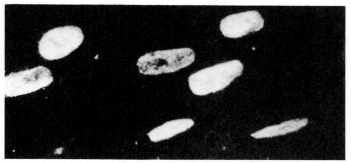

Fig. 4. Intranuclear antigen detected in human embryo lung cells infected with cytomegalovirus by the anticomplement indirect-fluorescent antibody test. The cells were reacted with antibody to cytomegalovirus, human complement (C3), and anti-human-complement globulin labeled with fluorescein isothiocyanate.

were present in virions and dense bodies. Four of the polypeptides were glycosylated and three of these were associated with virions and dense bodies. Gupta *et al.* (1977) detected 32 polypeptides with molecular weights ranging from 13,500 to 235,000 using polyacrylamide gel electrophoresis. Gupta and Rapp (1978) reported that synthesis of most host cell proteins is more sensitive to inhibition by a hypertonic condition than is synthesis of virus-induced proteins; they also observed that CMV-induced proteins are synthesized in a cyclic manner. Stinski (1976) detected eight glycopolypeptides associated with the membranes of CMV as well as with dense bodies. A later study by Stinski (1977) reported two peak periods of protein synthesis in CMV-infected cells. One period is early in infection and is host specific; the other is late in infection and is mainly virus specific. Even late in infection, approximately 50% of total protein synthesis is due to host protein synthesis.

In 1973, Huang *et al.* completed their first study on the characterization of human CMV DNA. Using purified CMV DNA, they were able to establish the molecular weight of CMV DNA as 100×10^6 and the density as 1.716 g/cm^3. Sarov and Friedman (1976) also reported a molecular weight of 100×10^6, but Geelen *et al.* (1978) reported a molecular weight of approximately $147.1 \pm 6.2 \times 10^6$ and DeMarchi *et al.* (1978) reported a weight of 150×10^6. The studies by Geelen *et al.* and DeMarchi *et al.* used sucrose gradient sedimentation and contour measurements in the electron microscope to arrive at their very similar results. In contrast, Huang *et al.* (1973) used cosedimentation with HSV DNA and Sarov and Friedman (1976) used length measurements to arrive at their molecular weights for CMV DNA. A more recent study by Kilpatrick and Huang (1977) using contour-length measurements reported the molecular weight of the human CMV genome to be $150–155 \times 10^6$ daltons. This estimate is now generally accepted as the correct value for full-length CMV DNA.

Continuing the studies with purified DNA, Huang and Pagano (1974) investigated the relatedness of human CMV DNA to the DNAs of HSV type 1 (HSV1) and HSV type 2 (HSV2), EBV, and simian and murine CMV using DNA-DNA reassociation kinetics. The results of their experiments demonstrated less than 5% or no homology among the DNAs. Huang (1975*a*) reported the induction of a human CMV-induced DNA polymerase following infection of human fibroblasts with human CMV. A follow-up study (Huang, 1975*b*) established that this CMV-induced DNA polymerase is specifically inhibited by phosphonoacetic acid. Kierszenbaum and Huang (1978) identified a novel

TABLE 2

Physical Properties of Cytomegalovirus

Size of virion	100–150 nm
Number of capsomeres	162
Envelope	Present
Molecular weight of DNA	150×10^6 daltons
Configuration of DNA	Double-stranded, linear
Buoyant density of DNA in cesium chloride	1.716 g/cm^3
Percent guanine and cytosine content of DNA	57
Percent homology with DNA of other herpesviruses	0–<5

chromatin pattern during the infection of human embryonic lung cells with human CMV. This chromatin pattern consists of a chain of bipartite and oblate ellipsoid particles arranged along the chromatin fibers. The significance of this observation is not yet clear. Jean and colleagues (1978) described intracellular forms of human CMV DNA before and after the initiation of virus DNA synthesis. Circular, con-catemeric, and linear molecules were observed prior to replication of CMV DNA, and linear molecules and concatemers were observed after DNA synthesis began. These data suggest that CMV DNA molecules acquire single-stranded sequences and then form circles which most likely have reiterated sequences located at or near the termini of the CMV DNA molecule. Table 2 lists the important physical properties of cytomegalovirus.

3. DETECTION OF CYTOMEGALOVIRUS INFECTIONS

In the early 1950s, exfoliative cytological procedures were used to diagnose patients with CID; prior to this time, diagnosis was made post-mortem. The procedure, using stained urinary sediment to demonstrate large intranuclear inclusions in epithelial cells, was not always reliable as reported by Weller and Hanshaw (1962). In a study of renal transplant patients (Lee and Balfour, 1977), the investigators found that the best way to recover CMV from the urine was to use uncentrifuged urine. It is possible that cytomegalic cells are not demonstrable at all times in the urine. By 1963, attempts were underway to establish assays to facilitate laboratory studies with CMV. The test in use at the time was the 50% end-point dilution method that required 4–6 weeks for results. Goodheart and Jaross (1963) were successful in establishing an assay using Giemsa staining in which CMV-infected cells were counted and the assay was completed in 48 hr. Rapp *et al.* (1963) were also successful using the immunofluorescent focus technique. These methods were superseded in 1964 when Plummer and Benyesh-Melnick published their plaque reduction neutralization test. Hanshaw (1966*a*) used the complement-fixation test to detect CMV antibody in CID patients. Finally, in 1970, Wentworth and French devised a plaque assay using two sequential agarose overlays: this technique is still the method of choice and is a practical, reliable, and accurate way to quantitate CMV.

For diagnosis of congenital CMV infection, isolation of virus has remained the most important indicator. However, identification of CMV infections can be accomplished by examination of the urine sediment, isolation of the virus in cell culture, and serological techniques which include neutralization, complement fixation, and various fluorescent antibody tests. The indirect immunofluorescent (IF) method used to detect CMV IgM antibody is the most sensitive of the serological techniques (Hanshaw, 1969). Of 50 infants under 1 year with congenital CID, 48 had detectable CMV-specific IgM globulin. However, the test is not nearly as reliable in asymptomatic infants. The direct fluorescent antibody technique has been employed for rapid detection of CMV in urine (Anderson and Michaels, 1972). Stagno *et al.* (1975) studied infants with congenital and acquired CMV infection using several serological assays. They found that congenitally infected infants bear a greater antigenic burden than the natally infected. Diagnostically, the fluorescent antibody test to late antigen was the most sensitive assay, the indirect hemagglutination assay slightly less sensitive, and the complement-fixation test the least sensitive. Griffiths and associates (1978) compared the complement-fixation, indirect IF, and anticomplement immunofluorescence (ACIF) tests and found that, although the titers obtained using ACIF and indirect IF were eight times higher than those obtained by using complement fixation, the enhanced sensitivity of the former tests did not produce an increased rate of detection of CMV seropositive sera. Cremer *et al.* (1978*a*) have recently reported, using the indirect hemagglutination test, that IgM reactivity with CMV antigen usually increased earlier than IgM reactivity detected by the complement-fixation method. Results from a subsequent study by these same investigators (1978*b*) on the role of rheumatoid factor in the complement-fixation and indirect hemagglutination tests demonstrate that the IgM-rheumatoid factor may lead to false-positive reactions in the complement-fixation test for IgM CMV antibody and that some patients produce an IgM antibody which will fix complement. In the indirect hemagglutination test, the removal of rheumatoid factor has little or no effect on the reaction of the IgM fraction of sera with CMV. Two recent groups of investigators (Henry *et al.*, 1978; Lee *et al.*, 1978) have used electron microscopy to rapidly detect the presence of CMV in infected infants. Both groups detected virus in the urine, and Lee *et al.* (1978) were able to detect CMV particles from oral specimens as well. The time to detect CMV in the specimens ranged from 15 to 30 min (Lee *et al.*, 1978) to 4 hr (Henry *et al.*, 1978). Sophisticated molecular techniques such as cRNA-DNA membrane hybridization, cRNA-DNA cytohybridization *in situ*, DNA-DNA reassociation kinetics, and the ACIF test have been used to detect the presence of human CMV antigens and genomes (Huang *et al.*, 1976). These methods have been used to analyze strain variations. Differences seem to exist among CMV strains, but it is premature to classify the strains into types. Zablotney *et al.* (1978) have studied different strains of human CMV in an attempt to determine antigenic relatedness. Of the 17 strains they studied using the kinetic neutralization test, four antigenic groups seem to be represented. McAllister *et al.* (1964) observed CID in newborn twins, with one twin dying at day 3 and the other one surviving the infection. It is presumed from this investigation that one strain can produce both fatal and nonfatal disease. A recent report (Huang *et al.*, 1978) describes the isolation of a CMV from the brain biopsy of a child with encephalopathy. The results of the antigenic studies suggest that this isolate is genetically related to simian CMV.

4. CLINICAL DISEASE

Cytomegalovirus is now known to be responsible for a wide spectrum of diseases, particularly several causing severe damage to the fetus and newborn infant (Table 3). These infections are extremely serious in that they often affect the fetus of an asymptomatically infected expectant mother. The resulting damage can afflict the newborn infant, if it is not stillborn, with deafness, blindness, microcephaly, pneumonia, mental retardation, cerebral palsy, jaundice, thrombocytopenia, and hepatosplenomegaly (Hanshaw, 1964; Me-

TABLE 3

Diseases Due to Cytomegalovirus

Primary diseases	Associated diseases
Cytomegalic inclusion disease	Guillain-Barré syndrome
Abortion	Kaposi sarcoma
Heterophile-negative mononucleosis	Cancer of the prostate
Interstitial pneumonia	Cervical cancer
Microcephaly	
Mental retardation	
Deafness	
Congenital CMV	
Blindness	
Jaundice	
Cerebral palsy	
Hepatosplenomegaly	
Thrombocytopenia	

dearis, 1964). The consequences of congenital infection are devastating, with most surviving children suffering from extensive mental and motor dysfunction.

Today, in the United States, approximately 3000 children are born with severe retardation as a result of congenital infections, and an average of 1% of all infants are infected with CMV at birth (Marx, 1975).

The most infamous of all CMV-induced diseases is congenital CID. It is a dreaded infection during pregnancy since a woman can be asymptomatically infected and pass the disease to the fetus. In addition, the disease is often fatal; however, even when it is not, the consequences are not optimal. Controversy exists concerning the route and manner of infection during pregnancy. It is still unclear whether the fetus is infected *in utero* following a primary infection of the mother or whether infection is due to reactivation of latent virus. Gehrz *et al.* (1977) studied the cell-mediated immune response in young children and mothers with CMV infections. They found that four children had a CMV-specific cell-mediated immune defect; they had antibodies to CMV and were shedding the virus in the urine. Three of the four mothers had decreased cell-mediated immunity to CMV. They suggest from their study that an antigen-specific immune defect aids the transmission of CMV from the mother to the infant and allows for persistence in the child. Starr *et al.* (1977) concur with the 1977 report of Gehrz and colleagues and have observed that a diminished blasto-genic response to purified CMV antigen exists in congenitally CMV-infected infants and their mothers. They also noticed that immune defects are detectable even in asymptomatically infected children.

In addition to the more common clinical pictures resulting from congenital CMV infection, i.e., jaundice, pneumonia, and hepatosple-nomegaly, other clinical manifestations have been associated with postnatally acquired CMV. Children who acquire CMV infections after birth are usually healthy with inapparent signs of infection: exposure to the virus is high and infection is quite common. One study (Hanshaw et al., 1965) followed 20 asymptomatic but CMV-positive children. From this group, 14 had hepatomegaly, and abnormal results in liver-function tests were obtained 6 times more often in virus-positive children than in the controls. The presence of liver abnormalities may indicate an active role of CMV in the liver. Cytomegalovirus infection of the inner ear is known to occur in infants infected congenitally as well as postnatally. Davis et al. (1977) reported an endolymphatic labyrinthitis due to CMV infection, suggesting that infection of the inner ear is due to spread of the virus into the endolabyrinth through capillaries of the stria vascu-laris. Another study (Hart et al., 1978) has detailed the isolation of CMV from the eye of a 3-year-old child with juvenile iridocyclitis, a chronic disorder. The child was otherwise healthy, had not demonstrated any signs of congenital disease, and did not have chorioretinitis. Whitley et al. (1976) observed two infants who developed a protracted pneumonitis at the age of 1 month. They were able to detect CMV in the lung biopsies. They assume that CMV was acquired at birth from infected genital tracts of the mothers.

Cytomegalic inclusion disease has also been reported in child-ren with leukemia or lymphosarcoma (Gottmann and Beatty, 1962; Benyesh-Melnick et al., 1964; Bodey et al., 1965; Cox and Hughes, 1975b). However, association between CMV and the development of leukemias and lymphomas has not been established. More likely, CMV has been reactivated because of the immunosuppressive regimens that the patients are given. However, in the study by Bodey et al. (1965), they suggest that CID resulted from primary exposure to the virus in a group of highly susceptible patients. They proposed this idea since 11 CMV infections were diagnosed during a 13-month period and followed the pattern of epidemic spread.

Cytomegalic inclusion disease is extremely uncommon among adults and is usually a terminal complication of another serious disease. This disease, when localized, usually involves gastrointestinal ulcers

(Levine *et al.*, 1964) or the lungs, but as a generalized disease it is often unrecognizable clinically, masked by a second disease, and diagnosed as a CMV infection only at autopsy (Wong and Warner, 1962). An interesting case involving an adult with hypogammaglobulinemia and a thymoma was reported by Jacox *et al.* (1964). They were able to isolate CMV from the urine and sputum of this individual on several occasions, and a pulmonary infection in the patient was most probably due to CMV infection. Nakoneczna and Kay (1967) reported a fatal, generalized CID in an elderly woman with a lesion of the gastrointestinal tract, and Freeman *et al.* (1977) described a patient with late-onset immunodeficiency syndrome who developed intractable diarrhea due to a widespread CMV infection of the gastrointestinal tract. Other investigators (Chin *et al.*, 1973; Henson *et al.*, 1974; Behrens and Quick, 1974; Minars *et al.*, 1977; Murray *et al.*, 1977; Sahud and Bachelor, 1978) have reported adult cases of meningoencephalitis, hepatitis, interstitial pneumonitis, vasculitis, retinitis, and thrombocytopenia, respectively, which have been shown to be caused by CMV infection.

Another disease which is caused by CMV is a type of infectious mononucleosis. This disease was first reported by Klemola and Kääriäinen in 1965; they observed a significant rise in the titer of complement-fixing antibodies to CMV in patients who had a mononucleosis-like disease but did not react positively in the heterophile agglutination test. They also noticed a significant rise in the titer of CMV neutralizing antibodies. The disease is characterized by malaise, myalgia, fever, abnormal liver functions, and atypical lymphocytosis; occasional lymphadenopathy and splenomegaly are present but not as frequently as seen with EBV-induced infectious mononucleosis. Reports by Jordan *et al.* (1973), Causey (1976), and Rinaldo *et al.* (1977) have followed cases of CMV-caused mononucleosis: Jordan *et al.* (1973) suggest that the disease may be venereally transmitted. Rinaldo *et al.* (1977) observed that patients with CMV mononucleosis are infected with virus that may persist within the peripheral blood leukocytes and that the lymphocytes of the patients are less responsive to certain mitogens.

A recent study (Schmitz and Enders, 1977) has associated CMV with Guillain-Barré syndrome based on the presence of IgM antibodies. To date, this syndrome has been linked with a number of viruses including measles, mumps, rubella, HSV, and varicella-zoster. These investigators postulate that, although Guillain-Barré syndrome may result from many factors, the presence of high titers of CMV-specific IgM antibodies in nine out of ten patients may be important in demonstrating that CMV is responsible for some cases of Guillain-

Barré syndrome. Supporting this report is the observation by Dowling *et al.* (1977) that elevated complement-fixing antibody levels to CMV were detected in 33% of patients with Guillain-Barré syndrome, and that, although measles virus and adenovirus were also tested, there was no significant elevation in antibody levels to the other viruses.

5. LATENCY AND PERSISTENCE

Infection with CMV is followed by persistence of the virus in latent form, probably for life. From time to time, virus is known to reactivate from the latent state in response to an imbalance in the immunological integrity of the host. Although the conditions that trigger the reactivation of CMV may, in fact, seem quite diverse, they are closely related in that there is a compromise in the immune status of the individual. Clinical situations which allow for the reactivation of CMV include pregnancy, organ and bone marrow transplants, immunosuppressive therapies for the treatment of malignancies, and blood transfusions. All share common features: a change in the immune system and the presence of foreign antigens.

The type of cell in which CMV persists is unknown; however, there is some evidence that it exists in human lymphocytes as is the case with the EBV (Pagano, 1975*b*; St. Jeor and Weisser, 1977). Lang and Noren (1968) observed a postnatal cytomegaloviremia and -viruria in congenitally infected children and postulated that CMV is harbored in leukocytes in a latent state. *In vitro* experiments have utilized human embryo fibroblast (Gönczöl and Váczi, 1973) and epithelial (St. Jeor and Weisser, 1977) cells to study latency of CMV. CMV has also been detected in leukocytes (Fiala *et al.*, 1975). A report by Joncas *et al.* (1975) claimed that CMV DNA has persisted in an EBV-transformed human lymphoblastoid line; however, it is not known whether the presence of CMV in this line is fortuitous or is directly related to the transformation of the line. St. Jeor and Weisser (1977) observed that human CMV-infected lymphocytes produce an infection that resembles a persistent infection rather than the type of infection normally seen in human fibroblasts. Pagano (1975*b*) reported that CMV has been demonstrated in human kidney epithelial cells using cRNA-DNA hybridization *in situ* and that CMV may replicate in human spermatozoa. *In vitro*, CMV replicates preferentially in fibroblastoid cells, although *in vivo* replication may occur in a variety of cells including those of epithelial origin (Lang *et al.*, 1976).

Persistence is a state in which a host has been infected by a virus and has been unable to eradicate the virus infection. As a result, virus continues to replicate and is actively shed. Latency occurs when the host is no longer shedding virus but is harboring the virus in a "silent" condition. Sophisticated techniques have now demonstrated CMV genetic material in hosts where there was no evidence of whole virus or virus antigens. CMV latency is probably more prevalent than is realized since the virus can be harbored with no direct effect on its host.

6. TRANSMISSION

The way in which CMV can be transmitted is still not clear, although the virus is present in saliva and urine and it is likely that transmission occurs as a result of contact with these excretions. Acquisition of CMV will occur congenitally, natally, venereally, and through blood transfusions and organ and bone transplants. Individuals who are immunosuppressed are particularly susceptible to infection; however, a study of leukemic children demonstrated that standard isolation (quarantine) procedures are of no help in preventing CMV infection (Cox and Hughes, 1975*a*). Transmission of CMV is also possible by reactivation of latent virus. In addition, an asymptomatically infected individual may be able to transmit the virus.

6.1. Congenital Infection

6.1.1. Symptomatic

Congenital CMV infection is acquired by *in utero* transmission of CMV from mother to child. Congenital CMV infection produces a wide spectrum of clinical manifestations, including microcephaly, blindness, deafness, and mental retardation. It has been reported (Hanshaw, 1966*b*; Stern, 1975) that significant developmental problems exist even in children who have not been seriously affected by CID. These children have been congenitally infected but are asymptomatic at birth. In a report by Ahlfors *et al.* (1978), it was reported that prolonged CMV excretion can occur following congenital and postnatal infections. Symptomatic congenital CMV infection is manifested in the patient by the dreaded CID. Since CMV is known to cross the placenta, it would be interesting to know when central nervous system damage of the fetus due to CID occurs. Stern and Tucker (1973) observed that fetal infection occurred more commonly during the first or second trimester. It is currently held that the first trimester of pregnancy is the most critical period for contracting a CMV infection and for passing it on to the fetus. Hanshaw (1971) reported the results of retrospective and prospective studies on congenital CMV infection. Based on the results of the retrospective study he was unable to assess the amount of central nervous system damage due to CMV. In the prospective studies he observed that 17% of the infants followed had some type of central nervous system damage. Diosi *et al.* (1967) reported the recovery of CMV from a milk specimen and uterine discharge of a recently delivered mother and from uterine discharge of a patient who had just aborted, suggesting that offspring may be infected after birth by infected milk and that intrauterine infection of the fetus is highly likely.

In children who were congenitally infected with CMV, there is evidence (Lang and Noren, 1968) that viremia can persist for many months in the circulating leukocytes. A major study by MacDonald and Tobin (1978) in England tested over 6000 neonates for virus excretion. They found an excretion rate of approximately 2.4 per 1000, which is similar to the rate in the United States. In addition, they observed that, if characteristic central nervous system (CNS) signs are recognized neonatally, there is only a 7% chance of delivering a normal child; if CNS signs are present but not characteristic of CMV infection, then there is a 40% chance of the child developing normally; however, there may be an absence of neurological signs in the presence of a serious infection. A highly immune population of young women was studied (Stagno *et al.*, 1977) to determine whether the presence of antibodies to CMV would protect the fetus. They found that infection *in utero* occurred in 3.4% of the seroimmune women and suggest that maternal humoral antibody may not protect the fetus against congenital CMV infection and that recurrent maternal CMV infections may be responsible for transmission rather than a primary infection. Cox and Hughes (1974) studied children with CID and were able to isolate CMV from the feces. Particularly interesting is their observation that CMV was isolated from the feces of all CID cases, but, in patients who were excreting CMV from other areas, there was no evidence of CID. Several clinical studies have been conducted to determine the incidence of cytomegaloviruria in newborns. Two of these studies (Starr and Gold, 1968; Birnbaum *et al.*, 1969) revealed that, of the congenitally infected infants excreting virus in their urine, none showed any evidence of CID. Cytomegalovirus has also been isolated from the cerebrospinal fluid (Jamison and Hathorn, 1978) of a congenitally infected infant.

6.1.2. Asymptomatic

Asymptomatic congenital infections appear to be present among newborns. There is evidence (Starr *et al.*, 1970) that primipara younger mothers are more likely to give birth to infected infants and that their babies are more likely to have lower birth weights than uninfected controls. A later investigation by Kumar *et al.* (1973) extended this study by following the physical and mental development of the children described by Starr *et al.* (1970). They found that the children with inapparent congenital CMV infection at birth were indistinguishable from the controls at 4 years of age. It is unknown whether hearing difficulties and learning disabilities developed as the children matured. A 1974 study by Reynolds *et al.* demonstrated that a consequence of asymptomatic CMV infection may be auditory deficiency; this is often accompanied by subnormal intelligence. This is in contrast to the study by Kumar *et al.* (1973) in which the IQ of infected children was similar to that of the control children. In 1976, Hanshaw and his associates studied a group of asymptomatically infected children and found a decrease in the IQ of infected children as compared to controls, as well as a hearing loss. They are convinced that inapparent CMV infections can seriously disturb CNS development.

6.2. Natal Infection

Many infants contract a primary CMV infection after birth but during the first year of life (Numazaki *et al.*, 1970; Plotkin, 1977). It is not clear whether the infection is the result of transplacental transmission from the mother during pregnancy or by cervical infection during delivery. Reynolds *et al.* (1973) found that CMV infection of infants in the first 3 months of life could be correlated to cervical excretion of the virus by the mother late in the final trimester. They concur with Numazaki *et al.* (1970) that an infected cervix is a major route of natal transmission of CMV. Many infants exposed to CMV during birth or shortly after delivery are not protected by passive humoral antibody and contract a primary CMV infection (Reynolds *et al.*, 1978*b*). Studies have now shown that the incidence of sequelae following *in utero* infection is much greater than that for natal infection.

6.3. Venereal Transmission

Cytomegalovirus is capable of producing cervicitis and urethritis following venereal transmission (Evans, 1976). The first observation demonstrating CMV in semen appeared in 1972, when Lang and Kummer reported the presence of CMV replicating in the genital tract of a male recovering from CMV mononucleosis. CMV was detected in semen from the testicles, seminal vesicles, prostate, and accessory ducts and tissues. The male, at the time of virus isolation, was asymptomatic. CMV has also been recovered more frequently from the cervix of younger women with only one pregnancy than from women over 25 years with multiple births (Montgomery *et al.*, 1972); this may be directly related to sexual activity. A seroepidemiological study comparing women seen in a venereal disease clinic with nuns found that the prevalence of CMV antibodies in nuns was significantly lower than that in women from the clinic as well as from women from upper and lower socioeconomic backgrounds, suggesting that venereal or salivary contact may account for a transmission route in adults (Davis *et al.*, 1975). A later study by Lang and Kummer (1975) demonstrated additional cases of CMV present in semen; virus was detectable in semen even when it was undetectable in blood and urine. A recent and very interesting study (Chretien *et al.*, 1977) documents the development of CMV mononucleosis in two men following sexual contact with a woman who had a similar illness several months earlier. The woman presented with CMV in her urine and cervix. A new sexual contact of one of the men developed a CMV infection. Waner *et al.* (1977) isolated CMV from 10% of women who were seen at a venereal disease clinic; they found that CMV genital infections elicit a secretory IgA antibody response and have indirect evidence which associates secretory IgA antibody with a recent CMV infection.

The venereal transmission of CMV is extremely important and may be responsible for initiating some types of genital cancer in humans (for discussion, refer to Sections 8.1 and 8.4).

6.4. Blood Transfusions

Cytomegalovirus has been associated with an illness that develops in patients following cardiopulmonary bypass surgery. This illness is now known as CMV mononucleosis but is also referred to as the postperfusion syndrome. In addition, patients undergoing surgical procedures other than the bypass but receiving blood transfusions risk CMV infections. Stevens *et al.* (1970) reported that 32% of the patients studied had a fourfold or greater rise in CMV complement-fixing antibody titer following whole blood transfusions, although CMV could be isolated from only one patient. A study to determine the incidence of CMV isolated from peripheral blood leukocytes of healthy blood bank donors was completed by Mirkovic *et al.* (1971). They were unable to detect CMV in any of the specimens tested. Armstrong *et al.* (1971) were able to isolate CMV from the blood erythrocyte and leukocyte layers as well as plasma and serum of seven postsurgical patients. Monif *et al.* (1976) learned from their study that blood is a mode of transmission for CMV but that the inability to distinguish heterologous antibody from homologous antibody makes it extremely difficult to eliminate blood units that may contain CMV. A recent report (Bryan *et al.*, 1978) describes a postpartum CMV infection in a woman who had a history of blood transfusions. At the time, the woman was not immunosuppressed and not pregnant; yet a latent CMV, possibly transmitted from the transfused blood, caused a serious infection.

6.5. Organ and Bone Transplants

Cytomegalovirus infection is a known complication following hemodialysis and renal transplantation. The manifestation of CID in renal transplant recipients appears to occur coincidentally with the use of drugs to suppress the immunological rejection of the transplant. In a study of patients with CID following transplants, 32% had received immunosuppressive therapies (Kanich and Craighead, 1966). Only patients who survived the transplantation for 1 or more months contracted CID, and it was quite evident that the onset of disease was directly linked to the drug therapy. Craighead *et al.* (1967) also observed that CMV infection was present in 73% of patients who survived 1 or more months after transplantation. Infection was higher among patients (91%) with serological evidence of exposure to CMV before transplantation than in the group of patients (47%) with no detectable antibody at the time of surgery. It is possible that the CMV infection is a reactivation of latent virus or that there is exposure to CMV after the transplant (Craighead, 1969). There is also evidence which suggests that some patients who develop CMV undergo a change in their antibody response while on immunosuppressive therapy: the antibody levels decrease or fail completely (Craighead, 1969). Several groups of investigators (Lopez *et al.*, 1974; Fiala *et al.*, 1975; Ho *et al.*, 1975; Rubin *et al.*, 1977; Simmons *et al.*, 1977) have studied the epidemiology of CMV infections following transplantation and immunosuppressive therapy. Lopez and his colleagues have speculated that a CMV infection is responsible for triggering the rejection of a transplant or that the rejection of a transplant activates a latent virus. Ho and his colleagues, using complement-fixation tests, observed results similar to those of Craighead *et al.* (1967) and also noticed that antibody to CMV has little protective effect. CMV infection in a nonimmune renal recipient may be transmitted in the kidneys transplanted from latently infected seropositive donors. However, another report (Naraqi *et al.*, 1978) suggests that only 6% of the allograft kidneys studied were infected with CMV. A group of renal transplant patients were studied for development of CMV and HSV infections (Pass *et al.*, 1978). The investigators found that HSV infections occurred in the first month after transplant when immunosuppressive therapy was at its peak; CMV infection was more common in patients from 1 to 6 months and then the virus persisted in most patients. Two cases of CMV infection developing 2 years after kidney transplantation were reported (Linnemann *et al.*, 1978*a*), with one case presenting as a primary CMV infection and the other a reactivation of a latent infection. Linnemann *et al.* (1978*b*) also reported the results of a prospective study of 15 renal transplant recipients and the effect of the transplantation on the cellular immune response to CMV. They found a dissociation of the humoral and cellular immune response to CMV infection in these patients and also that cellular immunity, if present before transplantation, disappeared as a result of the immunosuppressive therapy. This was followed by reactivation of CMV infection with a normal humoral immune response. Pollard *et al.* (1978) studied the cell-mediated immune response of normal subjects and cardiac transplant patients to CMV infection and found that normal subjects with recent CMV infection have increased responses compared to the cardiac transplant recipients who have depressed responses even though many are suffering from overt CMV infection. Tests of the cellular immune response to CMV may help in identifying times of increased susceptibility to infection.

In addition to the complications of renal transplantations due to CMV, liver homograft recipients (Fulginiti *et al.*, 1968) and bone marrow recipients (Pagano, 1975*a*; Rinaldo *et al.*, 1976) also contract CMV infections. A high incidence of death in bone marrow recipients is due to the interstitial pneumonia caused by CMV (Neiman *et al.*, 1977). The failure to respond serologically to CMV infection apparently places a patient at an increased risk for development of interstitial pneumonia, often a fatal disease in these patients. Strong *et al.* (1978) studied the cellular immune response in a bone marrow transplantation patient. They found that lymphoid cells specifically recognize and respond *in vitro* by transformation to a CMV-infected cell line and by production of a macrophage migration-inhibition factor to CMV antigen. A blocking factor that inhibited these assays was contained in the plasma and spinal fluid of the patient. The blocking factor may be an antigen–antibody complex.

7. *IN VITRO* TRANSFORMATION OF MAMMALIAN CELLS

Several properties of human CMV are similar to certain characteristics associated with oncogenic DNA viruses (Table 4). These properties include the stimulation of cell DNA and RNA synthesis (St. Jeor *et al.*, 1974; Tanaka *et al.*, 1975). In 1973, Albrecht and Rapp were successful in transforming hamster embryo fibroblasts with ultraviolet-inactivated CMV to a malignant state. Properties of CMV-transformed cells are listed in Table 5. These studies followed the earlier experiments of Duff and Rapp (1971, 1973) in which HSV was used to transform hamster cells. Both the HSV- and CMV-transformed cells are oncogenic in hamsters. Since the etiology of prostate cells is unknown and there has been some evidence suggesting a role for CMV in the development of prostatic cancer, a project was initiated with normal human prostate cells (Rapp *et al.*, 1975). These prostate cells were originally infected with CMV *in vivo* (Webber *et al.*, 1974); *in*

TABLE 4

Properties of Cytomegalovirus Related to Oncogenesis

Large number of naturally defective particles
Persists in host for extended period in various tissues
Stimulates host DNA and RNA synthesis
Transforms cells to malignancy

TABLE 5

Properties of Cytomegalovirus-Transformed Cells

Changes in morphology
Extended lifetime in culture (immortal)
Retention of fragment(s) of virus DNA
Synthesis of virus antigens in nucleus, cytoplasm, and membrane of cells
Resistance to superinfection
Malignant with metastases

vitro they developed a long-term persistent infection followed by a latent infection and grew to passage levels that were significantly higher than those attained by normal cells. The virus could not be rescued in the latent stage, although CMV-specific antigens and nucleic acids could be detected. These cells were subsequently transformed *in vitro* by the human CMV isolate of prostatic origin (Geder *et al.*, 1976). These transformed cells are tumorigenic in nude mice (Geder *et al.*, 1977*a*), have detectable nuclear antigens (Geder and Rapp, 1977), exhibit lack of contact inhibition in cell culture (Figs. 5 and 6), and react positively with CMV-immune sera in indirect IF tests (Geder *et al.*, 1977*a*). The CMV-transformed cells are also resistant to superinfection with CMV (Fig. 7) but not to HSV, a possible indication that the CMV genome is present in the cells. Thus the transforming ability of

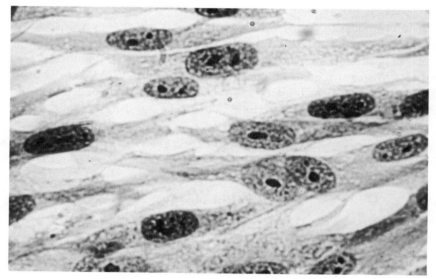

Fig. 5. Normal human embryo lung cells in culture. Stained with hematoxylin and eosin.

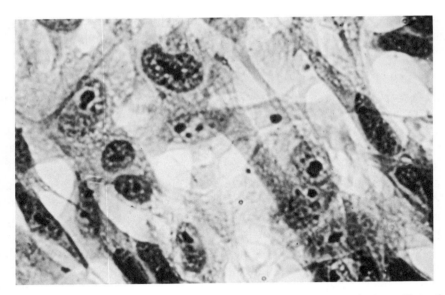

Fig. 6. Human embryo lung cells exposed *in vitro* to cytomegalovirus. Note the "criss-cross" pattern of growth. Stained with hematoxylin and eosin.

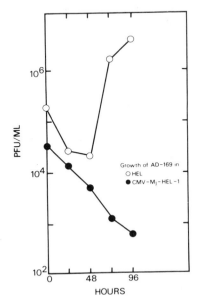

Fig. 7. Replication of cytomegalovirus (CMV) in human embryo lung (O) and CMV-transformed human embryo lung (●) cells. Multiplicity of infection was 5 plaque-forming units per cell. From Figueroa *et al.* (1978).

noninactivated CMV has been demonstrated and strengthens the argument that this virus may be reponsible for the development of neoplasias in humans under natural conditions (Rapp and Geder, 1978).

8. ASSOCIATION OF CYTOMEGALOVIRUS WITH CANCER IN HUMANS

The herpesvirus group has several members that produce naturally occurring neoplasias in nonhuman species. These include the Lucké frog virus, which produces renal adenocarcinomas in leopard frogs, and Marek's disease virus, which is responsible for a lymphoproliferative disease of chickens. Herpesvirus ateles and herpesvirus saimiri also produce malignancies but not in their natural hosts. For these reasons, the human herpesviruses have been carefully observed for many years for association with human neoplastic disease. Laboratory investigators, epidemiologists, and clinicians, as well as others, have followed and studied the pathogenesis of disease due to human herpesviruses. Today it is widely accepted that EBV plays a major role in the development of Burkitt lymphoma; less clear is the association of this virus with nasopharyngeal carcinoma. Herpes simplex virus is suspected of causing cervical cancer, but, although the evidence is now impressive, there is still much controversy over the etiology of the disease. Since CMV shares many properties with EBV and HSV and since many of these properties are characteristic of transforming viruses, CMV is now being studied for its possible role in certain malignant conditions of humans.

8.1. Prostatic Cancer

In the United States today, adenocarcinoma of the prostate is the second most common cause of mortality from cancer. The prostate is the repository for CMV which is transmitted venereally (Lang and Kummer, 1972), and persistent viruria and viremia can be detected in asymptomatic patients following CMV infection (Lang *et al.*, 1975). Centifanto *et al.* (1973) demonstrated the presence of herpesvirus antigens in the nuclei of prostatic cancer cells of primary explants, and Rapp *et al.* (1975) reported the presence of CMV in normal prostate tissue from a 3-year-old donor at autopsy. In a preliminary experiment Geder *et al.* (1977*b*) reported that sera from patients with prostatic cancer reacted twice as frequently in IF tests with CMV-transformed human cells than did sera from the control group. Sanford *et al.* (1977) detected significant humoral antibody titers against CMV and found that a greater percentage of prostatic cancer patients had higher titers against CMV than the other groups tested and that patients with non-genitourinary tumors had lower titers. A later study by Sanford *et al.* (1978) reported that a high percentage of patients with prostatic adenocarcinoma and with benign prostatic hyperplasia have high titers against a CMV-transformed human cell line. Moreover, when CMV-infected human cell lines were used, more prostatic cancer patients demonstrated high CMV antibody titers than did patients with benign prostatic hyperplasia.

It is possible that CMV plays a major role in the etiology of prostatic cancer; however, it is likely that a cofactor(s) is required to produce a malignancy in the human host.

8.2. Kaposi Sarcoma

Kaposi sarcoma is primarily a skin cancer as evidenced by a multiple pigmented hemangiosarcoma. It is a disease that affects predominantly the native population of equatorial Africa, with low incidence in Europe and America. Immunological studies (Giraldo *et al.*, 1972) demonstrated soluble antigens in extracts of cells tested against CMV and EBV sera. It was not clear whether CMV and EBV were both infecting the Kaposi sarcoma lines or whether a new herpesvirus was present. European and African patients with Kaposi sarcoma were studied to determine whether the disease was associated with the presence of high titers of antibodies to CMV, EBV, HSV1, or HSV2 (Giraldo *et al.*, 1975). An increased incidence of high anti-CMV titers in European but not African cases and no specific serological association with HSV1, HSV2, or EBV was reported. Giraldo *et al.* (1978) extended the earlier seroepidemiological studies by following larger groups of Kaposi sarcoma patients. They used sera from American patients since the clinical behavior and expression of the disease is indistinguishable between American and European patients. They detected a specific serological association of CMV with American patients and speculate that CMV may be involved in the development of Kaposi sarcoma in a manner analogous to EBV and its role in Burkitt lymphoma. Glaser *et al.* (1977) reported the characterization of a herpes-type virus isolated from a cell culture that had been derived from biopsy material from a Kaposi sarcoma patient. Complement-fixation and IF tests confirmed the presence of CMV antigens, and the density of the virus DNA was consistent with CMV DNA. It is still not clear whether CMV is responsible for the initiation of Kaposi sarcoma, and only more sophisticated experiments will be able to answer this question.

8.3. Adenocarcinoma of the Colon

Two recent reports (Roche and Huang, 1977; Huang and Roche, 1978) have associated CMV with bowel disease and adenocarcinoma of the colon. In some patients with inflammatory bowel disease, a high incidence of antibody to CMV has been demonstrated in serological studies (Farmer *et al.*, 1973); however, the presence of virus in diseased tissue has not been detected by electron microscopy. Using membrane cRNA-DNA hybridization, Roche and Huang (1977) failed to demonstrate consistently the presence of CMV DNA in histologically normal or abnormal bowels from patients with inflammatory bowel disease; this included patients with Crohn's disease. The results from patients with ulcerative colitis were also inconsistent. In 1978 Huang and Roche reported the results of their investigations on CMV DNA and adenocarcinoma of the colon. Using membrane cRNA-DNA hybridization, they detected CMV DNA in four of seven tumors of the colon. Normal and abnormal colon tissues from Crohn's patients were negative for CMV DNA; however, in patients with conditions predisposing to adenocarcinoma of the colon, such as familial polyposis and ulcerative colitis, CMV DNA was detected. The studies in this area are still in their infancy, but the association is extremely interesting and the observation is important since it links CMV with another human neoplasia.

8.4. Cervical Cancer

Cervical cancer is a major cause of death due to cancer in women. Many studies have linked the etiology of this neoplasia to HSV2. Two reports (Pacsa *et al.*, 1975; Muñoz, 1976) speculate that CMV, since it is known to reside in the semen and is spread venereally, may be responsible for the induction of cervical cancer. The study by Pacsa *et al.* (1975) is based on the detection of antibodies and antigens in cervical anaplasia patients and controls. They found that, in sera of women with cervical atypia (61%), antibodies to CMV were detected more frequently than in sera of women with cervical disorders other than atypia (42%) or in sera from healthy controls (33%). However, they also observed the presence of antibodies to HSV in sera of patients with cervical atypia (58%) vs. the matched controls (23%). It is possible that CMV may be acting as a cofactor with HSV in the development of cervical cancer. Cytomegalovirus has been isolated from cell cultures derived from biopsies of advanced cervical cancers (Melnick *et al.*, 1978). All cervical cancer patients studied had higher antibody titers to the CMV isolates from the biopsy material than to the CMV AD169 prototype strain. Very few studies have investigated the possible involvement of CMV in the initiation of cervical cancer. It is possible that this virus may, in fact, play a major etiological role in this disease considering the venereal transmission of CMV and the current evidence linking CMV to cancer of the prostate.

9. VACCINES AND ANTIVIRAL AGENTS

Congenital CMV infection is a serious complication of pregnancy, and natally acquired CMV infections are quite common. Interest in controlling virus infections by the use of vaccines has grown in recent years, particularly in the area of herpesvirus vaccines. The reason, in part, is due to the absence of a safe, efficient therapeutic agent to prevent or control infections due to herpesviruses. As a result, there has been considerable controversy over the issues involved with the use of a herpesvirus vaccine. Since several members of the herpesvirus group are oncogenic and since at least two animal herpesviruses (Lucké and Marek's disease virus) are known to produce naturally occurring tumors in their hosts, the voices urging caution in the use of herpesvirus vaccines can be understood. However, Marek's disease is being controlled by an attenuated vaccine, which thus fuels the controversy concerning possible control of some human malignancy by vaccination. The development of a live attenuated CMV vaccine may be of great benefit but it must be approached conservatively since much needs to be learned about the pathogenesis and epidemiology of CMV infections. Reviews on viral vaccines have been prepared by Hanshaw (1974), Melnick (1977, 1978), and Phillips (1977).

In 1974, Elek and Stern reported the development of a CMV vaccine against mental retardation. They subcutaneously inoculated 26 volunteers with a live cell-culture-adapted strain of CMV and observed mild reactions in 12 individuals. Ninety-five percent seroconverted and there was no virus excreted in saliva or urine up to 8 weeks after vaccination. Seroconversion by oral administration was unsuccessful, and intradermal inoculations strong enough to produce seroconversion resulted in severe reactions. To date, there has been no reported follow-up of the volunteers used in this study. Plotkin *et al.* (1975) also developed a live attenuated vaccine using the Towne strain of CMV which is resistant to trypsin and releases high amounts of extracellular virus. The vaccine was administered to adult volunteers by intranasal and subcutaneous routes: no infection resulted in 18 volunteers who received intranasal inoculation, although antibody responses were produced in ten volunteers subcutaneously inoculated. No virus excretion was detectable, and all volunteers remained healthy. A study involving live attenuated measles-mumps-rubella vaccine was undertaken by Reynolds *et al.* (1978*a*) to investigate the antibody response to this live vaccine in congenitally and natally CMV-infected infants. They found that humoral immunity to heterologous virus antigens is intact in infants with congenital and natal CMV infections even when excretion of the virus is detectable. This evidence suggests that infection with CMV does not have a negative effect on antibody production. Glazer *et al.* (1978) reported the study of the first renal transplant patient who received the live Towne strain CMV vaccine prior to the transplant. The transplant was rejected but before it would have been most susceptible to a CMV infection: virus reactivation did not occur although the patient was on immunosuppressive therapy. A second transplant recipient who received the vaccine has had a successful course without excretion of CMV while on immunosuppressive therapy.

It is still too early to know how safe these vaccines are and whether they will be effective. Four important safety considerations include immediate reactions, markers for attenuation, possible oncogenicity, and persistence of the CMV vaccine in a latent state. If a safe, effective CMV vaccine can be produced, it will be possible that CID of infants can be prevented by administering the vaccine to adolescent females. Further controlled and cautious studies in humans are required to determine the safety of a CMV vaccine.

Antiviral agents including cytosine arabinoside, adenine arabinoside, and interferon have also been used to treat CMV infections but with little or no success (Ch'ien *et al.*, 1974; O'Malley *et al.*, 1975; Alford and Whitley, 1976; Arvin *et al.*, 1976; Cheeseman *et al.*, 1977; Kraemer *et al.*, 1978; Pollard and Merigan, 1978). It appears that the virological and clinical responses to adenine arabinoside are determined to some extent by the condition of the infected host. The effect of interferon on CMV replication is greatly influenced by the input multiplicity and the nature of the inoculum (Holmes *et al.*, 1978).

Cheeseman *et al.* (1977) have also reported on the use of interferon in CMV infections in man. Although CMV is sensitive to interferon *in vitro*, its use as a therapeutic agent in controlling CMV infections in humans is still in the early stages. Vidarabine was used by Phillips *et al.* (1977) to treat two adult cases of CMV encephalitis; both patients showed dramatic improvement after treatment with the compound.

Antiviral chemotherapy is an undeveloped area of research at the present time. There is a great need for the development of safe, effective drugs to treat virus infections. It is to be hoped that the next few years will see the availability of safe compounds which will prevent and control infections due to herpesviruses.

10. LOOKING AHEAD

As acute microbial infections are better controlled by vaccines and chemotherapeutic agents, the chronic and latent infections of man will assume increasing prominence. This will become even more pronounced as the geriatric population increases and growing drug usage for medical problems immunocompromises the host during critical periods of illness. The consequent sequelae due to chronic and latent virus infections will be all the more damaging because they are unexpected and generally uncontrollable.

It remains unlikely that antimetabolites or interferon will serve to eradicate these infections; at best, they will help control selected disease syndromes. It also seems unlikely that transmission of cytomegalovirus will be changed without massive and unexpected changes in life style (i.e., sexual habits). Thus the rationale for effective control will rest primarily on immunopreventive or immunotherapeutic measures, possibly coupled with selected antiviral substances.

The earlier concepts of vaccination as a disease-preventive measure are probably not appropriate for viruses causing latent infection and recurrent disease as a consequence of reactivation. Attenuation of viruses known to cause latency is a myth, as most are measured for attenuation by injection into animals via unnatural routes (i.e., intracerebrally, subcutaneously). Even this crutch is not possible for human cytomegalovirus, which does not cause disease in any species tested except its natural host.

What solutions remain? One approach would be to determine those virus proteins responsible for eliciting protective reactions via humoral and cell-mediated mechanisms. The use of recombinant DNA technology could allow replication of the responsible gene(s) and large scale synthesis of the gene product(s) sought. Such a purified product(s) might safely prevent primary infection and even ameliorate or prevent recurrences. Again, caution will be needed in widespread use of such therapy in the human population and an experimental model for human CMV remains a desirable objective for preliminary evaluation. Failure to achieve this goal will probably mean that herpes simplex viruses, for which models exist, should be given priority in attempts to prevent disease with selected virus-specific gene products.

A species that has sent men to the moon, has learned to control and eradicate smallpox, and has doubled its own longevity within this century should be capable of devising measures to neutralize the hazards represented by a genome of 150 million daltons.

ACKNOWLEDGMENTS

I wish to thank Nancy Kain and Melissa Reese for their secretarial and editorial assistance, respectively. This chapter bears the special imprint of Barbara A. McCarthy, to whom I am very grateful. This work was supported in part by Contract NO1-CP-53516 within the Virus Cancer Program of the National Cancer Institute and by Grant CA 18450 awarded by the National Cancer Institute, DHEW.

11. REFERENCES

Ahlfors, K., Ivarsson, S.-A., Johnsson, T., and Svensson, I., 1978, Congenital and acquired cytomegalovirus infections. Virological and clinical studies on a Swedish infant population, *Acta Paediatr. Scand.* **67**:321.
Albrecht, T., and Rapp, F., 1973, Malignant transformation of hamster embryo fibroblasts following exposure to ultraviolet-irradiated human cytomegalovirus, *Virology* **55**:53.
Albrecht, T., Nachtigal, M., St. Jeor, S. C., and Rapp, F., 1976, Induction of cellular DNA synthesis and increased mitotic activity in Syrian hamster embryo cells abortively infected with human cytomegalovirus, *J. Gen. Virol.* **30**:167.
Alford, C. A., Jr., and Whitley, R. J., 1976, Treatment of infections due to herpesvirus in humans: A critical review of the state of the art, *J. Infect. Dis.* **133**:A101.
Anderson, C. H., and Michaels, R. H., 1972, Cytomegalovirus infection: Detection by direct fluorescent-antibody technique, *Lancet* **2**:308.
Armstrong, D., Ely, M., and Steger, L., 1971, Post-transfusion cytomegaloviremia and persistence of cytomegalovirus in blood, *Infect. Immun.* **3**:159.
Arvin, A. M., Yeager, A. S., and Merigan, T. C., 1976, Effect of leukocyte interferon on urinary excretion of cytomegalovirus by infants, *J. Infect. Dis.* **133**:A205.

Behrens, H. W., and Quick, C. A., 1974, Bronchoscopic diagnosis of cytomegalovirus infection, *J. Infect. Dis.* **130**:174.

Benyesh-Melnick, M., Dessy, S. I., and Fernbach, D. J., 1964, Cytomegaloviruria in children with acute leukemia and in other children, *Proc. Soc. Exp. Biol. Med.* **117**:624.

Birnbaum, G., Lynch, J. I., Margileth, A. M., Lonergan, W. M., and Sever, J. L., 1969, Cytomegalovirus infections in newborn infants, *J. Pediatr.* **75**:789.

Bodey, G. P., Wertlake, P. T., Douglas, G., and Levin, R. H., 1965, Cytomegalic inclusion disease in patients with acute leukemia, *Ann. Intern. Med.* **62**:899.

Bryan, C. S., Foster, C. M., and Edwards, W. G., 1978, Postpartum cytomegalovirus infection. A hazard of multiple transfusions, *Obstet. Gynecol.* **52**:68.

Causey, J. Q., 1976, Spontaneous cytomegalovirus mononucleosis-like syndrome and aseptic meningitis, *South. Med. J.* **69**:1384.

Centifanto, Y. M., Kaufman, H. E., Zam, Z. S., Drylie, D. M., and Deardourff, S. L., 1973, Herpesvirus particles in prostatic carcinoma cells, *J. Virol.* **12**:1608.

Cheeseman, S. H., Rinaldo, C. R., Jr., and Hirsch, M. S., 1977, Use of interferon in cytomegalovirus infections in man, *Tex. Rep. Biol. Med.* **35**:523.

Chi'en, L. T., Cannon, N. J., Whitley, R. J., Diethelm, A. G., Dismukes, W. E., Scott, C. W., Buchanan, R. A., and Alford, C. A., Jr., 1974, Effect of adenine arabinoside on cytomegalovirus infections, *J. Infect. Dis.* **130**:32.

Chin, W., Magoffin, R., Frierson, J. G., and Lennette, E. H., 1973, Cytomegalovirus infection. A case with meningoencephalitis, *J. Am. Med. Assoc.* **225**:740.

Chretien, J. H., McGinnis, C. G., and Muller, A., 1977, Venereal causes of cytomegalovirus mononucleosis, *J. Am. Med. Assoc.* **238**:1644.

Cox, F., and Hughes, W. T., 1974, Fecal excretion of cytomegalovirus in disseminated cytomegalic inclusion disease, *J. Infect. Dis.* **129**:732.

Cox, F., and Hughes, W. T., 1975a, The value of isolation procedures for cytomegalovirus infections in children with leukemia, *Cancer* **36**:1158.

Cox, F., and Hughes, W. T., 1975b, Cytomegaloviremia in children with acute lymphocytic leukemia, *J. Pediatr.* **87**:190.

Craighead, J. E., 1969, Immunologic response to cytomegalovirus infection in renal allograft recipients, *Am J. Epidemiol.* **90**:506.

Craighead, J. E., Hanshaw, J. B., and Carpenter, C. B., 1967, Cytomegalovirus infection after renal allotransplantation, *J. Am. Med. Assoc.* **201**:725.

Cremer, N. E., Hoffman, M., and Lennette, E. H., 1978a, Analysis of antibody assay methods and classes of viral antibodies in serodiagnosis of cytomegalovirus infection, *J. Clin. Microbiol.* **8**:153.

Cremer, N. E., Hoffman, M., and Lennette, E. H., 1978b, Role of rheumatoid factor in complement fixation and indirect hemagglutination tests for immunoglobulin M antibody to cytomegalovirus, *J. Clin. Microbiol.* **8**:160.

Davis, G. L., Spector, G. J., Strauss, M., and Middlekamp, J. N., 1977, Cytomegalovirus endolabyrinthitis, *Arch. Pathol. Lab. Med.* **101**:118.

Davis, L. E., Stewart, J. A., and Garvin, S., 1975, Cytomegalovirus infection: A seroepidemiologic comparison of nuns and women from a venereal disease clinic, *Am. J. Epidemiol.* **102**:327.

DeMarchi, J. M., and Kaplan, A. S., 1977, The role of defective cytomegalovirus particles in the induction of host cell DNA synthesis, *Virology* **82**:93.

DeMarchi, J. M., Blankenship, M. L., Brown, G. D., and Kaplan, A. S., 1978, Size and complexity of human cytomegalovirus DNA, *Virology* **89**:643.

Diosi, P., Babusceac, L., Nevinglovschi, O., and Kun-Stoicu, G., 1967, Cytomegalovirus infection associated with pregnancy, *Lancet* **1**:1063.

Dowling, P., Menonna, J., and Cook, S., 1977, Cytomegalovirus complement fixation antibody in Guillain-Barré syndrome, *Neurology* **27**:1153.

Duff, R., and Rapp, F., 1971, Properties of hamster embryo fibroblasts transformed *in vitro* after exposure to ultraviolet-irradiated herpes simplex virus type 2, *J. Virol.* **8**:469.

Duff, R., and Rapp, F., 1973, Oncogenic transformation of hamster embryo cells after exposure to inactivated herpes simplex virus type 1, *J. Virol.* **12**:209.

Edwards, R. L., 1976, Structural proteins of human cytomegalovirus, *Yale J. Biol. Med.* **49**:65.

Elek, S. D., and Stern, H., 1974, Development of a vaccine against mental retardation caused by cytomegalovirus infection *in utero*, *Lancet* **1**:1.

Estes, J. E., and Huang, E.-S., 1977, Stimulation of cellular thymidine kinases by human cytomegalovirus, *J. Virol.* **24**:13.

Evans, T. N., 1976, Sexually transmissible diseases, *Am. J. Obstet. Gynecol.* **125**: 116.

Farmer, G. W., Vincent, M. M., Fuccillo, D. A., Horta-Barbosa, L., Ritman, S., Sever, J. L., and Gitnick, G. L., 1973, Viral investigations in ulcerative colitis and regional enteritis, *Gastroenterology* **65**:8.

Fiala, M., Payne, J. E., Berne, T. V., Moore, T. C., Henle, W., Montgomerie, J. Z., Chatterjee, S. N., and Guze, L. B., 1975, Epidemiology of cytomegalovirus infection after transplantation and immunosuppression, *J. Infect. Dis.* **132**:421.

Fiala, M., Honess, R. W., Heiner, D. C., Heiner, J. W., Murnane, J., Wallace, R., and Guze, L. B., 1976, Cytomegalovirus proteins. I. Polypeptides of virions and dense bodies, *J. Virol.* **19**:243.

Figueroa, M. E., Geder, L., and Rapp, F., 1978, Replication of herpesviruses in human cells transformed by cytomegalovirus, *J. Gen. Virol.* **40**:391.

Freeman, H. J., Shnitka, T. K., Piercey, J. R. A., and Weinstein, W. M., 1977, Cytomegalovirus infection of the gastrointestinal tract in a patient with late onset immunodeficiency syndrome, *Gastroenterology* **73**:1397.

Fulginiti, V. A., Scribner, R., Groth, C. G., Putnam, B. A., Brettschneider, L., Gilbert, S., Porter, K. A., and Starzl, T. E., 1968, Infections in recipients of liver homografts, *N. Engl. J. Med.* **279**:619.

Furukawa, T., Fioretti, A., and Plotkin, S., 1973, Growth characteristics of cytomegalovirus in human fibroblasts with demonstration of protein synthesis early in viral replication, *J. Virol.* **11**:991.

Furukawa, T., Jean, J.-H., and Plotkin, S. A., 1978, Enhanced poliovirus replication in cytomegalovirus-infected human fibroblasts, *Virology* **85**:622.

Geder, L., 1976, Evidence for early nuclear antigens in cytomegalovirus-infected cells, *J. Gen. Virol.* **32**:315.

Geder, L, and Rapp, F., 1977, Evidence for nuclear antigens in cytomegalovirus-transformed human cells, *Nature (London)* **265**:184.

Geder, L., Lausch, R. N., O'Neill, F. J., and Rapp, F., 1976, Oncogenic transformation of human embryo lung cells by human cytomegalovirus, *Science* **192**:1134.

Geder, L., Kreider, J., and Rapp, F., 1977*a*, Human cells tranformed *in vitro* by human cytomegalovirus: Tumorigenicity in athymic nude mice, *J. Natl. Cancer Inst.* **58**:1003.

Geder, L., Sanford, E. J., Rohner, T. J., and Rapp, F., 1977*b*, Cytomegalovirus and cancer of the prostate: *In vitro* transformation of human cells, *Cancer Treat. Rep.* **61**:139.

Geelen, J., Walig, C., Wertheim, P., and van der Noordaa, J., 1978, Human cytomegalovirus DNA. I. Molecular weight and infectivity, *J. Virol.* **26**:813.

Gehrz, R. C., Marker, S. C., Knorr, S. O., Kalis, J. M., and Balfour, H. H., Jr., 1977, Specific cell-mediated immune defect in active cytomegalovirus infection of young children and their mothers, *Lancet* **1**:844.

Giraldo, G., Beth, E., and Haguenau, F., 1972, Herpes-type virus particles in tissue culture of Kaposi's sarcoma from different geographic regions, *J. Natl. Cancer Inst.* **49**:1509.

Giraldo, G., Beth, E., Kourilsky, F. M., Henle, W., Henle, G., Miké, V., Huraux, J. M., Andersen, H. K., Gharbi, M. R., Kyalwazi, S. K., and Puissant, A., 1975, Antibody patterns to herpesviruses in Kaposi's sarcoma: Serological association of European Kaposi's sarcoma with cytomegalovirus, *Int. J. Cancer* **15**:839.

Giraldo, G., Beth, E., Hämmerling, U., Tarro, G., and Kourilsky, F. M., 1977, Detection of early antigens in nuclei of cells infected with cytomegalovirus or herpes simplex virus type 1 and 2 by anti-complement immunofluorescence, and use of a blocking assay to demonstrate their specificity, *Int. J. Cancer* **19**:107.

Giraldo, G., Beth, E., Henle, W., Henle, G., Miké, V., Safai, B., Huraux, J. M., McHardy, J., and de Thé, G., 1978, Antibody patterns to herpesviruses in Kaposi's sarcoma. II. Serological association of American Kaposi's sarcoma with cytomegalovirus, *Int. J. Cancer* **22**:126.

Glaser, R., Geder, L., St. Jeor, S., Michelson-Fiske, S., and Haguenau, F., 1977, Partial characterization of a herpes-type virus (K9V) derived from Kaposi's sarcoma, *J. Natl. Cancer Inst.* **59**:55.

Glazer, J. P., Friedman, H. M., Grossman, R. A., Barker, C. F., Starr, S. E., and Plotkin, S. A., 1978, Cytomegalovirus vaccination and renal tranplantation, *Lancet* **1**:90.

Gönczöl, E., and Váczi, L., 1973, Cytomegalovirus latency in cultured human cells, *J. Gen. Virol.* **18**:143.

Goodheart, C. R., and Jaross, L. B., 1963, Human cytomegalovirus. Assay by counting infected cells, *Virology* **19**:532.

Goodheart, C. R., Filbert, J. E., and McAllister, R. M., 1963, Human cytomegalovirus. Effects of 5-fluorodeoxyuridine on viral synthesis and cytopathology, *Virology* **21**:530.

Gottmann, A. W., and Beatty, E. C., Jr., 1962, Cytomegalic inclusion disease in children with leukemia or lymphosarcoma, *Am. J. Dis. Child.* **104**:180.

Griffiths, P. D., Buie, K. J., and Heath, R. B., 1978, A comparison of complement fixation, indirect immunofluorescence for viral late antigens, and anti-complement immunofluorescence tests for the detection of cytomegalovirus specific serum antibodies, *J. Clin. Pathol.* **31**:827.

Gupta, P., and Rapp, F., 1978, Cyclic synthesis of human cytomegalovirus-induced proteins in infected cells, *Virology* **84**:199.

Gupta, P., St. Jeor, S., and Rapp, F., 1977, Comparison of the polypeptides of several strains of human cytomegalovirus, *J. Gen. Virol.* **34**:447.

Hanshaw, J. B., 1964, Clinical significance of cytomegalovirus infection, *Post. Med.* **35**:472.

Hanshaw, J. B., 1966a, Cytomegalovirus complement-fixing antibody in microcephaly, *N. Engl. J. Med.* **275**:476.

Hanshaw, J. B., 1966b, Congenital and acquired cytomegalovirus infection, *Pediatr. Clin. North Am.* **13**:279.

Hanshaw, J. B., 1969, Congenital cytomegalovirus infection: Laboratory methods of detection, *J. Pediatr.* **75**:1179.

Hanshaw, J. B., 1971, Congenital cytomegalovirus infection: A fifteen year perspective, *J. Infect. Dis.* **123**:555.

Hanshaw, J. B., 1974, A cytomegalovirus vaccine? *Am. J. Dis. Child.* **128**:141.

Hanshaw, J. B., Betts, R. F., Simon, G., and Boynton, R. C., 1965, Acquired cytomegalovirus infection. Association with hepatomegaly and abnormal liver-function tests, *N. Engl. J. Med.* **272**:602.

Hanshaw, J. B., Scheiner, A. P., Moxley, A. W., Gaev, L., Abel, V., and Scheiner, B., 1976, School failure and deafness after "silent" congenital cytomegalovirus infection, *N. Engl. J. Med.* **295**:468.

Hart, W. M., Jr., Reed, C. A., Freedman, H. L., and Burde, R. M., 1978, Cytomegalovirus in juvenile iridocyclitis, *Am. J. Ophthalmol.* **86**:329.

Henry, C., Hartsock, R. J., Kirk, Z., and Behrer, R., 1978, Detection of viruria in cytomegalovirus-infected infants by electron microscopy, *Am. J. Clin. Pathol.* **69**:435.

Henson, D. E., Grimley, P. M., and Strano, A. J., 1974, Postnatal cytomegalovirus hepatitis. An autopsy and liver biopsy study, *Hum. Pathol.* **5**:93.

Ho, M., Suwansirikul, S., Dowling, J. N., Youngblood, L. A., and Armstrong, J. A., 1975, The transplanted kidney as a source of cytomegalovirus infection, *N. Engl. J. Med.* **293**:1109.

Holmes, A. R., Rasmussen, L., and Merigan, T. C., 1978, Factors affecting the interferon sensitivity of human cytomegalovirus, *Intervirology* **9**:48.

Huang, E.-S., 1975a, Human cytomegalovirus. III. Virus-induced DNA polymerase, *J. Virol.* **16**:298.

Huang, E.-S., 1975b, Human cytomegalovirus. IV. Specific inhibition of virus-induced DNA polymerase activity and viral DNA replication by phosphonoacetic acid, *J. Virol.* **16**:1560.

Huang, E.-S., and Pagano, J. S., 1974, Human cytomegalovirus. II. Lack of related-ness to DNA of herpes simplex I and II, Epstein-Barr virus, and nonhuman strains of cytomegalovirus, *J. Virol.* **13**:642.

Huang, E.-S., and Roche, J. K., 1978, Cytomegalovirus DNA and adenocarcinoma of the colon: Evidence for latent viral infection, *Lancet* **1**:957.

Huang, E.-S., Chen, S.-T., and Pagano, J. S., 1973, Human cytomegalovirus. I. Purification and characterization of viral DNA, *J. Virol.* **12**:1473.

Huang, E.-S., Kilpatrick, B. A., Huang, Y.-T., and Pagano, J. S., 1976, Detection of human cytomegalovirus and analysis of strain variation, *Yale J. Biol. Med.* **49**:29.

Huang, E.-S., Kilpatrick, B., Lakeman, A., and Alford, C. A., 1978, Genetic analysis of a cytomegalovirus-like agent isolated from human brain, *J. Virol.* **26**:718.

Ihara, S., Hirai, K., and Watanabe, Y., 1978, Temperature-sensitive mutants of human cytomegalovirus: Isolation and partial characterization of DNA-minus mutants, *Virology* **84**:218.

Jack, I., and Wark, M. C., 1972, Immunofluorescent studies of the infection of fibro-blastoid cells within human cytomegaloviruses, in: *Oncogenesis and Herpesviruses*, (P. M. Biggs, G. de Thé and L. W. Payne, eds.), pp. 339–340, Lyon, France.

Jacox, R. F., Mongan, E. S., Hanshaw, J. B., and Leddy, J. P., 1964, Hypogammaglobulinemia with thymoma and probable pulmonary infection with cytomegalovirus, *N. Engl. J. Med.* **271**:1091.

Jamison, R. M., and Hathorn, A. W., Jr., 1978, Isolation of cytomegalovirus from cerebrospinal fluid of a congenitally infected infant, *Am. J. Dis. Child.* **132**:63.

Jean, J.-H., Yoshimura, N., Furukawa, T., and Plotkin, S. A., 1978, Intracellular forms of the parental cytomegalovirus genome at early stages of the infective process, *Virology* **86**:281.

Joncas, J. H., Menezes, J., and Huang, E.-S., 1975, Persistence of CMV genome in lymphoid cells after congenital infection, *Nature (London)* **258**:432.

Jordan, M. C., Rousseau, W. E., Stewart, J. A., Noble, G. R., and Chin, T. D. Y., 1973, Spontaneous cytomegalovirus mononucleosis. Clinical and laboratory observations in nine cases, *Ann. Intern. Med.* **79**:153.

Kanich, R. E., and Craighead, J. E., 1966, Cytomegalovirus infection and cytomegalic inclusion disease in renal homotransplant recipients, *Am. J. Med.* **40**:874.

Kierszenbaum, A. L., and Huang, E.-S., 1978, Chromatin pattern consisting of repeating bipartite structures in WI-38 cells infected with human cytomegalovirus, *J. Virol.* **28**:661.

Kilpatrick, B. A., and Huang, E.-S., 1977, Human cytomegalovirus genome: Partial denaturation map and organization of genome sequences, *J. Virol.* **24**:261.

Klemola, E., and Kääriäinen, L., 1965, Cytomegalovirus as a possible cause of a disease resembling infectious mononucleosis, *Br. Med. J.* **2**:1099.

Kraemer, K. G., Neiman, P. E., Reeves, W. C., and Thomas, E. D., 1978, Prophylactic adenine arabinoside following marrow transplantation, *Transplant. Proc.* **10**:237.

Krugman, R. D., and Goodheart, C. R., 1964, Human cytomegalovirus. Thermal inactivation, *Virology* **23**:290.

Kumar, M. L., Nankervis, G. A., and Gold, E., 1973, Inapparent congenital cytomegalovirus infection: A follow-up study, *N. Engl. J. Med.* **288**:1370.

Laing, A. C., 1974, Comparison of antiglobulin, direct and anti-complement immunofluorescent staining for the identification of cytomegalovirus in cultured human fibroblasts, *Can. J. Microbiol.* **20**:1353.

Lang, D. J., and Kummer, J. F., 1972, Demonstration of cytomegalovirus in semen, *N. Engl. J. Med.* **287**:756.

Lang, D. J., and Kummer, J. F., 1975, Cytomegalovirus in semen: Observations in selected populations, *J. Infect. Dis.* **132**:472.

Lang, D. J., and Noren, B., 1968, Cytomegaloviremia following congenital infection, *J. Pediatr.* **73**:812.

Lang, D. J., Kummer, J. F., and Hartley, D. P., 1975, Cytomegalovirus in semen, *N. Engl. J. Med.* **291**:121.

Lang, D. J., Cheung, K. S., Schwartz, J. N., Daniels, C. A., and Harwood, S. E., 1976, Cytomegalovirus replication and the host immune response, *Yale J. Biol. Med.* **49**:45.

Lee, F. K., Nahmias, A. J., and Stagno, S., 1978, Rapid diagnosis of cytomegalovirus infection in infants by electron microscopy, *N. Engl. J. Med.* **299**:1266.

Lee, M. S., and Balfour, H. H., Jr., 1977, Optimal method for recovery of cytomegalovirus from urine of renal transplant patients, *Transplantation* **24**:228.

Levine, R. S., Warner, N. E., and Johnson, C. F., 1964, Cytomegalic inclusion disease in the gastro-intestinal tract of adults, *Ann. Surg.* **159**:37.

Linnemann, C. C., Jr., Dunn, C. R., First, M. R., Alvira, M., and Schiff, G. M.,

1978*a*, Late onset of fatal cytomegalovirus infection after renal transplantation. Primary or reactivation infection? *Arch. Intern. Med.* **138:**1247.

Linnemann, C. C., Jr., Kauffman, C. A., First, M. R., Schiff, G. M., and Phair, J. P., 1978*b*, Cellular immune response to cytomegalovirus infection after renal transplantation, *Infect. Immun.* **22:**176.

Lopez, C., Simmons, R. L., Mauer, S. M., Najarian, J. S., Good, R. A., and Gentry, S., 1974, Association of renal allograft rejection with virus infections, *Am. J. Med.* **56:**280.

MacDonald, H., and Tobin, J. O'H. 1978, Congenital cytomegalovirus infection: A collaborative study on epidemiological, clinical and laboratory findings, *Dev. Med. Child Neurol.* **20:**471.

Marx, J. L., 1975, Cytomegalovirus: A major cause of birth defects, *Science* **190:**1184.

McAllister, R. M., Straw, R. M., Filbert, J. E., and Goodheart, C. R., 1963, Human cytomegalovirus. Cytochemical observations of intracellular lesion development correlated with viral synthesis and release, *Virology* **19:**521.

McAllister, R. M., Wright, H. T., Jr., and Tasem, W. M., 1964, Cytomegalic inclusion disease in newborn twins, *J. Pediatr.* **64:**278.

McGavran, M. H., and Smith, M. G., 1965, Ultrastructural, cytochemical, and microchemical observations on cytomegalovirus (salivary gland virus) infection of human cells in tissue culture, *Exp. Mol. Pathol.* **4:**1.

Medearis, D. N., Jr., 1964, Observations concerning human cytomegalovirus infection and disease, *Bull. Johns Hopkins Hosp.* **114:**181.

Melnick, J. L., 1977, Viral vaccines, *Progr. Med. Virol.* **23:**158.

Melnick, J. L., 1978, Viral vaccines: New problems and prospects, *Hosp. Pract.*, July, 1978, pp. 104–112.

Melnick, J. L., Lewis, R., Wimberly, I., Kaufman, R. H., and Adam, E., 1978, Association of cytomegalovirus (CMV) infection with cervical cancer: Isolation of CMV from cell cultures derived from cervical biopsy, *Intervirology* **10:**115.

Michelson-Fiske, S., Horodniceanu, F., and Guillon, J.-C., 1977, Immediate early antigens in human cytomegalovirus infected cells, *Nature (London)* **270:**615.

Miller, R. L., Iltis, J. P., and Rapp, F., 1977, Differential effect of arabinofuranosylthymine on the replication of human herpesviruses, *J. Virol.* **23:**679.

Minars, N., Silverman, J. F.,, Escobar, M. R., and Martinez, A. J., 1977, Fatal cytomegalic inclusion disease, *Arch. Dermatol.* **113:**1569.

Mirkovic, R., Werch, J., South, M. A., and Benyesh-Melnick, M., 1971, Incidence of cytomegaloviremia in blood-bank donors and in infants with congenital cytomegalic inclusion disease, *Infect. Immun.* **3:**45.

Monif, R. G., Daicoff, G. I., and Flory, L. L., 1976, Blood as a potential vehicle for the cytomegaloviruses, *Am. J. Obstet. Gynecol.* **126:**445.

Montgomery, R., Youngblood, L., Medearis, D. N., Jr., 1972, Recovery of cytomegalovirus from the cervix in pregnancy, *Pediatrics* **49:**524.

Muñoz, N., 1976, Model systems for cervical cancer, *Cancer Res.* **36:**792.

Murray, H. W., Knox, D. L., Green, W. R., and Susel, R. M., 1977, Cytomegalovirus retinitis in adults. A manifestation of disseminated viral infection, *Am. J. Med.* **63:**574.

Nakoneczna, I., and Kay, S., 1967, Fatal disseminated cytomegalic inclusion disease in an adult presenting with a lesion of the gastrointestinal tract, *Am. J. Clin. Pathol.* **47:**124.

Naraqi, S., Jackson, G. G., Jonasson, O., and Rubenis, M., 1978, Search for latent cytomegalovirus in renal allografts, *Infect. Immun.* **19**:699.

Neiman, P. E., Reeves, W., Ray, G., Flournoy, N., Lerner, K. G., Sale, G. E., and Thomas, E. D., 1977, A prospective analysis of interstitial pneumonia and opportunistic viral infection among recipients of allogeneic bone marrow grafts, *J. Infect. Dis.* **136**:745.

Numazaki, Y., Yano, N., Morizuka, T., Takal, S., and Ishida, N., 1970, Primary infection with human cytomegalovirus: Viral isolation from healthy infants and pregnant women, *Am. J. Epidemiol.* **91**:410.

O'Malley, J. A., Al-Bussam, N., Beutner, K., Wallace, H. J., Gailani, S., Henderson, E. S., and Carter, W. A., 1975, Cytomegalovirus infection with acute myelocytic leukemia. Antiviral (interferon and antibody) responses, *N.Y. State J. Med.* **75**:738.

Pacsa, A. S., Kummerländer, L., Pejtsik, B., and Pali, K., 1975, Herpesvirus antibodies and antigens in patients with cervical anaplasia and in controls, *J. Natl. Cancer Inst.* **55**:775.

Pagano, J. S., 1975*a*, Infections with cytomegalovirus in bone marrow transplantation: Report of a workshop, *J. Infect. Dis.* **132**:114.

Pagano, J. S., 1975*b*, Diseases and mechanisms of persistent DNA virus infection: Latency and cellular transformation, *J. Infect. Dis.* **132**:209.

Pass, R. F., Long, W. K., and Whitley, R. J., Soong, S.-J., Diethelm, A. G., Reynolds, D. W., and Alford, C. A., Jr., 1978, Productive infection with cytomegalovirus and herpes simplex virus in renal transplant recipients: Role of source of kidney, *J. Infect. Dis.* **137**:556.

Phillips, C. A., Fanning, W. L., Gump, D. W., and Phillips, C. F., 1977, Cytomegalovirus encephalitis in immunologically normal adults. Successful treatment with vidarabine, *J. Am. Med. Assoc.* **238**:2299.

Phillips, C. F., 1977, Congenital cytomegalovirus diseases. Is prevention possible? *Prog. Med. Virol.* **23**:62.

Plotkin, S. A., 1977, Perinatally acquired viral infections, *Curr. Top. Microbiol. Immunol.*, **78**:111.

Plotkin, S. A., Furukawa, T., Zygraich, N., and Huygelen, C., 1975, Candidate cytomegalovirus strain for human vaccination, *Infect. Immun.* **12**:521.

Plummer, G., and Benyesh-Melnick, M., 1964, A plaque reduction neutralization test for human cytomegalovirus, *Proc. Soc. Exp. Biol. Med.* **117**:145.

Plummer, G., and Lewis, B., 1965, Thermoinactivation of herpes simplex virus and cytomegalovirus, *J. Bacteriol.* **89**:671.

Pollard, R. B., and Merigan, T. C., 1978, Perspectives for the control of cytomegalovirus infections in bone marrow transplant recipients, *Transplant. Proc.* **10**:241.

Pollard, R. B., Rand, K. H., Arvin, A. M., and Merigan, T. C., 1978, Cell-mediated immunity to cytomegalovirus infection in normal subjects and cardiac transplant patients, *J. Infect. Dis.* **137**:541.

Rapp, F., and Geder, L., 1978, Persistence and transformation by human cytomegalovirus, in: *Persistent Viruses*, ICN-UCLA Symposia on Molecular and Cellular Biology (J. G. Stevens, G. J. Todaro and C. F. Fox, eds.), pp. 767–785, Academic Press, New York.

Rapp, F., Rasmussen, L. E., and Benyesh-Melnick, M., 1963, The immunofluorescent focus technique in studying the replication of cytomegalovirus, *J. Immunol.* **91**:709.

Rapp, F., Geder, L., Murasko, D., Lausch, R., Ladda, R., Huang, E.-S., and Webber, M., 1975, Long-term persistence of cytomegalovirus genome in cultured human cells of prostatic origin, *J. Virol.* **16**:982.

Reynolds, D. W., Stagno, S., Hosty, T. S., Tiller, M., and Alford, C. A., 1973, Maternal cytomegaloviruses excretion and perinatal infection, *N. Engl. J. Med.* **289**:1.

Reynolds, D. W., Stagno, S., Stubbs, K. G., Dahle, A. J., Livingston, M. M., Saxon, S. S., and Alford, C. A., 1974, Inapparent congenital cytomegalovirus infection with elevated cord IgM levels. Causal relation with auditory and mental deficiency, *N. Engl. J. Med.* **290**:291.

Reynolds, D. W., Stagno, S., Herrman, K. L., and Alford, C. A., 1978a, Antibody response to liver virus vaccines in congenital and neonatal cytomegalovirus infections, *J. Pediatr.* **92**:738.

Reynolds, D. W., Stagno, S., Reynolds, R., and Alford, C. A., Jr., 1978b, Perinatal cytomegalovirus infection: Influence of placentally transferred maternal antibody, *J. Infect. Dis.* **137**:564.

Rinaldo, C. R., Jr., Hirsch, M. S., and Black, P. H., 1976, Activation of latent viruses following bone marrow transplantation, *Transplant. Proc.* **8**:669.

Rinaldo, C. R., Jr., Black, P. H., and Hirsch, M. S., 1977, Interaction of cytomegalovirus with leukocytes from patients with mononucleosis due to cytomegalovirus, *J. Infect. Dis.* **136**:667.

Roche, J. K., and Huang, E.-S., 1977, Viral DNA in inflammatory bowel disease. CMV-bearing cells as a target for immune-mediated enterocytolysis, *Gastroenterology* **72**:228.

Roizman, B., and Furlong, A., 1974, The replication of herpesviruses, in: *Comprehensive Virology*, Vol. 3 (H. Fraenkel-Conrat and R. R. Wagner, eds.), pp. 229–403, Plenum Press, New York.

Rowe, A. P., Hartley, J. W., Waterman, S., Turner, H. C., and Huebner, R. J., 1956, Cytopathogenic agent resembling human salivary gland virus recovered from tissue cultures of human adenoids, *Proc. Soc. Exp. Biol. Med.* **92**:418.

Rubin, R. H., Cosimi, A. B., Tolkoff-Rubin, N. E., Russell, P. S., and Hirsch, M. S., 1977, Infectious disease syndromes attributable to cytomegalovirus and their significance among renal transplant recipients, *Transplantation* **24**:458.

Sahud, M. A., and Bachelor, M. M., 1978, Cytomegalovirus-induced thrombocytopenia. An unusual case report, *Arch. Intern. Med.* **138**:1573.

St. Jeor, S., and Rapp, F., 1973, Cytomegalovirus: Conversion of nonpermissive cells to a permissive state for virus replication, *Science* **181**:1060.

St. Jeor, S., and Weisser, A., 1977, Persistence of cytomegalovirus in human lymphoblasts and peripheral leukocyte cultures, *Infect. Immun.* **15**:402.

St. Jeor, S. C., Albrecht, T. B., Funk, F. D., and Rapp, F., 1974, Stimulation of cellular DNA synthesis by human cytomegalovirus, *J. Virol.* **13**:353.

Sanford, E. J., Geder, L., Laychock, A., Rohner, T. J., Jr., and Rapp, F., 1977, Evidence for the association of cytomegalovirus with carcinoma of the prostate, *J. Urol.* **118**:789.

Sanford, E. J., Geder, L., Dagen, J. E., Laychock, A., Rohner, T. J. Jr., and Rapp, F., 1978, Humoral and cellular immune response of prostatic cancer patients to cytomegalovirus-related antigens of cytomegalovirus-transformed human cells, *J. Surg. Res.* **24**:404.

Sarov, I., and Abady, I, 1975, The morphogenesis of human cytomegalovirus: Isolation and polypeptide characterization of cytomegalovirions and dense bodies, *Virology* **66**:464.

Sarov, I., and Friedman, A., 1976, Electron microscopy of human cytomegalovirus DNA, *Arch. Virol.* **50**:343.

Schmitz, H., and Enders, G., 1977, Cytomegalovirus as a frequent cause of Guillain-Barré syndrome, *J. Med. Virol.* **1**:21.

Simmons, R. L., Matas, A. J., Rattazzi, L. C., Balfour, H. H., Jr., Howard, R. J., and Najarian, J. S., 1977, Clinical characteristics of the lethal cytomegalovirus infection following renal transplantation, *Surgery* 82:537.

Smith, J. D., and deHarven, E., 1973, Herpes simplex virus and human cytomegalovirus replication in WI-38 cells. I. Sequence of viral replication, *J. Virol.* **12**:919.

Smith, J. D., and deHarven, E., 1974, Herpes simplex virus and human cytomegalovirus replication in WI-38 cells. II. An ultrastructural study of viral penetration, *J. Virol.* **14**:945.

Smith, J. D., and deHarven, 1978, Herpes simplex virus and human cytomegalovirus replication in WI-38 cells. III. Cytochemical localization of lysosomal enzymes in infected cells, *J. Virol.* **26**:102.

Smith, K. O., and Rasmussen, L., 1963, Morphology of cytomegalovirus (salivary gland virus), *J. Bacteriol.* **85**:1319.

Smith, M. G., 1956, Propagation in tissue cultures of a cytopathogenic virus from human salivary gland virus (SGV) disease, *Proc. Soc. Exp. Biol. Med.* **92**:424.

Stagno, S., Reynolds, D. W., Tsiantos, A., Fuccillo, D. A., Long, W., and Alford, C. A., 1975, Comparative serial virologic and serologic studies of symptomatic and subclinical congenitally and natally acquired cytomegalovirus infections, *J. Infect. Dis.* **132**:568.

Stagno, S., Reynolds, D. W., Huang, E.-S., Thames, S. D., Smith, R. J. and Alford, C. A., Jr., 1977, Congenital cytomegalovirus infection. Occurrence in an immune population, *N. Engl. J. Med.* **296**:1254.

Starr, J. G., and Gold, E., 1968, Screening of newborn infants for cytomegalovirus infection, *J. Pediatr.* **73**:820.

Starr, J. G., Bart, R. D., Jr., and Gold, E., 1970, Inapparent congenital cytomegalovirus infection, *N. Engl. J. Med.* **282**:1075.

Starr, S. E., Tolpin, M. D., Friedman, H. M., Plotkin, S. A., and Paucker, K., 1977, Immune responses in children with congenital cytomegalovirus and their mothers, *Lancet* **1**:1357.

Stern, H., 1975, Intrauterine infection with cytomegalovirus, *Proc. R. Soc. Med.* **68**:367.

Stern, H., and Tucker, S. M., 1973, Prospective study of cytomegalovirus infection in pregnancy, *Br. Med. J.* **2**:268.

Stevens, D. P., Barker, L. F., Ketcham, A. S., and Meyer, H. M., Jr., 1970, Asymptomatic cytomegalovirus infection following blood transfusion in tumor surgery, *J. Am. Med. Assoc.* **211**:1341.

Stinski, M. F., 1976, Human cytomegalovirus: Glycoproteins associated with virions and dense bodies, *J. Virol.* **19**:594.

Stinski, M. F., 1977, Synthesis of proteins and glycoproteins in cells infected with human cytomegalovirus, *J. Virol.* **23**:751.

Strong, D. M., Ahmed, A., Knudsen, R. C., Curry, J. L., Fleisher, T. A., Cahill, R. A., Hartzman, R. J., and Sell, S. W., 1978, Cellular immunity to cytomegalovirus in a patient following bone marrow transplantation, *Transplantation* **26**:99.

Tanaka, S., Furukawa, T., and Plotkin, S. A., 1975, Human cytomegalovirus stimulates host cell RNA synthesis, *J. Virol.* **15**:297.

Tanaka, S., Ihara, S., and Watanabe, Y., 1978, Human cytomegalovirus induces DNA-dependent RNA polymerases in human diploid cells, *Virology* **89**:179.

The, T. H., Klein, G., and Langenhuysen, M. M. A. C., 1974, Antibody reactions to virus-specific early antigens (EA) in patients with cytomegalovirus (CMV) infection, *Clin. Exp. Immunol.* **16**:1.

Vonka, V., Anisimová, E., and Macek, M., 1976, Replication of cytomegalovirus in human epithelioid diploid cell line, *Arch. Virol.* **52**:283.

Waner, J. L., Hopkins, D. R., Weller, T. H., and Allred, E. N., 1977, Cervical excretion of cytomegalovirus: Correlation with secretory and humoral antibody, *J. Infect. Dis.* **136**:805.

Webber, M. M., Stonington, O. G., and Poché, P. A., 1974, Epithelial outgrowth from suspension cultures of human prostatic tissue, *In Vitro* **10**:196.

Weller, T. H., 1970, Cytomegalovirus: The difficult years, *J. Infect. Dis.* **122**:532.

Weller, T. H., and Hanshaw, J. B., 1962, Virologic and clinical observations on cytomegalic inclusion disease, *N. Engl. J. Med.* **266**:1233.

Weller, T. H., Macaulay, J. C., Craig, J. M., and Wirth, P., 1957, Isolation of intranuclear inclusion producing agents from infants with illnesses resembling cytomegalic inclusion disease, *Proc. Soc. Exp. Biol. Med.* **94**:4.

Wentworth, B. B., and French, L., 1970, Plaque assay of cytomegalovirus strains of human origin, *Proc. Soc. Exp. Biol. Med.* **135**:253.

Whitley, R. J., Brasfield, D., Reynolds, D. W., Stagno, S., Tiller, R. E., and Alford, C. A., 1976, Protracted pneumonitis in young infants associated with perinatally acquired cytomegaloviral infection, *J. Pediatr.* **89**:16.

Wong, T.-W., and Warner, N. E., 1962, Cytomegalic inclusion disease in adults, *Arch. Pathol.* **74**:403.

Zablotney, S. L., Wentworth, B. B., and Alexander, E. R., 1978, Antigenic relatedness of 17 strains of human cytomegalovirus, *Am. J. Epidemiol.* **107**:336.

Závada, V., Erban, V., Rezácová, D., and Vonka, V., 1976, Thymidine kinase in cytomegalovirus infected cells, *Arch. Virol.* **52**:333.

CHAPTER 5

Aleutian Disease of Mink: A Model for Persistent Infection

David D. Porter

Department of Pathology
University of California School of Medicine
Los Angeles, California 90024

and

H. J. Cho

Animal Diseases Research Institute (Western)
Agriculture Canada
Lethbridge, Alberta T1J 3Z4, Canada

1. INTRODUCTION

Mink (*Mustela vison*) are members of the order Carnivora and family Mustelidae (Ewer, 1973). Other generally familiar members of the family include the wolverine, marten, badger, fisher, ferret, weasel, skunk, and otter. Mink are raised in large numbers on ranches for their valuable fur. The animals mate once a year in the early spring, and an average of four kits are born after a 50-day gestation period. The kits are usually weaned at 6–8 weeks of age and reach adult size at 7 months of age, at which time all except the breeding stock are sacrificed for their pelts on commercial ranches.

Aleutian disease (AD) was first described (Hartsough and Gorham, 1956) in mink homozygous for the recessive Aleutian coat color gene, but subsequently the disease has been shown to affect all colors of mink (Porter and Larsen, 1964). AD is the major health problem of commercial mink ranching, and we estimate that it causes the loss of $10 million annually in North America. Marked variation in the prevalence of AD on ranches in the same area has been found, and the disease frequently causes death before pelting season in mink of the Aleutian genotype. Early deaths in mink with other coat colors are relatively infrequent.

Aleutian disease virus (ADV) is temperature sensitive in its replication as isolated from persistently infected mink (Porter *et al.*, 1977*a*). *In vivo* viral replication is not associated with lesions but induces an extreme immune response in mink to the viral antigens. The disease associated with ADV infection results from the formation and tissue deposition of viral–antibody complexes, and can be prevented by immunosuppression. AD is a favorable model for the study of systemic persistent viral infections since large numbers of genetically defined (but outbred) animals of a sufficiently small size to allow large-scale experimentation are readily available.

2. THE VIRUS

2.1. Viral Etiology of Aleutian Disease

Evidence for the infectious nature of AD was first reported in 1962 by several groups of investigators who reproduced the disease by inoculating mink with suspensions of diseased tissue or cell-free filtrates (Henson *et al.*, 1962; Karstad and Pridham, 1962; Trautwein and Helmboldt, 1962). These findings indicated that the causative agent of AD was probably a virus. During the intervening years significant advances have been made in confirming the viral etiology of ADV. These include the development of specific serological tests (Porter *et al.*, 1969; McGuire *et al.*, 1971; Cho and Ingram, 1972), the adaptation of virus purification procedures and visualization of the virus (Cho and Ingram, 1973*a*; Kenyon *et al.*, 1973), and successful propagation of the virus *in vitro* (Porter *et al.*, 1977*a*). The behavior of the virus in cell culture (Porter *et al.*, 1977*a*) and its biochemical properties (Shahrabadi *et al.*, 1977) suggest that ADV is an autonomous parvovirus.

2.2. *In Vivo* Replication

The virus is readily recovered from the serum, whole blood, feces, urine, saliva, and various tissues of infected mink (Eklund *et al.*, 1968; Gorham *et al.*, 1964; Kenyon *et al.*, 1963). Although ADV is regarded as a slow virus, initial replication in mink is rapid, and peak viral titers of 10^8–10^9 ID_{50} per gram of spleen, liver, and lymph nodes are found 10 days after intraperitoneal inoculation (Fig. 1) coincident with the development of antiviral antibody (Porter *et al.*, 1969). Subsequently, the virus titers in tissues slowly fall so that 2 or more months after infection spleen titers of 10^5 ID_{50}/g and serum titers of 10^4 ID_{50}/ml are commonly found. Using the Utah-1 strain of ADV, Porter *et al.* (1969) did not find a difference in the degree of virus replication in mink of different genotypes. However, Eklund *et al.* (1968) have shown that when a stock suspension of the Pullman strain was titrated in mink of different genotypes much higher virus titers were obtained in mink homozygous for the Aleutian gene that in non-Aleutian mink. It has been recognized that the Pullman strain is markedly less virulent than the Utah strain (Bloom *et al.*, 1975).

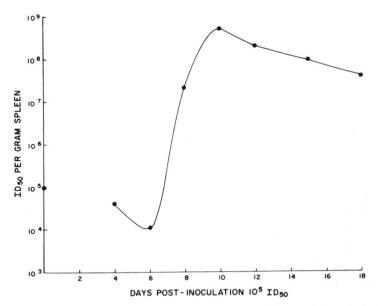

Fig. 1.   Growth curve of Aleutian disease virus in the spleen of mink. Viral yields were quantitated by *in vivo* infectivity in mink. From Porter *et al.* (1969).

It appears that ADV replicates *in vivo* in macrophages. By immunofluorescence, Porter *et al.* (1969) showed viral antigen mainly in the cytoplasm of macrophages in spleen and lymph node or Kupffer cells in the liver. Subsequently, antigen has been seen in the nuclei of macrophages (unpublished). Numerous viruslike particles (20–22 nm diameter) have been detected by electron microscopy in macrophages and in Kupffer cells (Shahrabadi and Cho, 1977). The particles were principally present in cytoplasmic vacuoles and occasionally in the nucleus. Furthermore, it was shown that areas containing the viruslike particles reacted with ADV antibody conjugated to horse ferritin.

2.3. Replication in Cell Culture

The highly virulent Utah-1 strain of ADV recovered from mink tissue was found to produce viral antigen and infectious virus in a continuous line of feline renal cells (CRFK) or in primary feline renal cells when the cultures were incubated at 31.8°C; no infectious virus was produced at 37°C or 39°C in primary isolation attempts (Porter *et al.*, 1977a). The body temperature of mink is 39°C. The cells must be rapidly dividing to permit viral replication. The virus did not produce plaques and has been quantitated by an immunofluorescence focus assay. The viral antigen first appears in the nucleus of cultured cells, and shortly thereafter some antigen can be seen in the cytoplasm as well (Fig. 2). After 10 passages at 31.8°C, the temperature optimum for ADV replication was found to be 37°C (Fig. 3). The virus is markedly

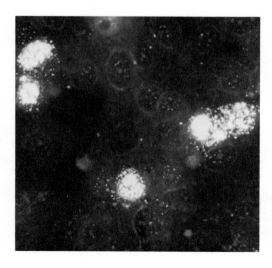

Fig. 2. A continuous line of feline renal cells were infected for 3 days with Aleutian disease virus at 31.8°C, and the fixed cells were stained with fluorescein-conjugated mink antiviral antibody. Both nuclear antigen and cytoplasmic antigen are present. ×1180. From Porter *et al.* (1977a).

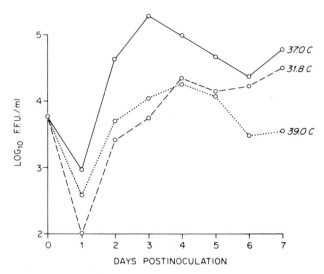

Fig. 3. The effect of temperature on yields of Aleutian disease virus, Utah-1 strain, in a continuous line of feline renal cells after ten passages in these cells at 31.8°C. From Porter *et al.* (1977*a*).

cell associated. The cultured virus has equal infectivity for cell cultures and mink, and can be reisolated from mink at all times after infection. No hemagglutination by ADV could be demonstrated. Although ADV will induce antigen in mink cells, little or no infectious virus is produced.

Less virulent ADV strains such as the Pullman and Guelph isolates are difficult to passage at 31.8°C, but they can be serially passaged if the incubation temperature is further reduced to 28°C. Persistently infected cell cultures are easily developed, especially when the virulent Utah-1 strain of ADV is used, but the cultures permanently lose the virus after one or two passages at 37°C (unpublished observations). The Connecticut strain of ADV has been found to produce antigen without infectivity in feline cells (Hahn *et al.*, 1977).

2.4. Purification and Properties

2.4.1. Purification of the Virus

The ADV infectivity titer can be increased 3–4 logs over that found in chronically infected mink by rapid serial intraperitoneal passages of the virus in mink (Porter *et al.*, 1969). This strategy is necessary for viral purification studies using mink organs as the starting material.

For virus purification, mink tissues from animals infected for 10 days, at the peak of viral proliferation, are homogenized and subjected to stepwise fluorocarbon extraction and concentration by sedimentation at 105,000*g* for 2 hr. The partially purified ADV is present in the form of complexes with antibody. Such complexes can be dissociated and the virus further purified by three or four additional fluorocarbon extractions. After dissociation, the AD virion antigen can be detected by counterimmunoelectrophoresis (CIEP) (Cho and Ingram, 1974). Further purification of the virion may be done using CsCl gradient centrifugation (Cho, 1977).

The CIEP technique is performed by placing antigen (such as the ADV virion) in one well of an agarose slide and antibody in an adjacent well. The antigen and antibody are moved through each other by an electrical field, and a precipitin line forms. The direction and degree of movement of the antigen are largely determined by its isoelectric point, and antibody movement is largely the result of endosmotic effects. The technique is suited for handling large numbers of samples, and is both faster and more sensitive than the Ouchterlony type of double diffusion in agar.

2.4.2. Properties of the Virus

Table 1 summarizes the known properties of ADV. Many of these properties are quite similar to other parvoviruses. Several ADV characterization studies have been performed using virus prepared from chronically infected mink which is complexed with antibody. Because of recent successful virus growth in cell culture and the advances in purification of the virus, it is now possible to characterize antibody-free ADV. In general, similar results have been obtained when antibody-free and complexed virus were compared.

By electron microscopy, negatively stained ADV had an icosahedral structure with a diameter of 23–25 nm (Cho and Ingram, 1973*a*; Chesebro *et al.*, 1975; Porter *et al.*, 1977*a*). With optimal resolution, hollow tubular-shaped capsomers 4.5 nm in diameter with a 1–2-nm central hole are visible. The virion probably has 32 capsomers. ADV from crude tissue extracts is filterable through a 50-nm Millipore membrane (Eklund *et al.*, 1968), but the virus cannot pass through an intact dialyzing membrane (Tabel and Ingram, 1970*a*).

TABLE 1

Physicochemical Properties of Aleutian Disease Virus

Description	Properties	Reference
Size	23–25 nm	Chesebro et al. (1975), Cho and Ingram (1973a), Porter et al. (1977a)
Morphology	Icosahedral	Cho and Ingram (1973a), Porter et al. (1977a)
Buoyant density in CsCl	1.41–1.43 g/ml	Cho (1977), Porter et al. (1977a)
Sedimentation constant	125 S	Cho et al. (unpublished)
Particle molecular weight	5.4–6.9×10^6	Calculated
Replication site	Nuclear	Hahn et al. (1977), Porter et al. (1977a)
Nucleic acid		
Strandedness	Single stranded	Cho and Ingram (1974), Shahrabadi et al. (1977)
Type	DNA	Porter et al. (1977a), Shahrabadi et al. (1977)
Density in CsCl	1.733 g/ml	Shahrabadi et al. (1977)
Molecular weight	1.2×10^6	Shahrabadi et al. (1977)
Structural protein	3 or 4 polypeptides	Shahrabadi et al. (1977)
Classification	Parvovirus	Chesebro et al. (1975), Cho and Ingram (1974), Porter et al. (1977a), Shahrabadi et al. (1977)
Dialysis	Not dialyzable	Tabel and Ingram (1970a)
Ether	Stable	Eklund et al. (1968), Porter et al. (1977a)
Chloroform	Stable	Porter (unpublished)
Fluorocarbon	Stable	Burger et al. (1965)
pH 3	Stable	Haagsma (1969)
Ultraviolet light	Inactivated	Goudas et al. (1970)
Heat		
56°C—30 min	Stable	Eklund et al. (1968), Porter et al. (1977a)
60°C—30 min	Partially inactivated	Eklund et al. (1968), Porter et al. (1977a)
80°C—30 min	Inactivated	Eklund et al. (1968), Porter et al. (1977a)
Deoxycholate	Stable	Burger et al. (1965), Porter et al. (1977a)
Protease enzymes	Stable	Burger et al. (1965)
Nuclease enzymes	Stable	Burger et al. (1965)
2.5 M KI, pH 7.0	Stable	Porter et al. (1977a)
2.0 M KSCN, pH 7.0	Partially inactivated	Porter et al. (1977a)
0.05 N NaOH	Inactivated	Burger et al. (1965)
0.5 N HCl	Inactivated	Burger et al. (1965)
0.5% iodine	Inactivated	Burger et al. (1965)
0.5% NaOCl	Inactivated	Porter (unpublished)

ADV infectivity of frozen, thawed, and sonicated cultures applied to CsCl gradients was broadly distributed over a density range of 1.26–1.43 gm/ml. After a single fluorocarbon extraction a major peak of infectivity was observed at 1.41–1.43 g/ml, as shown in Fig. 4 (Porter *et al.*, 1977*a*). Highly concentrated ADV preparations from infected mink tissues yielded three visible bands at buoyant densities of 1.295, 1.332, and 1.405–1.416 g/ml in CsCl (Cho, 1977). The lightest band contains mainly empty particles, while the other two bands contain both complete and empty particles (Fig. 5). In the heaviest-density band many smaller ring-shaped particles measuring 10–12 nm, which are believed to be mink ferritin, were also present. The different density populations of AD virions showed identical immunological specificity and polypeptide composition. The standard particles (ρ = 1.405–1.416) had CIEP antigen and infectivity titers 16 and 10,000 times higher, respectively, than the middle-band ADV (ρ = 1.332). The middle-band ADV had a particle-to-CIEP antigen ratio comparable with the standard ADV but possessed much lower infectivity, indicating that it is markedly defective in terms of infectivity. At present it is not known if these middle-band virions represent defective interfering particles of ADV, but such particles have been observed in other parvovirus preparations such as H1 (Rhode, 1978) and adeno-associated virus type 2 (Myers *et al.*, 1978). The defective ADV could play a significant role in relation to the persistence of the virus *in vivo*. In addition to the particles of the three densities discussed above, small amounts of infectivity may be detected at a density of 1.48 g/ml (Porter *et al.*, 1977*a*). Similar very heavy infectious particles are often seen in other parvovirus preparations (Rose, 1974).

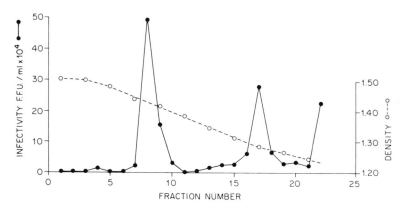

Fig. 4. Distribution of Aleutian disease viral infectivity in a CsCl equilibrium density gradient after extraction with Freon 113. From Porter *et al.* (1977*a*).

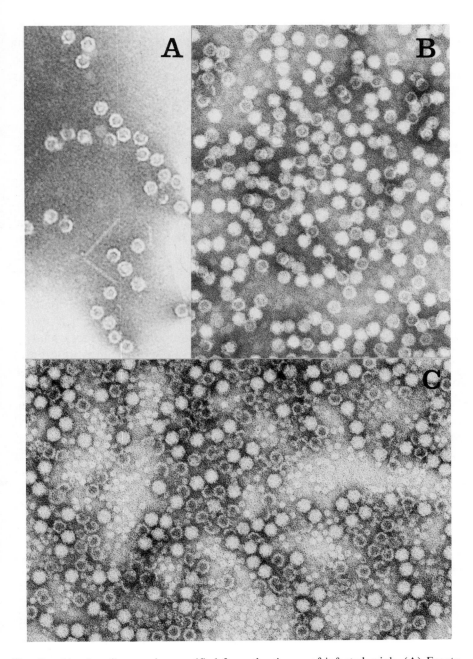

Fig. 5. Aleutian disease virus purified from the tissues of infected mink. (A) Empty particles, $\rho = 1.295$. (B) Full and empty particles, $\rho = 1.332$. (C) Full and empty particles and mink ferritin, $\rho = 1.405–1.416$. Infectivity is principally in this band. From Cho (1977).

In common with other parvoviruses (Rose, 1974), ADV is more resistant to heat than most conventional viruses but is far less resistant than the scrapie agent. However, it is interesting to note that ADV is more resistant than the scrapie agent to chemical treatments such as fluorocarbon, ether, and cesium chloride.

2.5. Structure and Classification

2.5.1. Nucleic Acid

The single-stranded nature of ADV nucleic acid was suggested initially by the observation of a flame-red fluorescence reaction under UV light when purified ADV or ADV–antibody complexes formed in the CIEP immune precipitates were stained with 0.01% acridine orange (Cho and Ingram, 1974). Electron microscopic examination of the ADV nucleic acid (Fig. 6) showed the presence of large, intermediate, and small molecules with approximate molecular weights of 1.2×10^6, 0.5×10^6, and 0.23×10^6, respectively. It is not known whether each size class of DNA is present in all virions. After analytical centrifugation in CsCl, ADV nucleic acid banded at a buoyant density of 1.733 g/ml. When ADV nucleic acid was treated with pancreatic DNAse, no visible band was observed after analytical centrifugation in CsCl. In addition, ADV nucleic acid did not exhibit RNA characteristics when centrifuged in Cs_2SO_4. The reaction of 1.8% formaldehyde with intact ADV caused an increase in absorption and a shift of the absorption maximum to a longer wavelength, from 264 nm to 268 nm. A thermal denaturation study of ADV DNA showed no sharp rise in optical density when the sample was heated to 100°C. These results indicate that ADV contains a single-stranded DNA (Shahrabadi et al., 1977).

2.5.2. Viral Proteins

Electrophoretic analysis of purified ADV virions on polyacrylamide slab gels revealed the presence of four polypeptides with molecular weights of 30,000, 27,000, 20,500, and 14,000 (Fig. 7). These polypeptides were present in a ratio of 10:3:10:1. The minor polypeptides of molecular weight 27,000 may be a dimer of the polypeptide of molecular weight 14,000. There was no difference between the polypeptide patterns of standard ($\rho = 1.41$ g/ml) and inter-

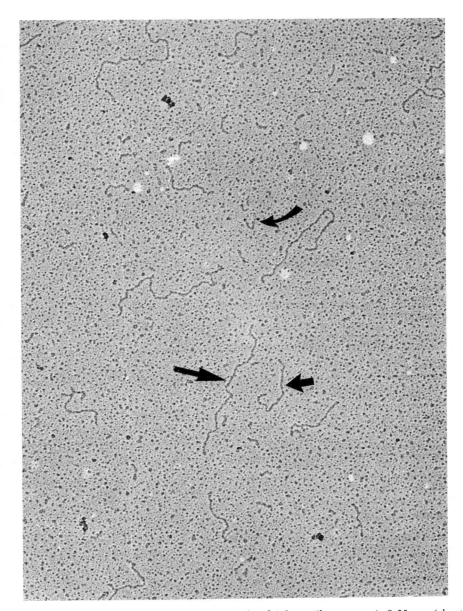

Fig. 6.   Aleutian disease viral DNA. Strands of 1.2 μm (long arrow), 0.55 μm (short arrow), and 0.25 μm (curved arrow) are present. ×50,000. From Shahrabadi *et al.* (1977).

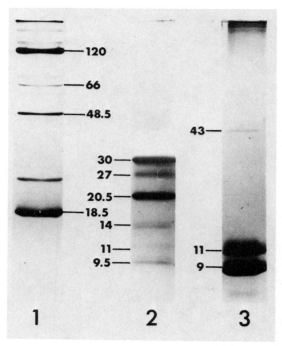

Fig. 7. SDS-polyacrylamide gel electrophoresis of (track 1) adenovirus type 2, (track 2) Aleutian disease virus purified from mink organs, and (track 3) purified mink ferritin. Aleutian disease virus contains polypeptides of molecular weight 30,000, 27,000, 20,500, and 14,000 in a ratio of 10:3:10:1, and is contaminated with a small quantity of mink ferritin. From Shahrabadi *et al.* (1977).

mediate-density (ρ = 1.33 g/ml) ADV. It is not known whether ADV codes for nonstructural proteins.

2.5.3. Classification

Many of the physicochemical properties of ADV are similar to those of described parvoviruses. These similarities include particle size and morphology, buoyant density and the heterogeneity of buoyant densities of the virions, and stability to heat, chemicals, and low pH. ADV replicates in the nucleus both *in vitro* and *in vivo*, it does not require helper virus in its multiplication, and, furthermore, it contains single-stranded DNA. Based on these properties, ADV can be tentatively classified as a member of the autonomous parvovirus group. However, the molecular weights of ADV polypeptides are approximately one-third those of other parvoviruses. It is possible that the purification of ADV fragments the polypeptides. No immunological relationship of ADV to 13 other parvoviruses could be demonstrated (Porter *et al.*, 1977*a*).

3. THE DISEASE PROCESS

3.1. Transmission

Both horizontal transmission and vertical transmission of ADV occur (Gorham *et al.*, 1964, 1976; Padgett *et al.*, 1967). When healthy, antibody-free mink were brought onto ADV-infected ranches, AD was occasionally observed in these animals. Since ADV has been found in saliva, urine, and feces (Kenyon *et al.*, 1963; Gorham *et al.*, 1964), it is possible that affected mink can transmit the disease to normal mink by bites, through excrement, or during handling with contaminated gloves (Larsen, 1969). Gorham *et al.* (1964) showed that two routes of natural transmission, fecal–oral and saliva–aerosol–respiratory, were possible. It appears that the latter is a more efficient route of infection since many mink remain ADV-antibody negative after being fed infected tissues, whereas ADV antibody was regularly detected in mink exposed to aerosols of virus (unpublished data).

Vertical transmission of infection appears to play an important role in perpetuating the disease in ranch mink and even more so in feral mink. The latter are quite territorial and do not have close and continuing contact with other mink after weaning (Gerell, 1970).

Porter *et al.* (1977*b*) demonstrated experimentally that transplacental ADV infection produced a disease with a marked reduction in severity of lesions. Mink infected in this fashion remain asymptomatic and live long enough to reproduce and could thus transmit infection to seronegative mink horizontally and also from one generation to the next vertically. Asymptomatic ADV infection has been observed in 39% of naturally infected pastel mink (An and Ingram, 1977) and in a much higher proportion (80%) of seropositive feral mink (Cho and Greenfield, 1978). Additionally, up to a quarter of mink of non-Aleutian genotypes may have self-limited nonpersistent infections by ADV (Larsen and Porter, 1975).

3.2. Pathology

A systemic plasmacytosis involving the bone marrow, spleen, lymph nodes, liver, and kidneys is the most consistent and striking lesion of AD (Helmboldt and Jungherr, 1958; Obel, 1959; Henson *et al.*, 1976). The degree of plasma cell proliferation is directly proportional to the serum γ-globulin levels and to the severity of the glomerular and arterial lesions (Porter and Larsen, 1964). Despite the occasional occurence of monoclonal immunoglobulins (Porter *et al.*, 1965*a*), no osteolytic lesions similar to those found in human and murine multiple myeloma have ever been noted.

Despite the rapid course of ADV replication in mink, the first morphological lesions are not seen until 3–4 weeks after infection, coincident with the onset of increased immunoglobulin levels (Hensen *et al.*, 1966). The persistently infected mink develop a severe glomerulonephritis. Immunofluorescence studies have shown IgG and C3 in a granular pattern along glomerular capillary walls, and, after acid elution of IgG, ADV antigen can be seen in the same location (Henson *et al.*, 1969; Porter *et al.*, 1969; Pan *et al.*, 1970; Johnson *et al.*, 1975). An acute and chronic arteritis affecting muscular arteries is found in a minority of severely diseased mink. Immunoglobulin, C3, and, after acid elution, ADV antigen can be found in the zone of fibrinoid necrosis in arteries (Porter *et al.*, 1973). Mink of the Aleutian genotype typically die of renal failure 3–5 months after infection, while non-Aleutian mink rarely die earlier than 5 months after infection, and half will still be alive after 1 year. An occasional mink with AD dies following the rupture of an inflamed artery or enlarged spleen.

Decreases in the platelet and fibrinogen levels and cyclic variation of clotting factors V and VIII in mink with Aleutian disease have been described (McKay *et al.*, 1967). The changes observed indicate that intravascular coagulation may contribute to the lesions of AD; however, no half-life studies have been performed to indicate the magnitude of consumption of these clotting components. A proliferation of small bile ducts, occasionally with cyst formation, has been noted in AD (Drommer and Trautwein, 1975), but the cause of this lesion is unknown.

3.3. Pathogenesis of Lesions

No clinical illness or pathological lesions are apparent in mink during the early phase of ADV growth when viral titers are maximal (Porter *et al.*, 1969). When cyclophosphamide is given to infected mink in doses which partially suppress antibody production to bovine serum albumin, the lesions of AD can be completely suppressed for a period of 13–16 weeks, although viral titers are not affected (Cheema *et al.*,

1972). If a large amount of ADV antibody is administered to acutely infected mink at the peak of viral proliferation, there is cytolysis of some of the infected cells in the liver and there are collections of polymorphonuclear leukocytes followed by lymphocytes around the infected cells (Porter *et al.*, 1972).

Immune complexes can be demonstrated in the serum of mink with AD by ultracentrifugation (Porter *et al.*, 1965*b*). The complexes seen were 9–14 S and 22–30 S; complexes of the latter size have been shown to localize in blood vessels (Cochrane and Hawkins, 1968). These complexes are smaller than virion size (125 S), and it is not known which antigen(s) of ADV participates in complex formation. Although all the mink with demonstrable immune complexes had such severe lesions that it was impossible to correlate the presence of complexes with specific lesions, it would appear that the arterial and glomerular lesions of AD are principally or totally caused by immune complex deposition.

3.4. Diagnosis and Control

AD cannot be prevented by immunizing mink with an inactivated crude tissue viral vaccine. In fact, pathological lesions of enhanced severity were observed in such vaccinated mink after challenge with live virus (Porter *et al.*, 1972). Therefore, control of this disease has been based on early detection of infection and culling of infected animals.

During the 1960s and early 1970s the simple iodine agglutination test (IAT) (Mallén *et al.*, 1950) was widely used to diagnose AD in the field and contributed significantly in reducing the incidence and mortality (Gorham *et al.*, 1976). This test gives a flocculant precipitate when a serum with an increased globulin-to-albumin ratio is mixed with an iodine–potassium iodide reagent. However, since this test is nonspecific and detects elevated γ-globulin levels irrespective of cause, it cannot be used to eradicate AD from mink ranches. The IAT detects only 16–65% of mink which have AD antibody by the CIEP tests (Greenfield *et al.*, 1973; Ingram and Cho, 1974; Gierloff and Thordal-Christensen, 1975). Serum protein electrophoresis has also been used (Larsen, 1965). Although this test is more accurate than the IAT, it is expensive and difficult to perform. AD can also be diagnosed on the basis of gross and microscopic lesions in mink tissues. Until the development of specific serological tests, histopathology was the most accurate method of making a definite diagnosis.

After Porter *et al.* (1969) described an immunofluorescence method for the detection of ADV antigen and antibody, several other specific serological tests were developed (McGuire et al., 1971; Cho and Ingram, 1972; Burger et al., 1978). Recently, the sensitivity, reproducibility, and specificity of immunofluorescence, complement fixation, and regular and modified counterimmunoelectrophoresis (CIEP) tests have been compared (Crawford et al., 1977). All of these tests were reliable and specific for ADV. Although CIEP is the least sensitive, it is the test of choice for large-scale application. It is easy to perform, reliable, and reasonably inexpensive, and commercial antigens are available. The CIEP test has been used on a large scale in several countries where mink are raised commercially, and the results show promise in controlling the disease. Recently Cho and Greenfield (1978) reported success in eliminating AD from three infected mink ranches using this test and subsequently pelting all animals which had ADV antibody. Using a similar procedure, Danish workers tested 125,000 mink by CIEP during the winter and spring of 1978. AD was eradicated from four farms, and subsequent litters showed improved pelts and increased size (M. Hansen, personal communication). Previously, about 250,000 breeding mink in Denmark were tested annually by IAT over a 10-year period without achieving successful control of AD.

It now appears that is may be possible to control and eliminate AD on infected mink ranches using specific serological tests and culling all mink that are positive for ADV antibody.

4. IMMUNOLOGICAL ASPECTS OF INFECTION

4.1. Hypergammaglobulinemia

There is a marked hypergammaglobulinemia in AD. Serum γ-globulin levels determined by electrophoresis were 0.74 g/100 ml for 570 histologically normal mink and 3.5 g/100 for 683 mink with tissue lesions of AD. The maximal levels of γ-globulin observed have been 11 g/100 ml. Both the percentage of γ-globulin and the total serum protein are elevated in AD. The serum albumin is decreased in hyperglobulinemic mink, probably as a physiological response to maintain a constant colloid osmotic pressure of the plasma (Porter and Larsen, 1964). The increased γ-globulin is nearly all 6.4 S IgG, and the increased amounts are caused by overproduction of the protein, since the half-life of IgG is decreased about one-third in hyperglobulinemic infected mink (Porter et al., 1965b). γ-Globulin, some of which is ADV antibody, may be produced by cell cultures of lymphoid tissues from infected mink (Bloom, 1976).

Elevated levels of IgG are found by 30 days after ADV infection. Some restriction of the heterogeneity of the elevated IgG levels may be found as early as 40 days after infection (Tabel and Ingram, 1970*b*), and in mink surviving 1 year after infection about 10% develop a monoclonal IgG (Porter *et al.*, 1965*a*). We regard the monoclonal IgG as a maximal immune response rather than transformation of a clone of lymphoid cells, and we have observed reversions to polyclonal IgG production (unpublished data). Some mink with markedly elevated levels of either heterogeneous or monoclonal IgG have Bence-Jones proteinuria.

A transient elevation of IgM and an elevation in IgA has been found in infected mink, and ADV antibody of these classes has been found in small amounts (Porter *et al.*, 1977*c*). Antibody of these classes may be involved in the glomerular lesions of AD (Johnson *et al.*, 1975; Portis and Coe, 1978).

4.2. Immune Complexes

Virus in the circulation of mink with chronic AD is in the form of infectious virus–antibody complexes, as indicated by precipitation of infectivity by antiserums to mink IgG (Porter and Larsen, 1967). Smaller complexes of 9–14 S and 22–30 S are readily demonstrated in the serum of mink with marked hypergammaglobulinemia by analytical ultracentrifugation (Porter *et al.*, 1965*b*). The complexes participate in the production of the tissue lesions of AD (see Section 3.2 and 3.3).

4.3. Viral-Specific Antibody

ADV antibody can be detected by the CIEP test occasionally as early as 4 days and consistently at 7 days after experimental infection (Cho and Ingram, 1973*b*). Immunofluorescence antibody is usually first detectable 9 or 10 days after infection and rapidly rises to much higher levels than in other viral infections (Porter *et al.*, 1969). The geometric mean ADV antibody titer measured by immunofluorescence rose from 3 on day 9 to 145 on day 15, and, on day 30, at which time hypergammaglobulinemia was evident, the antibody titer was 4400. On day 60 an extraordinarily high mean antibody titer of 100,000 was present. Complement-fixing antibody titers of 8000–260,000 were detected 6 weeks after infection (McGuire *et al.*, 1971). CIEP antibody titers of 5000–80,000 were observed in hypergammaglobulinemic sera collected 2 months or more after infection (Cho and Ingram, 1973*b*). Once the viral-specific antibody titers reach these high levels, they generally plateau. It has been shown that virion-specific antibody is detected by the CIEP and complement fixation tests. At present it is not known how much of the increased level in hypergammaglobulinemic mink sera represents the viral specific antibody; however, as little as 1 μg/ml of IgG from chronically infected mink will give a positive immunofluorescence reaction (Porter and Larsen, 1974), and it has been repeatedly observed that a general correlation exists between antibody titers and the increased level of γ-globulin (Porter *et al.*, 1969; McGuire *et al.*, 1971; Cho and Ingram, 1973*b*).

Despite the extremely high level of viral-specific antibody, the mink antibody does not neutralize ADV. The virus is infectious *in vivo* and in cell culture despite being complexed with antibody, and antibody can be demonstrated on the surface of agglutinated virions (Porter and Larsen, 1967; Porter *et al.*, 1969, 1977*a*). Serum from ADV infected mink without viremia (Larsen and Porter, 1975) and serum from ferrets with ADV antibody and no disease also will not neutralize ADV. No neutralization tests have been attempted with noncarnivore antisera.

4.4. Effect on Unrelated Immune Responses

At the time it was thought that AD might be an unrestrained proliferation of all plasma cells, a number of studies to assess the general immune responsiveness of normal and infected mink were carried out. Mink with AD make about one-quarter the humoral antibody response of normal mink to antigens such as keyhole limpet hemocyanin, peroxidase, or Brucella abortus; however, mink infected for 6 months or more responded normally to the latter antigen (Porter *et al.*, 1965*b*; Kenyon, 1966; Lodmell *et al.*, 1970; Trautwein *et al.*, 1974). If mink are immunized with various antigens and then challenged with ADV, the antibody response to the non-ADV antigens falls during the development of increased IgG levels. If ADV and another antigen are given at the same time, the initial response to the nonviral antigen is normal but falls rapidly with the development of hyperglobulinemia (Porter and Larsen, 1968; Tabel *et al.*, 1970). These results may be due to antigenic competition with ADV antigens which appear to have preempted the responsiveness of the immune system of the infected mink.

While no data are available on cellular immunity to ADV antigens, the nonspecific T-cell mitogen phytohemaglutinin P produces less than a normal response in peripheral blood lymphocytes of mink with AD (Perryman *et al.*, 1975).

5. GENETIC ASPECTS

5.1. Influence of Viral Strain on Disease

Viral strains of high virulence such as the Utah-1 and Guelph strains will produce progressive disease and death in all mink of the Aleutian genotype and in the majority of mink of non-Aleutian genotypes. ADV of low virulence, such as the Pullman strain, will produce disease and death only in mink of the Aleutian genotype. A number of additional ADV strains of each type are available, but they have not been widely used. Physicochemical or antigenic differences have not been found between ADV strains of high and low virulence, but only major differences could be noted with the techniques that have been used.

5.2. Influence of Host Genotype on Viral Persistence and Disease

Mink of the Aleutian genotype all die of AD when they are infected with a virus of either low or high virulence. Life table studies of Aleutian mink show that half will be dead of disease 120 days after infection with the Pullman strain of ADV (Eklund *et al.*, 1968). The Pullman strain of virus does replicate to some extent in non-Aleutian mink, but they fail to develop high ADV antibody titers or disease, although small amounts of virus may persist in lymph nodes for 22 months (Eklund *et al.*, 1968; Bloom *et al.*, 1975). Highly virulent ADV will kill Aleutian mink in about the same time as low-virulence virus; however, a viral strain such as Utah-1 will cause progressive disease in 75% of pastel (non-Aleutian) mink. Deaths in these mink reach 50% by 1 year, and a few mink with disease will survive for their full life span of 8 years. Analysis of pastel mink without disease has shown a group without viremia (Larsen and Porter, 1975) and another group with viremia (An and Ingram, 1977). Mink of the latter group had normal γ-globulin levels and could be recognized only by isolation of virus or the presence of ADV antibody. Breeding experiments with the mink which did not have viremia indicated that a single gene was not responsible for host resistance. The rate of progression of glomerulonephritis is much faster in Aleutian as compared with non-Aleutian mink (Johnson *et al.*, 1975), and this probably is the case with the other lesions.

6. DISCUSSION

ADV appears to be a member of the parvovirus group which does not require a helper virus for replication. The viral characterization that has been carried out has often used *in vivo*-grown virus since the yield of virus in feline cell cultures is relatively low and often erratic. Three size classes of viral DNA and the small size of the virion polypeptides suggest that ADV may differ substantially from other members of the autonomous parvovirus group. The temperature-sensitive nature of ADV replication in cell culture is of particular interest. Further characterization of ADV and examination of its replication in culture is urgently needed for the understanding of this interesting and economically important virus.

The disease produced in mink by ADV is now relatively well understood. Viral replication appears to be relatively innocuous for the host, but it provides a large amount of viral antigen. This results in a huge humoral antibody response to viral antigens, local antibody formation, and circulating immune complexes of virion size and smaller. The major lesions (glomerulonephritis and arteritis) are caused by deposition of complexes in the tissues and subsequent inflammation. The severity of the disease process is markedly influenced by the ADV strain used, the host genotype, and the age at which the mink is infected. Although it has not been possible to develop a useful vaccine for this virus, it appears that the disease can be controlled by eliminating all antibody-positive mink from commercial ranches.

The reason that ADV usually causes a persistent infection in mink is presently unknown. The temperature-sensitive nature of ADV replication might be responsible for *in vivo* persistence, since *in vitro* viral persistence has often been associated with the acquisition of a temperature-sensitive lesion in the viral genome (Preble and Youngner, 1975). ADV produces large amounts of light particles *in vivo* which are defective in terms of infectivity. This defective ADV could play a role in viral persistence. Phagocytosis of ADV–antibody complexes by macrophages, with reactivation and replication of the virus in these cells, might also be involved with viral persistence (Porter *et al.*, 1969). The failure of mink ADV antibody to neutralize viral infectivity might lead to persistence by means other than phagocytosis by macrophages. There are no data presently available which strongly suggest that one of these explanations for *in vivo* ADV persistence is correct. A search for viral mutants which fail to cause persistent infection might provide insight into the reason for viral persistence.

ACKNOWLEDGMENTS

The authors' work was supported by Grant AI-09476 from the National Institute of Allergy and Infectious Diseases, National Institutes of Health, by the Mink Farmers' Research Foundation, and by Agriculture Canada.

7. REFERENCES

An, S. H., and Ingram, D. G., 1977, Detection of inapparent Aleutian disease virus infection in mink, *Am. J. Vet. Res.* **38**:1619.

Bloom, M. E., 1976, Aleutian disease of mink: Production of ^{14}C-labeled antiviral antibodies by mink lymphoid cells *in vitro*, *Infect. Immun.* **13**:281.

Bloom, M. E., Race, R. E., Hadlow, W. J., and Chesebro, B., 1975, Aleutian disease of mink: The antibody response of sapphire and pastel mink to Aleutian disease virus, *J. Immunol.* **115**:1034.

Burger, D., Gorham, J. R., and Leader, R. W., 1965, Some physical and chemical characteristics of partially purified Aleutian disease virus, in: *Slow, Latent, and Temperate Virus Infections* (D. C. Gajdusek, C. J. Gibbs, and M. Alpers, eds.), pp. 307–313, NINDB Monograph No. 2, U.S. Government Printing Office, Washington, D.C.

Burger, D., Srironganathan, N., and Gorham, J. R., 1978, Detection of antibody and antigen in Aleutian disease virus infected mink with enzyme-linked immunosorbent assay (ELISA), *Abstr. Annu. Meet. Am. Soc. Microbiol.* **1978**:65.

Cheema, A., Henson, J. B., and Gorham, J. R., 1972, Aleutian disease of mink. Prevention of lesions by immunosuppression, *Am. J. Pathol.* **66**:543.

Chesebro, B., Bloom, M., Hadlow, W., and Race, R., 1975, Purification and ultrastructure of Aleutian disease virus of mink, *Nature (London)* **254**:456.

Cho, H. J., 1977, Demonstration of heavy and light density populations of Aleutian disease virus, *Can. J. Comp. Med.* **41**:215.

Cho, H. J., and Greenfield, J., 1978, Eradication of Aleutian disease of mink by eliminating positive counterimmunoelectrophoresis reactors, *J. Clin. Microbiol.* **7**:18.

Cho, H. J., and Ingram, D. G., 1972, Antigen and antibody in Aleutian disease in mink. I. Precipitation reaction by agar-gel electrophoresis, *J. Immunol.* **108**:555.

Cho, H. J., and Ingram, D. G., 1973a, Isolation, purification and structure of Aleutian disease virus by immunological techniques, *Nature (London) New Biol.* **243**:174.

Cho, H. J., and Ingram, D. G., 1973*b*, Antigen and antibody in Aleutian disease in mink. II. The reaction of antibody with the Aleutian disease agent using immunodiffusion and immunoelectroosmophoresis, *Can. J. Comp. Med.* **37**:217.

Cho, H. J., and Ingram, D. G., 1974, The antigen and virus of Aleutian disease in mink, *J. Immunol. Methods* **4**:217.

Cochrane, C. G., and Hawkins, D., 1968, Studies on circulating immune complexes. III. Factors governing the ability of circulating complexes to localize in blood vessels, *J. Exp. Med.* **127**:137.

Crawford, T. B., McGuire, T. C., Porter, D. D., and Cho, H. J., 1977, A comparative study of detection methods for Aleutian disease viral antibody, *J. Immunol.* **118**:1249.

Drommer, W., and Trautwein, G., 1975, Die pathogenese der Aleutenkrankheit der nerze. VII. Chronische hepatitis mit gallengangproliferation, *Vet. Pathol.* **12**:77.

Eklund, C. M., Hadlow, W. J., Kennedy, R. C., Boyle, C. C., and Jackson, T. A., 1968, Aleutian disease of mink. Properties of the etiologic agent and the host responses, *J. Infect. Dis.* **118**:510.

Ewer, R. F., 1973, *The Carnivores*, Cornell University Press, Ithaca.

Gerell, R., 1970, Home ranges and movements of the mink *Mustela vision* Schreber in southern Sweden, *Oikos* **21**:160.

Gierloff, B., and Thordal-Christensen, A., 1975, Aleutiansyge hos mink. Studie over infektionens forekomst og betygning ved pavisning af specifikt antistof v.h.a. modstrøselektroforese, *Dan. Vet. Tidsskr.* **58**:589.

Gorham, J. R., Leader, R. W., and Henson, J. B., 1964, The experimental transmission of a virus causing hypergammaglobulinemia in mink: Sources and modes of infection, *J. Infect. Dis.* **114**:341.

Gorham, J. R., Henson, J. B., Crawford, T. B., and Padgett, G. A., 1976, The epizootiology of Aleutian disease, in: *Slow Virus Diseases of Animals and Man* (R. H. Kimberlin, ed.), pp. 135–158, North-Holland, Amsterdam.

Goudas, P., Karstad, L., and Tabel, H., 1970, Ultraviolet inactivation of the infective agent of Aleutian disease of mink, *Can. J. Comp. Med.* **34**:118.

Greenfield, J., Walton, R., and MacDonald, K. R., 1973, Detection of Aleutian disease in mink: Serum-plate agglutination using iodine compared with precipitation by agar-gel electrophoresis, *Res. Vet. Sci.* **15**:381.

Haagsma, J., 1969, A study about the resistance of Aleutian disease agent against chemical and physical influences as to control the disease, *Tijdschr. Diergeneeskd.* **94**:824.

Hahn, E. C., Ramos, L., and Kenyon, A. J., 1977, Expression of Aleutian mink disease antigen in cell culture, *Infect. Immun.* **15**:204.

Hartsough, G. R., and Gorham, J. R., 1956, Aleutian disease in mink, *Natl. Fur News* **28**:10.

Helmboldt, C. F., and Jungherr, E. L., 1958, The pathology of Aleutian disease in mink, *Am. J. Vet. Res.* **19**:212.

Henson, J. B., Gorham, J. R., Leader, R. W., and Wagner, B. M., 1962, Experimental hypergammaglobulinemia in mink, *J. Exp. Med.* **116**:357.

Henson, J. B., Leader, R. W., Gorham, J. R., and Padgett, G. A., 1966, The sequential development of lesions in spontaneous Aleutian disease of mink, *Pathol. Vet.* **3**:289.

Henson, J. B., Gorham, J. R., and Padgett, G. A., 1969, Pathogenesis of the glomerular lesions in Aleutian disease of mink: Immunofluorescent studies, *Arch Pathol.* **87**:21.

Henson, J. B., Gorham, J. R., McGuire, T. C., and Crawford, T. B., 1976, Pathology and pathogenesis of Aleutian disease, in: *Slow Virus Diseases of Animals and Man* (R. H. Kimberlin, ed.), pp. 175–205, North-Holland, Amsterdam.

Ingram, D. G., and Cho, H. J., 1974, Aleutian disease in mink: Virology, immunology and pathogenesis, *J. Rheumatol.* **1**:74.

Johnson, M. I., Henson, J. B., and Gorham, J. R., 1975, The influence of genotype on the development of glomerular lesions in mink with Aleutian disease virus. A correlated light, fluorescent, and electron microscopic study, *Am. J. Pathol.* **81**:321.

Karstad, L., and Pridham, T. J., 1962, Aleutian disease of mink. I. Evidence of its viral etiology, *Can. J. Comp. Med.* **26**:97.

Kenyon, A. J., 1966, Immunologic deficiency in Aleutian disease of mink, *Am. J. Vet. Res.* **27**:1780.

Kenyon, A. J., Helmboldt, C. F., and Nielsen, S. W., 1963, Experimental transmission of Aleutian disease with urine, *Am. J. Vet. Res.* **24**:1066.

Kenyon, A. J., Gander, J. E., Lopez, C., and Good, R. A., 1973, Isolation of Aleutian mink disease virus by affinity chromatography, *Science* **179**:187.

Larsen, A. E., 1965, Electrophoresis, IAT and the elusive Aleutian disease, *Natl. Fur News* **37**:18.

Larsen, A. E., 1969, Immunological and viral studies of Aleutian disease in mink, Ph.D. Dissertation, University of Utah.

Larsen, A. E., and Porter, D. D., 1975, Pathogenesis of Aleutian disease of mink: Identification of nonpersistent infections, *Infect. Immun.* **11**:92.

Lodmell, D. L., Hadlow, W. J., Munoz, J. J., and Whitford, H. W., 1970, Hemagglutinin antibody response of normal and Aleutian disease-affected mink to keyhole limpet hemocyanin, *J. Immunol.* **104**:878.

Mallén, M. S., Ugalde, E. L., Balcazar, M. R., Bolívar, J. I., and Meyran, S., 1950, Precipitation of abnormal serums by Lugol's solution, *Am. J. Clin. Pathol.* **20**:39.

McGuire, T. C., Crawford, T. B., Henson, J. B., and Gorham, J. R., 1971, Aleutian disease of mink: Detection of large quantities of complement-fixing antibody to viral antigens, *J. Immunol.* **107**:1481.

McKay, D. G., Phillips, L. L., Kaplan, H., and Henson, J. B., 1967, Chronic intravascular coagulation in Aleutian disease of mink, *Am. J. Pathol.* **50**:899.

Myers, M., Laughlin, C., De La Maza, L. M., and Carter, B., 1978, Adeno-associated virus type 2 defective interfering particles, *Abstr. Annu. Meet. Am. Soc. Microbiol.* **1978**:229.

Obel, A.-L., 1959, Studies on a disease in mink with systemic proliferation of the plasma cells, *Am. J. Vet. Res.* **20**:384.

Padgett, G. A. Gorham, J. R., and Henson, J. B., 1967, Epizootiologic studies of Aleutian disease. I. Transplacental transmission of the virus, *J. Infect. Dis.* **117**:35.

Pan, I. C., Tsai, K. S., and Karstad, L., 1970, Glomerulonephritis in Aleutian disease of mink: Histological and immunofluorescence studies, *J. Pathol.* **101**:119.

Perryman, L. E., Banks, K. L., and McGuire, T. C., 1975, Lymphocyte abnormalities in Aleutian disease virus infection of mink: Decreased T lymphocyte responses and increased B lymphocyte levels in persistent viral infection, *J. Immunol.* **115**:22.

Porter, D. D., and Larsen, A. E., 1964, Statistical survey of Aleutian disease in ranch mink, *Am. J. Vet. Res.* **25**:1226.

Porter, D. D., and Larsen, A. E., 1967, Aleutian disease of mink: Infectious virus–antibody complexes in the serum, *Proc. Soc. Exp. Biol. Med.* **126**:680.

Porter, D. D., and Larsen, A. E., 1968, Virus–host interactions in Aleutian disease of mink, *Perspect. Virol.* **6**:173.

Porter, D. D., and Larsen, A. E., 1974, Aleutian disease of mink, *Prog. Med. Virol.* **18**:32.

Porter, D. D., Dixon, F. J., and Larsen, A. E., 1965a, The development of a myeloma-like condition in mink with Aleutian disease, *Blood* **25**:736.

Porter, D. D., Dixon, F. J., and Larsen, A. E., 1965b, Metabolism and function of gamma globulin in Aleutian disease of mink, *J. Exp. Med.* **121**:889.

Porter, D. D., Larsen, A. E., and Porter, H. G., 1969, The pathogenesis of Aleutian disease of mink. I. *In vivo* viral replication and the host antibody responses to viral antigen, *J. Exp. Med.* **130**:575.

Porter, D. D., Larsen, A. E., and Porter, H. G., 1972, The pathogenesis of Aleutian disease of mink. II. Enhancement of tissue lesions following the administration of a killed virus vaccine or passive antibody, *J. Immunol.* **109**:1.

Porter, D. D., Larsen, A. E., and Porter, H. G., 1973, The pathogenesis of Aleutian disease of mink. III. Immune complex arteritis, *Am. J. Pathol.* **71**:331.

Porter, D. D., Larsen, A. E., Cox, N. A., Porter, H. G., and Suffin, S. C., 1977a, Isolation of Aleutian disease virus of mink in cell culture, *Interviology* **8**:129.

Porter, D. D., Larsen, A. E., and Porter, H. G., 1977b, Reduced severity of lesions in mink infected transplacentally with Aleutian disease virus, *J. Immunol.* **119**:872.

Porter, D. D., Porter, H. G., and Larsen, A. E., 1977c, Immunoglobulin class of Aleutian disease viral antibody, *Fed. Proc.* **36**:1268 (abstr.).

Portis, J. L., and Coe, J. E., 1978, Predominant glomerular deposition of IgA and β_1C in Aleutian disease of mink, *Fed. Proc.* **37**:1558 (abstr.).

Preble, O. T., and Youngner, J. S., 1975, Temperature-sensitive viruses and the etiology of chronic and inapparent infections, *J. Infect. Dis.* **131**:467.

Rhode, S. L., III, 1978, Defective interfering particles of parvovirus H1, *J. Virol.* **27**:347.

Rose, J. A., 1974, Parvovirus reproduction, in: *Comprehensive Virology*, Vol. 3 (H. Fraenkel-Conrat and R. R. Wagner, eds.), pp. 1–61, Plenum Press, New York.

Shahrabadi, M. S., and Cho, H. J., 1977, Detection and localization of Aleutian disease virus and its antigens *in vivo* by immunoferritin technique, *Can. J. Comp. Med.* **41**:435.

Shahrabadi, M. S., Cho, H. J., and Marusyk, R. G., 1977, Characterization of the protein and nucleic acid of Aleutian disease virus, *J. Virol.* **23**:353.

Tabel, H., and Ingram, D. G., 1970a, Dialysis experiments with the infectious agent of Aleutian disease of mink, *Arch. Gesamte Virusforsch.* **32**:53.

Tabel, H., and Ingram, D. G., 1970b, The immunoglobulins in Aleutian disease (viral plasmacytosis) of mink. Different types of hypergammaglobulinemias, *Can. J. Comp. Med.* **34**:329.

Tabel, H., Ingram, D. G., and Fletch, S. M., 1970, Natural antibodies in sera of mink before and after the development of Aleutian disease (viral plasmacytosis), *Can. J. Comp. Med.* **34**:320.

Trautwein, G. W., and Helmboldt, C. F., 1962, Aleutian disease of mink. I. Experimental transmission of the disease, *Am. J. Vet. Res.* **23**:1280.

Trautwein, G., Schneider, P., and Ernst, E., 1974, Urtersuchugen über die Pathogenese der Aleutenkrankheit der Nerze. VIII. Depression der Antikorperbildung gegen Meerrettich-peroxydase, *Zbl. Vet. Med. B* **21**:467.

Role of Viruses in Chronic Neurological Diseases

Jerry S. Wolinsky and Richard T. Johnson

Departments of Neurology and Microbiology
The Johns Hopkins University School of Medicine
Baltimore, Maryland 21205

1. INTRODUCTION

Viruses play unique roles in a variety of chronic neurological diseases. The prototype slow infections of sheep (scrapie and visna) and the five established slow infections of man [kuru, Creutzfeldt-Jakob disease, subacute sclerosing panencephalitis (SSPE), progressive multifocal leukoencephalopathy, and progressive rubella panencephalitis] all are manifest primarily as neurological diseases. In those due to the spongiform encephalopathy agents, scrapie, kuru, and Creutzfeldt-Jakob disease, infectivity is found in many organs, but clinical and pathological abnormalities are confined to the CNS. In the slow infections associated with conventional viruses, infection may be generalized or limited to brain and spinal cord.

The persistence of infection in the CNS may be related in part to the brain and spinal cord structure. The CNS represents a relatively sequestered site with unique vasculature, tightly packed cellular components, and lack of a conventional lymphatic system. These structural barriers deter virus invasion of the CNS, yet, once invaded, the same barriers form an impediment to clearance of infection.

In addition to causing acute and chronic inflammatory disease, viral infections of the CNS in man and animals have been associated with malformation, degenerative disease, demyelinating disease, neo-plasms, and vascular disease. This extraordinary diversity of pathological reactions to viral infections can be explained by other unusual features of the CNS. The ontogeny of the CNS is complex, with proliferation, migration, and differentiation of varied cell populations at different times during gestation. Thus a constantly changing array of potential host cells evolves during embryogenesis. Conversely, the mature CNS represents an organ of extraordinarily high metabolic activity composed of a stable cell population that has only limited capacity to regenerate and little normal turnover of cells. Neurons, the major functional cell type of the brain, have no capacity for regeneration or mitotic division after the neonatal period. They are highly specialized for the transmission and reception of specific signals. This requires individualized membrane differentiation and metabolic activity within topographically and neurophysiologically discrete organizational units. Consequently, subpopulations of neurons have varying susceptibility to different viral infections. Considering these unique aspects of brain structure and function, it is possible to envision how a wide range of chronic pathological processes can result from viral infections.

We will first review the mechanisms by which viruses invade the CNS, how they can spread through a structure with a paucity of extracellular space, and how differences in cell susceptibility give rise to varied clinical and pathological syndromes. We will then discuss the mechanisms by which viruses are normally cleared from the CNS and the failures of clearance that occur either on the basis of defects in host response or on the basis of virus-specific mechanisms. The pathogenesis of virus-induced chronic neurological diseases will be addressed separately, since persistent infection and chronic disease often are not synonymous. Chronic disease can occur as a sequela of acute infection, and acute disease can be followed by virus persistence without the development of chronic disease. Since the discussions of virus invasion, clearance, and pathogenesis relate primarily to conventional viruses, the unique problem of the unconventional agents, the spongiform encephalopathy agents, will be summarized separately, followed by a brief discussion of the current status of studies of chronic human neurological disease of suspected viral etiology.

2. MECHANISMS OF VIRUS DISSEMINATION TO THE CNS

2.1. Systemic Barriers

Initial entry of virus into the animal host is impeded by a series of natural anatomical barriers. The most extensive of these is the skin. The intact epidermis is covered by the stratum corneum, a layer of dead, karytonized cells which cannot support virus replication. However, naked viable cells are exposed on the membranes of the respiratory, gastrointestinal, and genitourinary tracts. In immune hosts these membranes may be covered by specific secretory immunoglobulins (IgA), which can neutralize virus preventing attachment and cell penetration. In addition, the respiratory tract is normally coated by a mucous film, and the constantly beating cilia of epithelial cells move the mucous outward, sweeping particulate matter including viruses away from the epithelial cells. Even if virions are inspired into the pulmonary alveoli, these cavities are lined with macrophages which actively phagocytize particles reaching the lung. In the gastrointestinal tract the low pH of gastric acid and the presence of proteolytic enzymes inactivate most viruses. Bile of the upper intestine will dissociate the lipid membranes of enveloped viruses. Therefore, virus spread by direct contact, respiratory droplet, or contamination of food or water requires that particles breach these barriers to establish initial infection.

Viral penetration across the skin may occur with bites of arthropods or rabid or B-virus-infected animals. The skin is also penetrated by man during vaccinations, blood transfusions, or hypodermic injections. Respiratory or gastrointestinal infection may be dependent on dose of inoculum, specific properties of the virus, mode of presentation, such as droplet size, and presence of viral receptors on specialized cellular surfaces such as cilia of respiratory mucosal cells. Some infections remain confined to the surface of initial contact, such as the rhinoviruses which appear unable to replicate at core body temperatures and remain confined to the lower temperatures provided by the nasal and sinus mucosa. Similarly, wart virus remains confined to skin, and influenza virus only rarely spreads beyond the epithelial cells of the respiratory tract. In contrast, viruses which invade the CNS usually have the capacity to disseminate more widely (Johnson and Griffin, 1978).

Virus entry into the systemic circulation is normally followed by rapid removal of particles by the reticuloendothelial system (RES). As with other colloidal particles the rate of virus clearance is directly related to particle size. Thus large viruses are cleared rapidly, while small viruses are cleared more slowly; yet, even the relatively small togaviruses show 90% clearance within 1 hr. RES clearance can be circumvented when viruses circulated in blood are associated with cells. Many viruses can adsorb to red cells, a property utilized in the laboratory for serological studies, but one which may represent a selective genetic advantage in preventing clearance. Alternatively, viruses such as the paramyxoviruses and herpesviruses can replicate in white blood cells and are thus protected not only from RES clearance but also from circulating nonspecific inhibitors and specific immunoglobulins. Some small viruses such as togaviruses and picornaviruses produce a plasma viremia in the face of normal RES clearance. In some cases, this is related to virus replication in vascular endothelial cells or lymphatics, where a high input of virus into the circulation can exceed the capacity of the RES clearance mechanisms (Mims, 1964; Johnson and Mims, 1968).

2.2. CNS Barriers

The vasculature of the CNS has a unique structure correlating with its barrier function. The cerebral capillaries lack fenestrations seen in other vessels. Furthermore, adjacent endothelial cells are connected by tight junctions and are surrounded by a dense basement membrane against which are tightly apposed processes of cerebral astrocytes (Fig. 1). Within the choroid plexus where CSF is excreted, the endothelial cells more closely resemble those of extraneural tissues in that they contain fenestrae, lack basement membranes, and are surrounded by loosely arranged stromal cells. Although the capillaries in this area are clearly more permeable to large plasma molecules, free access to the CSF is impeded by apical tight junctions present between choroid plexus epithelial cells (Fig. 2). Similar tight junctions connect the pial cells surrounding the external surfaces of the brain (Peters *et al.*, 1976). These structural barriers explain the early observations that certain vital dyes injected into the general circulation stain virtually all tissues of the body but fail to stain the CSF or brain except in a few highly circumscribed regions (Katzman and Pappius, 1973).

2.3. Documented Pathways of Virus Entry

Viruses have been documented to enter the CNS along nerves and from the blood. For many years the neural route was considered the

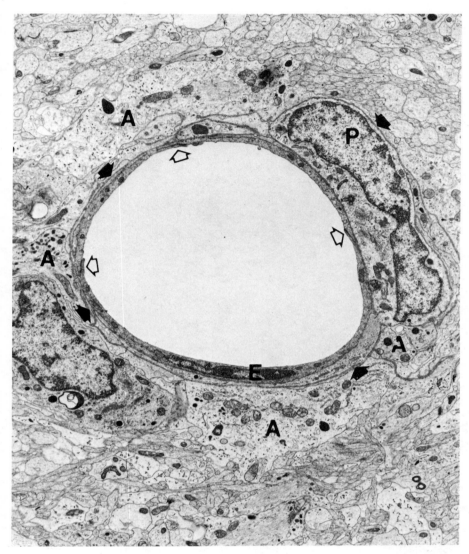

Fig. 1. Electron micrograph of a precapillary arteriole located in the cortex of an adult mouse. The vascular lumen has been cleared of blood and blood components by perfusion fixation. The portions of three endothelial cells are circumferentially sealed by tight junctions (open arrows). The nucleus of one of these endothelial cells (E) lies within the plane of section. Immediately adjacent to the endothelial cell is a pericyte (P); these cells are surrounded by a dense basement membrane (closed arrows). The foot processes of several astrocytes (A) form a final zone about the vascular complex separating it from the surrounding neuropil. These morphological structures correspond to the conceptual "blood–brain barrier." ×6850.

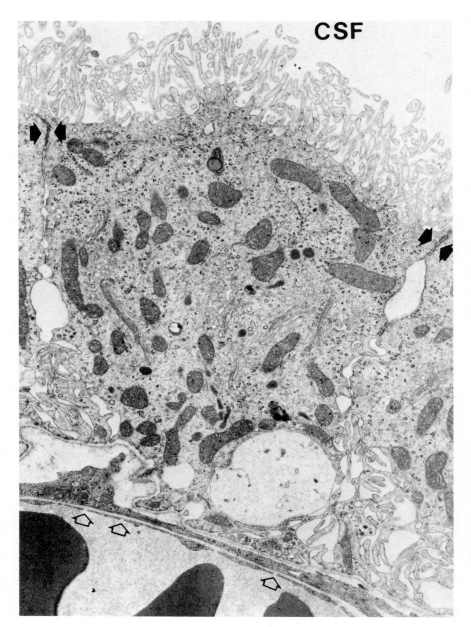

Fig. 2. Electron micrograph of a portion of the choroid plexus of an immature hamster. Portions of several red blood cells are seen as homogeneous dense structures at the bottom portion of the electron micrograph within a small venule consisting of fenestrated (open arrows) endothelial cells. The choroid plexus epithelial cells rest on a basement membrane and have a microvillous surface facing the CSF. Apical tight junctions (closed arrows) form an anatomical barrier to free diffusion between sera and CSF. ×13,700.

primary pathway, and early experimental studies documented the movement of rabies, herpes simplex, and polioviruses within peripheral nerves. Ascending infection of supporting cells within nerves or diffusion of viruses within extracellular spaces of nerves have been proposed as mechanisms for such centripetal spread of virus along nerves. However, in several instances experimental evidence now indicates that sensory or motor terminals of axons contain virus receptors, and that virus is probably carried within the axoplasm by a rapid transport system to the central cell body of the neuron (Kristensson *et al.*, 1971; Murphy, 1977; Johnson and Griffin, 1978).

In the nasal mucosa a unique relationship of nerve fibers to the external environment exists. The apical processes of receptor cells of the olfactory bulb of the CNS extend beyond the free margin of the nasal epithelium. This represents the only site where CNS fibers are exposed to the ambient environment. Colloidal particles placed on the olfactory mucosa have been found to move into the olfactory bulb in less than 1 hr (DeLorenzo, 1970). Several experimental studies have shown that viruses can enter directly into the CNS from the olfactory mucosa. Nevertheless, clinical and epidemiological observation indicate that this route is not important in most natural infections. It is, however, the suspected route of CNS invasion of togaviruses and rabies viruses in laboratory-acquired infections and is the likely mechanism by which rabies virus is transmitted to the brain from aerosols in bat-infested caves.

In most experimental and natural infections virus invades the CNS from the blood. In some togavirus infections and in murine retrovirus infections, viral replication in the vascular endothelial cells of brain precedes spread to adjacent astrocytes (Johnson and Mims, 1968; Swarz *et al.*, 1978). On the other hand, a number of viruses have been shown to infect neural cells adjacent to small vessels without electron microscopic or immunological evidence of endothelial cell infection (Albrecht, 1968). The mechanism of transport of viruses across the endothelial cell and basement membrane is unknown but may be similar to the limited passage of electron-dense tracer molecules which cross prearteriolar, capillary, and venular endothelial cells in pinocytotic vesicles with subsequent release into the intercellular space between adjacent astrocytes (Westergaard, 1977). The proposal that viruses may be carried across the endothelial cells by infected leukocytes at present seems unlikely in that leukocytes have not been shown to migrate freely into the CNS under normal circumstances.

Other viruses enter the CNS by infection of the choroid plexus cells, with seeding of virus into the CSF. Studies of rat virus and mumps virus infections of experimental animals have clearly shown a sequence of choroid plexus cell infection, followed by ependymal cell infection, followed by spread to parenchymal cells of the brain (Lipton and Johnson, 1972; Wolinsky *et al.*, 1976).

In summary, viruses usually invade the CNS via the blood, but the process requires a sequence of events involving the passage of extraneural barriers as well as those barriers unique to the CNS (Fig. 3). Along this route a variety of host defense mechanisms can be marshalled. The alveolar, epithelial, and subcutaneous phagocytic cells engulf and sometimes inactivate virus particles, barriers of nonsusceptible cells may be present in tissues where primary and secondary multiplication takes place, interferon is produced by infected cells, particles are cleared from blood by the RES, and the anatomical structure of the brain itself may exclude viruses. It is probable that the combination of these factors explains why viral infections of the brain are relatively rare, even though infection with viruses which are potential causes of CNS disease is common.

2.4. Spread of Viruses within the CNS

After a virus has entered the CNS via neural or hematogenous routes, disease can occur only if virus spreads within the nervous system and reaches and attaches to the cytoplasmic membrane of susceptible cells. Virus entering the CSF from the choroid plexus is readily dispersed throughout CSF pathways coming in contact with ependymal and meningeal cells. On the other hand, spread of virus through densely packed neuropil poses a theoretical problem. Ultrastructural studies of the CNS indicate that the extracellular gap between cells and processes measures only 10–15 nm, less than the diameter of any virion. These electron-lucent channels appear to represent a true pericellular space rather than hydrophobic lipid leaflets belonging to the plasma membranes of adjacent cells (Peters *et al.*, 1976). Viruses have been observed within these intracellular gaps in the neuropil, suggesting that these spaces may be more pliable in the vital state than when observed following perfusion-fixation for electron microscopy (Blinzinger and Muller, 1971). Nevertheless, unrestricted passage of viruses within the extracellular spaces of brain seems unlikely (Fig. 4).

In some infections sequential studies have indicated that virus appears to spread in contiguous fashion. For example, following the initial infection of the meningeal or ependymal surfaces there may be an apparent cell-to-cell spread causing focal or multifocal areas of

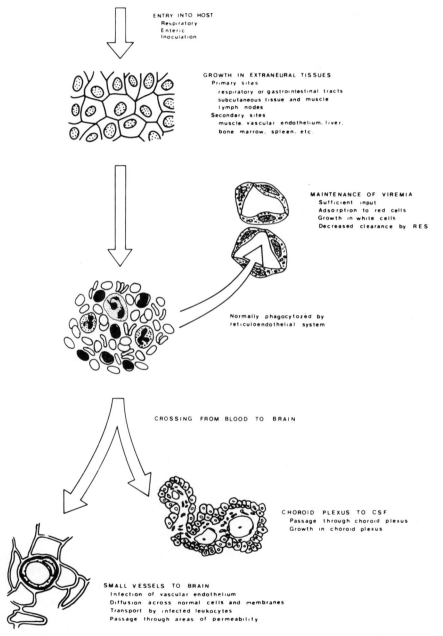

Fig. 3.   Schematic illustration of the steps in the hematogenous spread of virus to the CNS. From Johnson (1974).

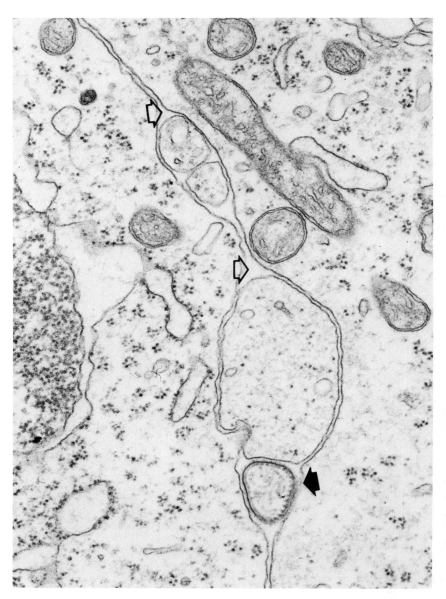

Fig. 4. A single mumps virus virion (closed arrow) is seen within the interstitial space between portions of three neurons of the hippocampal cortex of a newborn hamster. The interstitial space (open arrows) forms a small continuous network that extends between all cellular components of the CNS and freely communicates with the ventricular system. ×47,300.

infection. However, this is not true of viruses which infect only specific cell populations. The spread of viruses via the long dendritic and axonal cytoplasmic ramifications of neurons has long been suspected for rabies and polioviruses. Rabies virus appears to spread across the synaptic junction between neurons, suggesting that the virus may be transmitted along the long axonal ramifications of neurons to other susceptible neuron populations via axonal transport within the CNS (Murphy, 1977). Similarly, studies of poliovirus have suggested axonal transport of virus. Sequential histological studies showed both a restriction of virus within spinal cord following cordectomy and a correlation of speed of viral movement with age-related maturation of the fast transport system of axoplasm (Jubelt *et al.*, 1980). Spread of virus within axon transport systems would provide a mechanism for rapid movement of virus between widely separated but neurophysiologically coupled susceptible neurons.

2.5. Differential Susceptibility within the CNS

The diverse cell populations of the CNS show variable susceptibility to infection with viruses. Thus, although some viruses such as herpes simplex virus are capable of infecting a full range of CNS cell types, other viruses replicate only in ependymal or meningeal cells, only in glial cells, or only in neurons. Furthermore, susceptibility may be limited to very precise neuronal cell populations. For example, poliovirus infections appear to involve only motor neurons, and initial infection with rabies virus occurs within neurons localized in the limbic system, with relative sparing of neocortex. This selective vulnerability can explain the differences in the clinical features of encephalitis, which presents with somnolence and seizures, poliovirus infections, which cause flaccid paralysis without sensory abnormalities, and rabies infections, which cause the animal to be alert, with loss of normal timidity and aberrant behavior. The last appears to represent a diabolical selective adaptation of virus in which infection of specific neuronal cell populations modifies behavior, driving the host to bite and transmit virus to other animals.

In addition, the effect of a virus on different cells may vary. Cells may be lysed, transformed, or moderately infected, leading to slowly evolving disease or inhibition of specific cellular functions (Tamm, 1975; Robb, 1977). The same virus may even have different effects on different cell populations at the same time. This is best exemplified in progressive multifocal leukoencephalopathy in which each of the three major cell populations in the CNS appears to be affected differently. Neurons appear to escape infection. Oligodendrocytes, however, are lytically infected, resulting in demyelination, since their modified cyto-plasmic membranes which form the myelin sheaths surrounding axons can no longer be maintained. The third major cell population, the astrocytes, appears to be relatively nonpermissively infected. These cells proliferate and develop bizzare forms, mitotic figures, and multiple nuclei, suggesting that they have undergone transformation (Johnson *et al.*, 1974; Padgett and Walker, 1976).

Cellular susceptibility to virus infection may also change with maturation of the CNS. This appears to explain many of the malforma-tions which have been produced by viruses. For example, after late fetal or neonatal infection with parvoviruses, a specific loss of granular neurons of the cerebellum is found. Sequential histological studies have shown selective viral destruction of the external germinal cells of the cerebellum prior to their postnatal migration to form the granular cell layer. This abnormality has been related to rat virus infections in hamsters, minute virus in mice, and feline panleukopenia virus in cats or ferrets (Kilham and Margolis, 1975; Margolis and Kilham, 1975). Since these parvoviruses appear incapable of replication except in host cells actively engaged in DNA synthesis, involvement is limited to those cell populations actively dividing at the time of infection. Therefore, in the adult cat infected with feline panleukopenia virus, infection is manifest by leukopenia and diarrhea because the bone marrow and gas-trointestinal tract provide the susceptible cell pool. In the fetal cat the germinal cells of the cerebellum, a cell population that cannot be replenished, are also selectively destroyed (Kilham and Margolis, 1966).

Very different cerebral anomalies are produced by the vaccine strain of bluetongue virus inoculated into fetal lambs. This virus selec-tively infects the subventricular cells of the forebrain during their dif-ferentiation and migration. Once these precursor cells assume their mature position as neurons and glia of brain, they appear to be insus-ceptible to infection. Thus infection of the ovine fetus during the first trimester causes major destruction of the forebrain, an anomaly known as hydranencephaly. Infection at midgestation leads to multiple focal lesions within the brain substance, an anomaly known as porencephaly. Infection at the end of the second trimester produces no gross mal-formation of the brain, since at that time a majority of cells have already matured and differentiated. The type of malformation is age dependent, related to the availability of vulnerable, immature cells (Osburn *et al.*, 1971*a,b*). Therefore, not only is there selective vulnerability of specific cells to specific viruses, but also vulnerability may change with time during ontogeny.

3. MECHANISMS OF VIRAL CLEARANCE FROM THE CNS

3.1. Immune Responses in the CNS

Many factors which normally serve to limit viral replication and spread elsewhere in the body are not readily active within the CNS. Under normal conditions the CNS is believed to be devoid of lymphatics or immunocompetent cells. However, recent evidence suggests that lymphatic-like structures may be present and expand under the stimuli of some pathological conditions. Such development of lymphatic-like structures has been described anatomically in the region of multiple sclerosis plaques and would appear to provide a potential site for the local processing of viral antigens by macrophages (Prineas, 1979). However, the general applicability of such a system is unclear and such a system has not been directly documented in known viral infections.

Evidence for a locally active immune response in the CNS derives from clinicopathological observation of certain infections of man and animals. In some infections plasma cells can be demonstrated within Virchow-Robbin spaces surrounding blood vessel walls, and antibody of restricted electrophoretic migration presumably secreted from a limited number of plasma cell clones appears within CSF. Both features are well described in SSPE and progressive rubella panencephalitis, and the oligoclonal antibody response has also been found following mumps meningitis and other acute viral illnesses with CNS involvement (Vandvik et al., 1978a,b; Vandvik and Norrby, 1973). A remarkable example of this apparent expansion of immunocompetent cells in brain is seen in sheep chronically infected with visna virus; the intense inflammatory response has been found to organize into germinal centers, and levels of anti-visna antibody in CSF may exceed levels in serum (Griffin et al., 1978). A reversed brain or CSF:sera antibody ratio is also found in mice infected with Theiler's virus, and oligoclonal antibody patterns are seen in monkeys experimentally infected with measles virus (Lipton and Gonzalez-Scarano, 1978; Yamanouchi et al., 1979). Restricted B-cell responses have also been demonstrated by extracting cells from the brains of mice infected with parainfluenza virus and demonstrating

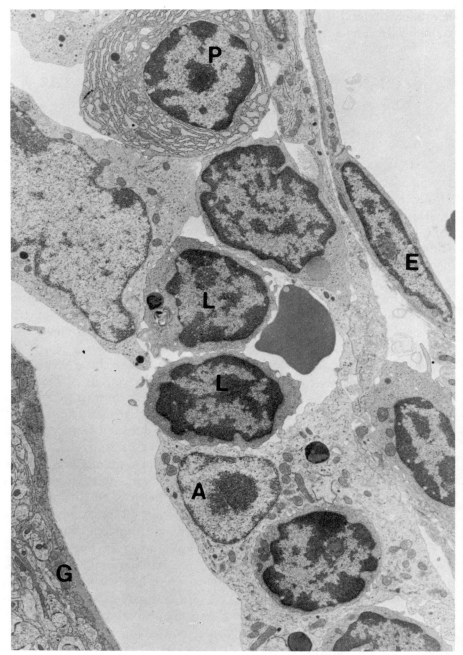

Fig. 5.   An inflammatory infiltrate is seen in the subarachnoid space of an adult mouse infected with parainfluenza-1 virus. A portion of the lumen of a meningeal blood vessel is seen at the upper right of the electron micrograph and is lined by endothelial cells

their ability to produce monoclonal antiviral antibody *in vitro* (Gerhard and Koprowski, 1977; Gerhard *et al.*, 1978).

Phagocytic cells also are not considered to be normally resident within the CNS. However, recently cells have been described in the Tegu lizard which lie scattered over the ependymal surface and are proposed to have a phagocytic function (Bleier *et al.*, 1975). Morphologically similar cells in the same topographic location have been shown to ingest viral particles which appear to be degraded within secondary phagolysosomes during experimental mumps meningoencephalitis in the hamster (Wolinsky *et al.*, 1974). With these exceptions, however, the evidence is compelling that most if not all mononuclear cells involved in inflammatory reactions of brain derive from blood (Fujita and Kitamura, 1976).

Therefore, under normal conditions the brain is relatively devoid of immunocompetent or phagocytic cells, leaving it initially rather vulnerable to viral infection. After infection is established, mononuclear cells appear to enter the CNS by transendothelial passage to form the inflammatory reaction (Fig. 5). Lymphocytes are probably the initial cells to respond, being attracted to brain by as yet unknown substances produced during the early phases of CNS infection. Studies of acute Sindbis virus encephalitis in mice have shown that the initial recruitment of mononuclear cells is immunologically specific (McFarland *et al.*, 1972). Once attracted to brain, such sensitized lymphocytes presumably serve to signal the recruitment of other cells by the secretion of lymphokines such as lymphocyte and macrophage migration inhibition factors. Continued antigenic stimulation by prolonged persistence of viral antigen in brain may result in local plasma cell differentiation and clonal expansion, giving rise to local antibody production as noted above.

The systemic humoral immune response is also rather ill suited for initial containment of virus replicating within the CNS. Large-molecular-weight constituents of blood such as antibody and complement are relatively excluded from the CNS compartment by the blood–brain barrier. Normally, these substances are present in the CSF at concentrations several hundredfold lower than that found in the

---

(E). Several lymphocytes (L) and a plasma cell (P) can be seen within the subarachnoid space. Arachnoid cells (A), normally found in this region, make up the fine network of tissue that characterizes the meninges. The clear spaces would normally be filled with CSF. A small portion of brain parenchyma is seen at the lower portion of the micrograph separated from the CSF by the glia limitans (G) composed of pial cells. ×6850.

systemic circulation (Fossan, 1977; Norrby, 1978). Further, while CSF circulates freely within the interstitial spaces of brain parenchyma, these pathways are sufficiently narrow even to impede the diffusion of large molecules. As tissue destruction and inflammatory reactions proceed, these barriers to the diffusion of large molecules into and within brain become less substantial. At such time, direct neutralization of virus by antibody or antibody and complement, as well as complement and antibody-dependent cell-mediated cytotoxicity, may effect of viral clearance from the CNS.

The role of complement in clearance of virus from CNS is undefined. Complement in the presence of antibody has been shown *in vitro* to induce membrane damage to some viral particles that results in their inactivation (Cooper *et al.*, 1976; Haukenes, 1977). *In vivo* the role of complement is ambiguous; Sindbis-virus-infected mice depleted of C3 complement by injections of cobra venom show substantially higher titers of virus in brain, possibly due to the prolongation of viremia. However, despite higher content of virus the complement-depleted animals survive longer (Hirsch *et al.*, 1978).

Interferon has been shown to develop in brain during infections. However, its role in clearance is also uncertain, since levels of interferon have been correlated with amount of virus replication but not with recovery from viral meningoencephalitis (Vilček, 1964). Postexposure treatment of rabies-virus-infected cynomolgus monkeys with interferon confers some protection but only for animals that never evidence symptoms of CNS infection (Weinmann *et al.*, 1979). Stimulation of adequate interferon levels would be expected to protect uninfected but otherwise susceptible cells adjacent to viral foci in brain, but this has not been shown for any CNS infection. Furthermore, clinical efficacy of interferon administration has been demonstrated in man only for non-CNS infections such as cutaneous herpes zoster and hepatitis B virus infections. Some viruses causing persistent infections fail to induce significant levels of interferon. This is characteristic of not only congenital rubella virus infections but also acquired rubella (Rawls, 1974). Recently, a circulating serum factor has been shown in sera of patients with progressive rubella panencephalitis which prevents normal donor leukocytes from secreting interferon in response to rubella viral antigens *in vitro* (Wolinsky *et al.*, 1979).

Other lymphokines may also be important in clearance of CNS infections. Macrophage chemotactic factor released by lymphocytes may serve to localize macrophages to a site of viral replication and might be expected to play a prominent role in attracting cells to brain.

Lymphocyte migration inhibition factor could be expected to play a similar role. Recent studies demonstrate an *in vitro* defect in gradient-purified blood mononuclear cells from patients with progressive multifocal leukoencephalopathy to generate lymphocyte migration inhibition factor on stimulation with JC virus antigen (Willoughby *et al.*, 1979). Such a defect might explain the lack of an inflammatory response usually seen in this infection.

3.2. Failure of Virus Clearance in Immunodeficient Hosts

Naturally occurring immune deficiencies in man and drug-induced immunosuppression of man and animals give insights into the role of humoral or cell-mediated immune responses in clearance of virus from the CNS. In general, patients with agammaglobulinemia are not predisposed to persistent viral infections, with the exception of enterovirus infections. Patients with agammaglobulinemia but intact cell-mediated immunity often fail to clear polioviruses or echoviruses. With CNS infection they can develop protracted clinical disease with virus recoverable from CSF and brain tissue for prolonged intervals (Davis *et al.*, 1977; Webster *et al.*, 1978; Wilfert *et al.*, 1977). Intense inflammatory responses accompany these chronic infections, but they are devoid of plasma cells. These observations suggest that either direct neutralization of virus by antibody or antibody-dependent cell-mediated cytotoxic reactions are of critical importance in effecting clearance of enteroviruses.

Defects in cell-mediated immunity have been associated with chronic CNS infections with a variety of viruses. Patients with lymphoproliferative diseases or receiving immunosuppressive therapy occasionally have opportunistic CNS infections with polyoma viruses, causing progressive multifocal leukoencephalopathy (see Chapter 4). Atypical CNS infections with varicella zoster (McCormick *et al.*, 1969), cytomegalovirus (Dorfman, 1973), adenovirus (Chou *et al.*, 1973), and measles have also complicated diseases or therapies suppressing cell-mediated immune responses.

Acute measles virus infections provide an interesting example of the problem of viral clearance. The acute systemic illness is normally associated with a transient impairment of cell-mediated immunity as measured by inhibition of delayed hypersensitivity reactions *in vivo* and depressed blastogenic responses to a variety of mitogens *in vitro*. However, humoral responses, antibody-dependent cell-mediated cytotoxicity responses, and recently haplotype specific T-lymphocyte killing responses have been shown to develop over a normal time course (Kreth et al., 1979). In a large proportion of children with acute primary measles, virus may well disseminate to brain as reflected by CSF pleocytosis and EEG changes (Johnson et al., 1978). However, these abnormalities are transient except in children with significant defects in cell-mediated immunity. These children may develop a subacute fatal CNS infection (Aicardi et al., 1977; Wolinsky et al., 1977). This pattern appears to have a reasonable counterpart in experimental animals. Mature hamsters can clear measles virus from brain without showing signs of CNS infection. However, if thymectomized at birth and then challenged with the same virus as adults, they develop fatal encephalitis without evidence of the expected inflammatory response in brain or development of antibody, presumably because of the accompanying defect of T-helper-cell function necessary to process antigen for recognition by B cells (Johnson et al., 1975).

3.3. Viral Persistence in Immunologically Intact Hosts

Viruses can persist and cause chronic disease in the face of normal immune responses if latency is established, if replication is restricted with a reduced rate of spread, or if the agent is not antigenic and fails to excite host responses. Examples of each of these strategies have been implicated in chronic neurological diseases.

Several of the herpes viruses (varicella zoster, herpes simplex viruses 1 and 2) appear to establish latency when virus reaches the sensory ganglia (Stevens, 1978). The viral genome is apparently sequestered in the nonreplicating neurons by unknown mechanisms. Latently infected cells do not express viral antigens and therefore are seen as normal uninfected cells by the host. These cells can serve as a potential reservoir for recurrent, albeit restricted, and usually acute disease when the viral genome is reactivated.

Visna virus of sheep provides an example of latency in which chronic disease does evolve. The DNA provirus of visna virus, a retrovirus, has been detected by in situ hybridization in neural cells (Haase, 1975). The immune response does not appear to induce restriction since no exponential growth of virus and little free infectious virus were observed in CNS of sheep after thymectomy and antilymphocyte treatment (Narayan et al., 1977). The pathogenesis of the chronic neurological disease is discussed in the next section.

Viruses other than DNA viruses or retroviruses do appear capable of persistence by mechanisms as yet undefined. One example is in SSPE, an uncommon complication of measles virus infection (see Chapter 5). In this condition as initial acute infection occurs in a normal although young host. Virus appears to be adequately cleared, but persistence of the genome must occur at some site since the late disease does not appear to result from reinfection. The late disease occurs in a reasonably intact host without consistent defects in cellular immune function and with a well-developed humoral immune response both in sera and within the CNS (Agnarsdóttir, 1977). While viral antigens are easily shown in brain tissue, it is possible that antigens at the surface of infected cells are only intermittently expressed, resulting in the slowly evolving syndrome. There is also supportive data to suggest that viral antigens critical for maturation of complete virus are altered in a way that enables virus persistence (Wechsler and Fields, 1978; Hall *et al.*, 1978).

Defective particles that interfere with the replication of the parent virus or temperature-sensitive mutants of parental virus would provide an additional viral "strategy" for contained infections. While animal models for CNS disease with prolonged courses compared to those seen with parental virus have been described using defective interfering particles (Doyle and Holland, 1973) and atypical neural disease patterns have been shown for certain temperature-sensitive mutants (Rabinowitz *et al.*, 1976; Haspel and Rapp, 1975), no clear role of these agents has yet been shown for either human or naturally occurring animal diseases. Indeed, in progressive multifocal leukoencephalopathy, the one human slow infection in which large numbers of virions are seen and in which defective interfering particles might be suspected, virions extracted directly from brain do not show a population of less dense defective particles as is routinely found when polyomaviruses are grown *in vitro* (Dörries *et al.*, 1979).

Finally, the virus may not provoke an immune response. Some viruses such as coronaviruses and retroviruses do not incite vigorous immune responses, possibly because of the preponderance of host lipids in the virus envelope. However, there is no evidence for antigenicity of the spongiform encephalopathy agents in either natural or experimentally infected hosts. Thus far, the only suggestion that the host recognizes these agents is by inference from the finding of amyloid-containing plaques in brains of selected mice infected with scrapie (Wisniewski *et al.*, 1975). These may or may not represent deposits of immunoglobulins.

4. MECHANISMS OF CHRONIC DISEASE INDUCTION

Chronic virus-induced neurological diseases need not be associated with chronic or persistent infection, nor does persistent infection always result in chronic disease. Chronic diseases have been associated with acute, chronic, or latent infections, and the pathological changes may be dependent on immune-mediated cell destruction, may evolve only in immunodeficient hosts, or the immune response may appear irrelevant in the evolution of the disease. The various relations of types of infection to disease are shown schematically in Fig. 6.

4.1. Chronic Neurological Diseases as Sequelae of Acute Infections

Acute infections are usually associated with acute disease resolved by either recovery or death of the host. However, many severe acute

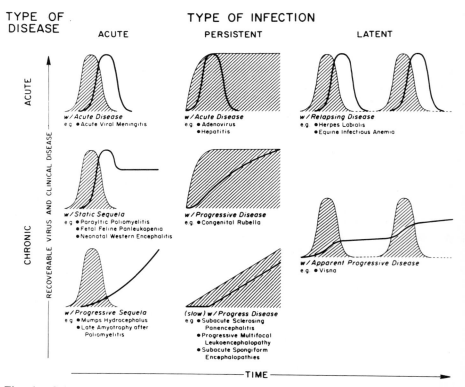

Fig. 6.   Schematic representation of patterns of infection (shaded areas) and disease (solid lines) characteristic of acute, persistent, and latent infections. From Johnson *et al.* (1978).

infections of the CNS leave permanent disabling sequelae, e.g., the static residual flaccid paralysis following acute spinal motor neuron destruction by polioviruses or the spastic paralysis and mental deficits following destruction of cortical motor cells by arthropod-borne encephalitis viruses. Subsequent to fetal or neonatal infection of the CNS, such static sequelae may give the clinical appearance of progressive disease. For example, parvovirus infections of the CNS of late fetal or neonatal animals cause selective destruction of the granule cells of the cerebellum (see Section 2.5). Immediately following the acute infection, infant animals appear normal, even though they lack the sole excitatory cell population of the cerebellum. However, they are subsequently incapable of developing the normal synaptic connections required for development of coordinated motor activity. Therefore, as they mature they fail to acquire coordination, giving the clinical appearance of suffering a progressive degenerative process. Similar situations occur in human infections, e.g., some patients appear to have progressive neurological dysfunction following Western equine encephalitis virus infections (Finley *et al.*, 1967). However, studies of these children indicate that acute destruction of neural cells in infancy simply leaves the child unable to achieve subsequent developmental milestones. Although neurological deficits appear to intensify over time, this does not necessarily represent a loss of further neural cells or persistence of virus.

On the other hand, progressive pathological changes can actually evolve following acute viral infection. This is exemplified in the progressive obstructive hydrocephalus which has been found to follow a variety of viral infections which are limited to ependymal cells lining the ventricles of the brain (Johnson, 1975*a*). This was first demonstrated with experimental mumps virus infections in neonatal hamsters. Young animals show no clinical signs of disease during the acute infection. Ependymal cells are destroyed, virus is cleared, the inflammatory response resolves, and immunity develops. However, over subsequent weeks the aqueduct of Sylvius, an ependymal-cell-lined channel connecting the third and fourth ventricles of the brain, becomes reduced in size, eventually becoming markedly stenotic or totally occluded. This leads to the obstruction of CSF flow, with enlargement of the ventricles, compression of the cerebral cortex, distortion of the skull, and paralysis. The progressive hydrocephalus usually causes death within 3 months after the initial infection. However, at the time of clinical disease there is no detectable free virus, viral antigen, or inflammation. Subsequent to the description of this phenomenon in experimental animals, a number of children have been described who developed hydrocephalus several months following mumps virus meningitis or encephalitis.

A different mechanism of late progressive disease following remote antecedent acute infection may occur following paralytic poliomyelitis in man. After poliomyelitis during childhood or early adult life most patients live with a static deficit for many years, but some develop progressive weakness and paralysis in late middle age (Mulder *et al.*, 1972). After loss of motor neurons in the spinal cord, distal axons of remaining motor neurons probably sprout and increase their peripheral field of innervation. This compensation may be lost over time, either because overloading of residual neurons causes their premature degeneration and death, or because motor neurons normally start undergoing natural attrition at approximately age 50 (Tomlinson and Irving, 1977). This natural loss may cause no disease in the normal individual, but may jeopardize the strength and motor control of the patient who has less reserve. Again, the chronic progressive disease need not depend on the persistence of poliovirus but can be explained by the effects of an anatomical residua of a remote acute infection.

4.2. Chronic Disease and Persistent Infection

Persistent infections can cause acute monophasic diseases followed by a chronic asymptomatic carrier state as recognized with adenoviruses and hepatitis viruses. Alternatively, a chronic carrier state can lead to chronic, progressive disease. This is probably best exemplified by the remarkable diseases which have been observed in man following fetal infection with rubella virus. The severity and frequency of congenital disease are related to the time of gestational infection. Thus maternal infection early during pregnancy causes more severe and more frequent disease in the fetus than infection late in pregnancy. The pathogenesis of the abnormalities produced by rubella appears to involve two different mechanisms. Infection of some cells leads to cell destruction, but possibly of greater importance is the noncytopathic infection with inhibition of mitosis. Children born with rubella syndrome are small for gestational age and have an actual decrease in cell numbers (Naeye and Blanc, 1975). Cells grown from children with congenital rubella show a decrease in mitotic activity. Furthermore, this noncytopathic infection may be focal or multifocal. Focal infections have been suggested by immunofluorescent staining of tissue from a child dying with rubella syndrome demonstrating focal collections of histologically normal cells containing viral antigen (Woods *et al.*, 1966).

Cloning cells from similar infants shows a comparatively small number of infected cells but when explanted *in vitro* the infected cell clones have retarded growth rates (Rawls and Melnick, 1966). Rawls's theory of clonal noncytopathic infection with mitotic inhibition can account for the majority of phenomena observed in the congenital rubella syndrome such as the asymmetrical and noninflammatory lesions of different organs, persistence of infection despite the presence of transplacental IgG and the fetal production of IgM, and the ultimate apparent clearance of virus from most children (Rawls, 1968, 1974). After the initial transplacental infection of embryonic cells, maternal antibody presumably prevents cell-to-cell spread of the infection. However, since virus fails to lyse cells, cell division would be slowed but each daughter cell would be infected. This mechanism of clonal infection could account for hypoplasia of one eye, arising from an infected cell clone despite a normal eye on the other side arising from an uninfected clone. Cells with a lower doubling time would eventually disappear in most organs, which would explain why children congenitally infected with rubella eventually clear the virus, and why virus might persist longer in nonreplicating corneal or neural cells.

Recently, a late complication of this congenital infection has been noted in a number of adolescents who had variable stigmata of congenital rubella infection. After clinical stability of 11–12 years, they began to have intellectual deterioration with the development of seizures, abnormal movements, and signs of progressive CNS disease (Wolinsky, 1978). CSF from these patients has an increased amount of γ-globulin which is directed against rubella virus. Rubella virus antibody in serum is also elevated. Autopsy has shown pathological changes only within the CNS, with inflammatory changes, microglial nodules, mineralization around vessels, and destruction of myelin. Rubella virus has been recovered from the brain biopsy of one of these patients. Therefore, it would appear that rubella virus has the capacity to persist in the CNS for greater than 12 years after fetal infection. Why this infection is rekindled with the development of progressive disease during adolescence is unknown.

Progressive rubella panencephalitis shares some common features clinically and pathologically with SSPE due to measles virus. However, in SSPE (see Chapter 5) there appears to be a mutation in the virus so that fully enveloped virions are not produced. This defect in assembly may lead to slow cell-to-cell spread of virus, and to a lack of clearance of virus despite the markedly accentuated immune response. Conversely, in progressive multifocal leukoencephalopathy (see Chapter 4) fully infectious virus is produced. Failure of clearance is apparently explained by the immune deficits in patients with the disease, but the chronic nature of the infection is not readily explained. It is difficult to envision a "slow" replication of papovaviruses in CNS cells. Possibly the slowness of disease results from delayed release of virions from the infected oligodendrocytes. If depression of cellular DNA and protein synthesis are the major factors leading to cell destruction by papovaviruses, this depression might have less impact on oligo-dendrocytes. These are nondividing cells with a slow turnover rate of highly specialized, stable membrane. Thus a long period of virus-induced depressed metabolic activity may be tolerated by this cell popu-lation before physical disruption of cell membranes releases virus to infect neighboring oligodendrocytes.

Subtle effects of virus on CNS host cells is dramatically seen in lymphocytic choriomeningitis virus infections (see Chapter 7). Con-genitally infected carrier mice appear to tolerate widespread infection, including infection of the CNS, for almost a normal life expectancy. Behavioral studies of these mice, however, have shown some limitation of CNS function. Infections of lines of mouse neuroblastomas have shown preservation of vital cell functions such as growth rates and pro-tein synthesis. However, the synthesis of acetylcholine, choline acetyl transferase, and acetycholine esterase were reduced (Oldstone et al., 1977). Although Oldstone termed these "luxury functions," suppression of these products in vivo might have marked functional effects, causing chronic disease even without discernible pathological changes.

4.3. Chronic Disease as a Manifestation of Latent or Recurrent Infections

Latent infections, where virus is harbored without continuous production of infectious virus, are expected to produce disease only with reactivation of the latent genomes. Recent studies of visna, one of the classic slow infections of sheep, have suggested novel mechanisms relating viral latency to chronic disease. Visna is a persistent infection of sheep characterized clinically by slowly evolving paralysis and his-tologically by multiple foci of inflammation and demyelination. The disease occurred naturally in Icelandic sheep and has been experi-mentally induced in other breeds. The incubation period may extend for several years, and disease may progress chronically over many months. After experimental infection of sheep, exponential replication of the agent has not been demonstrated. However, by in situ hybridization, sequestration of proviral DNA can be found in cells of the CNS (Haase *et al.*, 1977). Sufficient viral proteins are apparently produced to evoke an immune response. Early inflammatory lesions are found in the clinically asymptomatic sheep in the first few months after infection. By the time animals develop clinical disease, there are multiple lesions within the CNS. Histologically, these appear to be of different ages (Petursson *et al.*, 1976). The sequestering of virus as provirus may explain the persistence, but it would appear that the ultimate development of disease may be explained by exacerbations of virus replication.

The demonstration of antigenic mutation of visna virus in persistently infected sheep may provide a mechanism for the chronic disease (Narayan *et al.*, 1977). The mutants which have been found in chronically infected sheep are fully virulent when inoculated into other sheep (Narayan *et al.*, 1978). Furthermore, studies in cell culture suggest that mutant selection is enhanced by the presence of antibody in cultures. Thus the sequential evolution of virulent mutants within the same individual might result in exacerbations of acute disease but appear clinically as progressive disease as lesions accumulate. If this proves to be the mechanism, both competence of the immune response and presence of virulent nondefective viruses may be prerequisites to production of chronic disease. The virus would escape immune surveillance both by its ability to persist as provirus and by the formation of nonneutralizable mutant viruses which the immune response has selected or even helped to induce but which the immune responses cannot clear.

5. SUBACUTE SPONGIFORM ENCEPHALOPATHIES

The subacute spongiform encephalopathies are naturally occurring noninflammatory degenerative diseases of the CNS of man and animals. They appear closely related, with common clinical and histopathological features, a unique pathogenesis independent of any apparent host immune response, and similar physical and chemical properties of their causative agents. These diseases include kuru and Creutzfeldt-Jakob disease in man (Gibbs and Gajdusek, 1978), scrapie in sheep and goats, and transmissible mink encephalopathy. Under experimental conditions these diseases can be shown to cross wide species barriers; for example, Creutzfeldt-Jakob disease has been transmitted to mice and transmissible mink encephalopathy has been transmitted to subhuman primates (Table 1).

TABLE 1

Subactue Spongiform Encephalopathies—Known Host Ranges[a]

Natural host	Disease	Man	Apes	Old World monkeys	New World monkeys	Sheep	Goats	Mink	Mice	Guinea pigs	Hamsters	Ferrets
Man	Creutzfeldt-Jakob disease	×	×	×	×		×		×	×	×	×
	Kuru		×	×	×			×				×
Sheep, goats	Scrapie				×	×	×	×	×	×	×	×
Mink	Transmissible mink encephalopathy			×	×	×	×	×			×	×

[a] Isolated transmissions to cat (CJD); rat, gerbil, vole (scrapie); racoon, skunk (TME) are also reported.

5.1. Clinical Diseases

Scrapie has been recognized as a clinical entity for over a century. Affected sheep are identified by the appearance of progressive ataxia, tremor, and hyperexcitability or lethargy; excessive thirst, weakness, and wasting are also seen. The course is progressive to death within 2–6 months. Successful transmission of the disease by inoculation of brain and spinal cord tissue from affected animals into healthy sheep was accomplished more than 40 years ago. Passage of the disease into small laboratory animals, especially mice and hamsters, has enabled extensive although tedious pathogenesis studies in experimental animals.

Transmissible mink encephalopathy was first observed in 1947, but the nature of the illness was not well appreciated until it was successfully transmitted experimentally. The clinical and pathological abnormalities are very similar to those of scrapie, and evidence suggests that the disease originated in mink being fed on scrapie-infected sheep carcasses. Consistent with the suspected sheep origin of the agent is that transmissible mink encephalopathy has been successfully transmitted back to sheep and goats.

Kuru was first described in 1957 as an epidemic disease of the Fore natives of the Eastern New Guinea Highlands. The disorder was most common in adult women and children of both sexes. The clinical disorder is initially characterized by a mild tremor which presages a severe symmetrical gait ataxia and proceeds to eventual immobilization. Death from inanition occurs within 3–6 months. Similarities of the clinical disease and pathology to scrapie led to the successful attempts to transmit the disease to subhuman primates. These transmissions demonstrated incubation periods up to 8 years. Subsequent epidemiological observations focused attention on ritualistic cannibalism practiced by the Fore as a probable mechanism of disease transmission within the tribe. Kuru has shown progressive disappearance with the discontinuation of this rite (Gajdusek, 1977).

Creutzfeldt-Jakob disease is an uncommon sporadic "degenerative" CNS disease of man. It is worldwide in distribution with a probable incidence between one and two cases per million population (Masters *et al.*, 1978). It is clinically characterized by a rapidly progressive dementia with myoclonus and variable presence of other neurological signs (Roos *et al.*, 1973). The disease was first described in 1920, but demonstration of its transmissible nature awaited the unraveling of the nature of kuru. Although clinically and epidemiologically very distinct from kuru, similar spongiform pathological changes in the CNS gray matter sparked successful attempts to transmit Creutzfeldt-Jakob disease to subhuman primates. Recent transmission to small laboratory animals should facilitate the study of the agent (Brownell *et al.*, 1975; Manuelidis, 1975). As the result of several unfortunate accidental transmissions of this disease from man to man, Koch's postulates now appear fulfilled for Creutzfeldt-Jakob disease (Duffy *et al.*, 1974; Bernoulli *et al.*, 1977).

In each of these diseases transmission has been possible with extraneural tissues, but clinical and pathological changes are confined to the CNS. Pathological studies show widespread neuronal loss and status spongiosis. The latter change, which typifies the spongiform encephalopathies as a group, is the result of membrane-bound vacuoles which develop in dendrites and axons of the neuropil and may appear in neuronal cell bodies. The vacuoles are variably filled with complex curled membranous debris or amorphous osmiophilic material, or they may appear empty (Lampert *et al.*, 1972). In scrapie and kuru this change is especially prominent in the cerebellum. There is usually an attendant striking astrogliosis but no inflammatory response. Focal deposits of amyloid referred to as kuru plaques are also found in kuru, some strains of scrapie, and some cases of Creutzfeldt-Jakob disease.

5.2. Pathogenesis of Spongiform Encephalopathies

A composite picture of the pathogenesis of these diseases can be proposed based largely on extensive studies of scrapie in mice. However, even scrapie in mice has shown marked variation in incubation period, topography of pathological changes, and infectivity titers dependent on strain variations of both the agent and host (Dickinson and Fraser, 1977). The spongiform encephalopathies can occur sporadically in nature or as endemic foci. Such foci may have varied explanations such as ritualistic cannibalism for kuru, food sources for transmissible mink encephalopathy, or increased genetic susceptibility for familial Creutzfeldt-Jakob disease or scrapie. The mode of sporadic transmission of these diseases in nature is unknown. However, normal skin and mucosal barriers may need to be breached, since experimental disease cannot be transmitted by simple aerosols or nasogastric feedings of infected material. The earliest replication after inoculation appears to be in spleen and other lymphoreticular organs (Ecklund *et al.*, 1967). However, initial replication of the agent in spleen is not mandatory since disease is only delayed and not prevented after infection of splenectomized or genetically asplenic mice with scrapie agent. The agent appears neither to induce interferon nor to be sensitive to its action (Katz and Koprowski, 1968). Further, disease proceeds in an unaltered fashion in both immunosuppressed and nude mice (McFarlin *et al.*, 1971). While replication in systemic organs can readily be demonstrated, pathological changes are not seen outside of the CNS.

Recovery of the agent from brain is not possible until months after experimental infection. With the development of demonstrable virus in brain, early neuronal vacuolization may be seen and electrophysiological evidence of neural dysfunction becomes apparent even though clinical behavior appears unaltered. As brain titers slowly increase, vacuolization proceeds, neuronal loss increases, and astrogliosis may become marked. With the progression of neuronal loss, shrinkage or atrophy of the brain occurs. Inflammatory changes are not observed at any time during the disease process. The pathological hallmarks of disease are usually well developed by the time clinical illness appears. The latency from inoculation to clinical disease varies but is usually not less than 7 months and may possibly require decades. The most accelerated clinical disease appears to occur in hamsters receiving concentrated intracerebral inocula.

The spongiform change that serves to link these diseases has received considerable attention (Fig. 7). It has been proposed that membranous fragments and debris associated with the vacuoles may harbor the disease agent. Attempts to purify scrapie agent from brain have lead to the speculation that it is highly membrane associated (Hunter, 1972; Clarke and Millson, 1976). However, it now appears that infectivity can be dissociated from plasma membranes (Prusiner *et al.*, 1977). Further, the spongiform change can be seen in animals given toxic doses of cuprizone, supporting the possibility that it may be a secondary phenomena. Indeed, development of vacuolization may be a transient phenomenon that does not appear to be an invariable feature of the late pathology of the transmissible dementias (Masters and Richardson, 1978). Finally, varying degrees of spongiform change are seen in experimental infections with conventional viral agents (Brooks *et al.*, 1979).

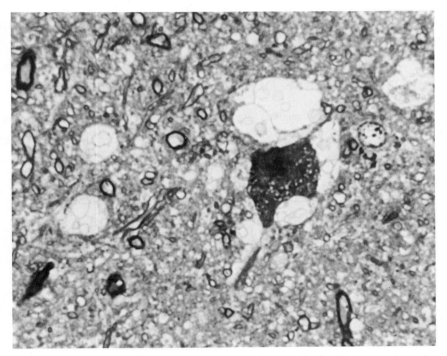

Fig. 7. Vacuolization of the neuropil in a photomicrograph of a biopsy specimen from a patient with Creutzfeldt-Jakob disease. Multiple curled membranes can be seen within vacuoles surrounding the degenerating cortical neuron. Several enlarged dendritic processes are present (left) containing similar vacuoles and curled membranes. ×1250.

5.3. Nature of the Spongiform Encephalopathy Agents

Identification of the agents by electron microscopy has not been possible. Freeze-fracture investigations of scrapie and Creutzfeldt-Jakob disease vacuoles show a diminished number of otherwise normal-appearing intramembranous protein particles rather than unusual particles or unique patterns (Dubois-Dalcq *et al.*, 1977). Standard ultrastructural investigations have generally been equally unrewarding. However, there is some renewed interest in a 23-nm spherical or icosahedral particle seen in paracrystalline arrays within dilated postsynaptic processes of scrapie-infected mice (Baringer and Pruisner, 1978).

Attempts to characterize the physical-chemical properties of these agents must be qualified by the present failure to purify the agents of homogeneity. Nonetheless, infected brain homogenates and partially purified preparations show unusual properties which include a relative resistance to heat, irradiation, alkylating agents, RNase and DNase, and certain organic solvents (Table 2). The size of the transmissible agent is < 200 nm and in the case of kuru probably < 50 nm.

6. HUMAN DISEASE OF SUSPECTED VIRAL ETIOLOGY

The isolation of viruses from SSPE, progressive multifocal leukoencephalopathy, and progressive rubella panencephalitis, and the

TABLE 2

Selected Physicochemical Properties of Scrapie

Particle size (filtration)	30–50 nm
Sedimentation coefficient	400–1200 S
Genome size (UV irradiation)	10^6 daltons
UV adsorption maxima	2370 Å
Not inactivated by:	Triton X-100
	Sodium dodecyl sulfate
	Sodium periodate
	Acetone
	Ether
	80°C × 30 min
	Formaldehyde
	β-Propiolactone
	Sodium deoxycholate
	Lysolecithin
	Ribonuclease
	Deoxyribonuclease

transmission of kuru and Creutzfeldt-Jakob disease to subhuman primates have demonstrated that viruses can cause slowly progressive neurological diseases of man with diverse pathological findings. This has led to speculation and preliminary studies of a variety of other human neurological diseases where viral involvement is suspected.

6.1. Multiple Sclerosis

Multiple sclerosis is a chronic human demyelinating disease with a remitting and relapsing course. Epidemiological studies have suggested an infectious etiology. There is a marked geographic gradient in the disease, and people who migrate from high- to low-risk zones after adolescence tend to maintain a high risk, suggesting that disease is dependent on childhood exposure to an external factor. Early-life environmental factors are also suggested by somewhat higher familial incidence yet a low conjugal incidence, indicating a lack of importance of adult exposure. The failure to find higher concordance in monozygotic than dizygotic twins suggests little genetic influence, although there is a higher incidence of certain histocompatibility antigens among multiple sclerosis patients. Serological studies from many independent investigations have shown that multiple sclerosis patients have higher antibody levels against measles virus than do controls and a higher frequency of measles antibody in CSF. Some studies have shown significant but smaller increases in antibody against herpes simplex, vaccinia, varicella zoster, influenza, parainfluenza, mumps, and rubella in the CSF of multiple sclerosis patients. The significance of these higher antibody titers, however, still remains unknown. A number of claims of transmission of disease or virus isolation have also been made, including the recovery of a rabieslike virus from patients in the Soviet Union, recovery of herpes simplex virus from the brain of a patient in Iceland, reported induction of scrapie in sheep inoculated with brain of a patient, recovery of parainfluenza type I from brain cell cultures derived from two patients, recovery of measles virus, and the recent recovery of coronaviruses. However, none of these virus recoveries has been independently corroborated in other laboratories (Johnson, 1975b).

6.2. Amyotrophic Lateral Sclerosis

Amyotrophic lateral sclerosis is a chronic degenerative disease characterized by the progressive loss of motor neurons. The selective involvement of motor neurons is reminiscent of the selectivity of poliovirus infections, and the observation of a late-life lower motor neuron disease in patients with sequelae of poliomyelitis (see Section 4.1) first led to speculation of a viral etiology. Transmission of amyotropic lateral sclerosis to monkeys was claimed in the Soviet Union, but these studies have not been confirmed by others despite extensive attempts (Johnson, 1976). In addition, an analogy can be drawn to the slowly progressive motor neuron disease in mice induced by naturally occurring ecotropic retrovirus (Gardner *et al.*, 1976). Although the murine disease is characterized by progressive upper and lower motor neuron signs similar to those seen in amyotropic lateral sclerosis, the pathological changes are much more characteristic of the vacuolization and curled membranes seen in the spongiform encephalopathies.

6.3. Parkinson's Disease

Parkinson's disease is a common progressive neurological disease in which the neurotransmitter deficit is known but the pathogenesis of the neuronal loss of the substantia nigra is not. The disease is occasionally seen following viral encephalitis and was a common sequela of Von Economo's disease, which occurred in pandemic form between 1916 and 1926. However, the causal agent of Von Economo's disease is unknown. The demonstration of influenzelike antigen in the brains of patients with postencephalitic parkinsonism has renewed interest in the possible viral etiology of other cases (Gamboa *et al.*, 1974), but attempts to transmit Parkinson's by inoculation of primates or to recover viruses have been uniformly unsuccessful (Gibbs and Gajdusek, 1972). Further, persistent infection of mice with neuro-adapted strains of influenza virus has not resulted in alteration of levels of neurotransmitter in the brains of these animals.

6.4. Continuous Focal Epilepsy

In some cases of continuous focal motor epilepsy in the Soviet Union it has been possible to recover tick-borne viruses from brain obtained during the surgical removal of epileptic foci long after resolution of the acute encephalitis. This has been verified in several different institutions. Furthermore, a strain of tick-borne encephalitis virus has been found to produce a nonfatal infection of rhesus monkeys followed by chronic movement disorder. The virus has been recovered from the monkey brain 9 months after inoculation. Studies have been carried out on a number of patients with chronic focal epilepsy with chronic inflammatory changes in North America, but no virus has been recovered from these cases (Asher, 1975). Additionally, Russian spring-summer encephalitis virus has been associated with a slowly evolving generalized neural disease with features similar to SSPE and progressive rubella panencephalitis in several patients (Ogawa *et al.*, 1973).

6.5. Alzheimer's Disease

Alzheimer's disease is the most common form of presenile dementia, and similar pathological changes of neurofibrillary tangles and senile plaques are the major pathological substrates of the majority of patients with senile dementia. Three lines of evidence have recently suggested the possibility of a transmissible agent in this disease. First, brain tissue from two patients with familial forms of Alzheimer's disease has induced neurological disease in chimpanzees. However, the pathological lesions in these animals have been those of spongiform encephalopathy typical of Creutzfeldt-Jakob disease without the pathological features of Alzheimer's disease (Gajdusek and Gibbs, 1975). Second, it has been shown with some strains of scrapie virus that amyloid-containing plaques can be produced in mouse brain reminiscent of the senile plaques of Alzheimer's disease (Wisniewski *et al.*, 1975). Finally, homogenates of the brains of patients with Alzheimer's disease have been shown to induce neurofibrillary changes in organotypic cultures of CNS similar to those seen in the disease (DeBoni and Crapper, 1978). All of these studies require further confirmation.

7. CONCLUSIONS

To fully understand the role of viruses in chronic neurological diseases, one must consider complex interactions involving varied viral replication strategies, virus–cell interactions, systemic barriers to viral spread, the complexities of nervous system structure and function, and host immune function. Chronic neurological diseases have been associated with viruses of many families, and very few generalizations regarding pathogenesis are possible. Viruses can enter the CNS by one or more different routes, and, indeed, the same virus may utilize different pathways in different hosts. Viral spread within the CNS and selective vulnerability of specific neural cell populations to viruses are still poorly understood phenomena, each with at least several divergent underlying mechanisms. Similarly, the contribution of the immune responses to the prevention, enhancement, or causation of chronic CNS disease is diverse, and a response of benefit to the host at one point during the infectious process may have adverse effects later in the same infection. Problems in defining the role of the immune response are compounded by our paucity of knowledge of compartmentalization of immune responses in the CNS.

In chronic CNS disease clear distinctions must be drawn between infection and replication, clinical disease and pathological change. Chronic clinical disease does not imply either chronic infection or a stereotyped pathological reaction. Neither does chronic infection necessarily lead to chronic disease. Furthermore, the mechanisms of chronic infection and chronic disease are almost as numerous as the number of virus–host systems studied.

Advances in molecular virology have been greatly enhanced by the use of *in vitro* and simplified continuous cell culture systems which reduce the number of confounding variables when dissecting mechanisms of viral replication and virus–cell interactions. Further, the use of more complex organ cultures has been invaluable in isolating certain components of viral pathogenesis for effective study. It is not always possible to extrapolate from *in vitro* systems, and the complexities of the CNS can certainly not be simulated in culture. Studies of the contribution of crucial anatomical factors and complex human responses to disease pathogenesis necessitate experimental study in animals and careful clinicopathological observations in man. The wealth of virological knowledge accumulated through handsome *in vitro* experimentation must continue to be extended to complex studies in animal hosts. The recognition of viral causation of five chronic albeit rare human neurological diseases has opened a window onto the possible extraordinary contributions that virology might have in the study of common chronic neurological diseases—diseases which, in both economic and human terms, represent some of our most important health problems.

ACKNOWLEDGMENTS

Studies by the authors have been supported by grants from the National Institute of Neurological and Communicative Disorders and

Stroke, The National Foundation–March of Dimes, and the Amyotrophic Lateral Sclerosis Society of America. Dr. Wolinsky is a recipient of a Research Career Development Award (1 KO4 NS 00443).

8. REFERENCES

Agnarsdóttir, G., 1977, Subacute sclerosing panencephalitis, *Recent Adv. Clin. Virol.* **1**:21.

Aicardi, J., Goutieres, F., Arsenio-Nunes, M., and Lebon, P., 1977, Acute measles encephalitis in children with immunosuppression, *Pediatrics* **59**:232.

Albrecht, P., 1968, Pathogenesis of neurotropic arbovirus infections, *Curr. Top. Microbiol. Immunol.* **43**:44.

Asher, D. M., 1975, Movement disorders in rhesus monkeys after infection with tick-borne encephalitis virus, *Adv. Neurol.* **10**:277.

Baringer, J. R., and Prusiner, S. B., 1978, Experimental scrapie in mice: Ultrastructural observations, *Ann. Neurol.* **4**:205.

Bernoulli, C., Siegfried, J., Baumgartner, G., Regli, F., Rabinowicz, T., Gajdusek, D. C., and Gibbs, C. J., Jr., 1977, Danger of accidental person-to-person transmission of Creutzfeldt-Jakob disease by surgery, *Lancet* **1**:478.

Bleier, R., Albrecht, R., and Cruce, J. A. F., 1975, Supraependymal cells of hypothalamic third ventricle: Identification as resident phagocytes of brain, *Science* **189**:299.

Blinzinger, K., and Muller, W., 1971, The intercellular gaps of the neuropil as possible pathways for virus spread in viral encephalomyelitides, *Acta Neuropathol.* **17**:37.

Brooks, B. R., Swarz, J. R., Narayan, O., and Johnson, R. T., 1979, Murine neurotropic retrovirus spongiform polioencephalomyelopathy: Accleration of disease by virus inoculum concentration, *Infect. Immun.* **23**:540.

Brownell, B., Campbell, M. J., Greenham, L. W., and Peacock, D. B., 1975, Experimental transmission of Creutzfeldt-Jakob disease, *Lancet* **2**:186.

Chou, S. M., Ross, R., Burrell, R., Gutmann, L., and Harley, J. B., 1973, Subacute focal adenovirus encephalitis, *J. Neuropathol. Exp. Neurol.* **32**:34.

Clarke, M. C., and Millson, G. C., 1976, The membrane location of scrapie infectivity, *J. Gen. Virol.* **31**:441.

Cooper, N. R., Jensen, F. C., Welsh, R. M., Jr., and Oldstone, M. B. A., 1976, Lysis of RNA tumor viruses by human serum: Direct antibody-independent triggering of the classical complement pathway, *J. Exp. Med.* **144**:970.

Davis, L. E., Bodian, D., Price, D., Butler, I. J., and Vickers, J. H., 1977, Chronic progressive poliomyelitis secondary to vaccination of an immunodeficient child, *New Engl. J. Med.* **297**:241.

DeBoni, U., and Crapper, D. R., 1978, Paired helical filaments of the Alzheimer's type in cultured neurones, *Nature (London)* **271**:566.

DeLorenzo, A. J. D., 1970, The olfactory neuron and the blood–brain barrier, in: *Ciba Foundation Symposium on Taste and Smell in Vertebrates* (G. E. W. Wolstenholme and J. Knight, eds.), pp. 151–176, Churchill, London.

Dickinson, A. G., and Fraser, H., 1977, Scrapie: Pathogenesis in inbred mice: An assessment of host control and response involving many strains of agent, in: *Slow*

Virus Infections of the Central Nervous System (V. ter Meulen and M. Katz, eds.), pp. 3–14, Springer-Verlag, New York.

Dorfman, L. J., 1973, Cytomegalovirus encephalitis in adults, *Neurology* **23**:136.

Dörries, K., Johnson, R. T., and ter Meulen, V., 1979, Detection of polyoma virus DNA in PML-brain tissue by (*in situ*) hybridization, *J. Gen. Virol.* **43**:49.

Doyle, M., and Holland, J. J., 1973, Prophylaxis and immunization in mice by use of a virus-free defective T particle to protect against intracerebral infection by vesicular stomatitis virus, *Proc. Natl. Acad. Sci. USA* **70**:2105.

Dubois-Dalcq, M., Rodriguez, M., Reese, T. S., Gibbs, C. J., Jr., and Gajdusek, D. C., 1977, Search for a specific marker in the neural membranes of scrapie mice: A freeze fracture study, *Lab. Invest.* **36**:547.

Duffy, P., Wolf, J., Collins, G., DeVoe, A. G., Streeten, B., and Cowen, D., 1974, Possible person-to-person transmission of Creutzfeldt-Jakob disease, *New Engl. J. Med.* **290**:692.

Eklund, C. M., Kennedy, R. C., and Hadlow, W. J., 1967, Pathogenesis of scrapie virus infection in the mouse, *J. Infect. Dis.* **117**:15.

Finley, F. H., Fitzgerald, L. H., Richter, R. W., Riggs, N., and Shelton, J. T., 1967, Western encephalitis and cerebral ontogenesis, *Arch. Neurol.* **16**:140.

Fossan, G. O., 1977, The transfer of IgG from serum to CSF, evaluated by means of a naturally occurring antibody, *Eur. Neurol.* **15**:231.

Fujita, S., and Kitamura, T., 1976, Origin of brain macrophages and the nature of the microglia, in: *Progress in Neuropathology*, Vol. 3 (H. M. Zimmerman, ed.), pp. 1–50, Grune and Stratton, New York.

Gajdusek, D. C., 1977, Unconventional viruses and the origin and disappearance of kuru, *Science* **197**:943.

Gajdusek, D. C., and Gibbs, C. J., Jr., 1975, Familial and sporadic chronic neurological degenerative disorders transmitted from man to primates, *Adv. Neurol.* **10**:291.

Gamboa, E. T., Wolf, A., Yahr, M. D., Harter, D. H., Duffy, P. E., Barden, H., and Hsu, K. C., 1974, Influenza virus antigen in post-encephalitis Parkinsonism brain detection by immunofluorescence, *Arch. Neurol.* **31**:228–232.

Gardner, M. B., Rasheed, S., Klement, V., Rongey, R. W., Brown, J. C., Dworsky, R., and Henderson, B. E., 1976, Lower motor neuron disease in wild mice caused by indigenous type C virus and search for a similar etiology in human amyotrophic lateral sclerosis, in: *Amyotrophic Lateral Sclerosis. Recent Research Trends* (J. M. Andrews, R. T. Johnson, and M. A. B. Brazier, eds.), pp. 217–234, Academic Press, New York.

Gerhard, W., and Koprowski, H., 1977, Viral immunology—B cells in CNS, *Nature (London)* **266**:360.

Gerhard, W., Iwasaki, Y., and Koprowski, H., 1978, The central nervous system associated immune response to parainfluenza type I virus in mice, *J. Immunol.* **120**:1256.

Gibbs, C. J., Jr., and Gajdusek, D. C., 1972, Amyotrophic lateral sclerosis, Parkinson's disease and the amyotrophic lateral sclerosis-Parkinsonism-dementia complex on Guam: A review and summary on attempts to demonstrate infection as the etiology, *J. Clin. Pathol. Suppl.* **25**:132.

Gibbs, C. J., Jr., and Gajdusek, D. C., 1978, Atypical viruses as cause of sporadic, epidemic, and familial chronic diseases in man: Slow viruses and human diseases, *Perspect. Virol.* **10**:161.

Griffin, D. E., Narayan, O., Bukowski, J., Adams, R. J., and Cohen, S., 1978, The cerebrospinal fluid in visna, a slow viral disease of sheep, *Ann. Neurol.* **4**:212.

Haase, A. T., 1975, The slow infection caused by visna virus, *Curr. Top. Microbiol. Immunol.* **72**:101.

Haase, A. T., Stowring, L., Narayan, O., Griffin, D., and Price, D., 1977, Slow persistent infection caused by visna virus: Role of host restriction, *Science* **195**:175.

Hall, W. W., Kiessling, W., and ter Meulen, V., 1978, Membrane proteins of subacute sclerosing panencephalitis and measles virus, *Nature (London)* **272**:460.

Haspel, M. V., and Rapp, E., 1975, Measles virus: An unwanted variant causing hydrocephalus, *Science* **187**:450.

Haukenes, G., 1977, Demonstration of host antigens in the myxovirus membrane: Lysis of virus by antibody and complement. *Acta Pathol. Microbiol. Scand.* **85**:125.

Hirsch, R. L., Griffin, D. E., and Winkelstein, J. A., 1978, The effect of complement depletion on the course of Sindbis virus infection in mice, *J. Immunol.* **121**:1276.

Hunter, G. D., 1972, Scrapie: A prototype slow infection, *J. Infect. Dis.* **125**:427.

Johnson, K. P., Feldman, E. G., and Byington, D. P., 1975, Effect of neonatal thymectomy on experimental subacute sclerosing panencephalitis in adult hamsters, *Infect. Immun.* **12**:1463.

Johnson, K. P., Wolinsky, J. S., and Ginsberg, A. H., 1978, Immune mediated syndromes of the nervous system related to virus infections, in: *Handbook of Clinical Neurology*, Vol. 34 (P. J. Vinken and G. W. Bruyn, eds.), pp. 391–434, North-Holland, New York.

Johnson, R. T., 1974, Pathophysiology and epidemiology of acute viral infections of the nervous system, *Adv. Neurol.* **6**:30.

Johnson, R. T., 1975a, Hydrocephalus and viral infections, *Dev. Med. Child Neurol.* **17**:807.

Johnson, R. T., 1975b, The possible viral etiology of multiple sclerosis, *Adv. Neurol.* **13**:1.

Johnson, R. T., 1976, Virological studies of amyotrophic lateral sclerosis: An overview, in: *Amyotrophic Lateral Sclerosis* (J. M. Andrews, R. T. Johnson, and M. A. B. Brazier, eds.), pp. 173–180, Academic Press, New York.

Johnson, R. T., and Griffin, D. E., 1978, Pathogenesis of viral infections, in: *Handbook of Clinical Neurology*, Vol. 34 (P. J. Vinken and G. W. Bruyn, eds.), pp. 15–37, North-Holland, Amsterdam.

Johnson, R. T., and Mims, C. A., 1968, Pathogenesis of viral infections in the nervous system, *New Engl. J. Med.* **278**:23, 84.

Johnson, R. T., Narayan, O., and Weiner, L. P., 1974, The relationship of SV40 related viruses to progressive multifocal leukoencephalopathy, in: *Mechanisms of Virus Disease* (W. S. Robinson and C. F. Fox, eds.), pp. 187–197, Benjamin, Menlo Park, California.

Johnson, R. T., Narayan, O., and Clements, J., 1978, Varied role of viruses in chronic neurologic diseases, in: *Persistent Viruses* (J. G. Stevens, G. J. Todaro, and C. F. Fox, eds.), pp. 551–561, Academic Press, New York.

Jubelt, B., Narayan, O., and Johnson, R. T., 1980, Pathogenesis of human poliovirus infection in mice. II. Age-dependency of paralysis, *J. Neuropathol. Exp. Neurol.* **39**:149.

Katz, M., and Koprowski, H., 1968, Failure to demonstrate a relationship between scrapie and production of interferon in mice, *Nature (London)* **219**:639.

Katzman, R., and Pappius, H. M., 1973, *Brain Electrolytes and Fluid Metabolism*, Williams and Wilkins, Baltimore.

Kilham, L., and Margolis, G., 1966, Viral etiology of spontaneous ataxia of cats, *Am. J. Pathol.* **48**:991.

Kilham, L., and Margolis, G., 1975, Problems of concern arising from animal models of intrauterine and neonatal infections due to viruses: A review, *Prog. Med. Virol.* **20**:113.

Kreth, H. W., ter Meulen, V., and Eckert, G., 1979, Demonstration of HLA restricted killer cells in patients with acute measles, *Med. Microbiol. Immunol.* **165**:203.

Kristensson, K., Lycke, E., and Sjöstrand, J., 1971, Spread of herpes simplex virus in peripheral nerves, *Acta Neuropathol.* **17**:44.

Lampert, P. W., Gajdusek, D. C., and Gibbs, C. J., Jr., 1972, Subacute spongiform virus encephalopathies: Scrapie, kuru and Creutzfeldt-Jakob disease: A review, *Am. J. Pathol.* **68**:626.

Lipton, H. L., and Gonzalez-Scarano, F., 1978, Central nervous system immunity in mice infected with Theiler's virus. I. Local neutralizing antibody response, *J. Infect. Dis.* **137**:145.

Lipton, H. L., and Johnson, R. T., 1972, The pathogenesis of rat virus infections in the newborn hamster, *Lab. Invest.* **27**:508.

Manuelidis, E. E., 1975, Transmission of Creutzfeldt-Jakob disease from man to guinea pig, *Science* **190**:571.

Margolis, G., and Kilham, L., 1975, Problems of concern arising from animal models of intrauterine and neonatal infections due to viruses: A review, *Prog. Med. Virol.* **20**:144.

Masters, C. L., and Richardson, E. P., Jr., 1978, Subacute spongiform encephalopathy (Creutzfeldt-Jakob disease): The nature of progression of spongiform change, *Brain* **101**:333.

Masters, C., Harris, J. O., Gajdusek, D. C., Gibbs, C. J., Jr., Bernoulli, C., and Asher, D. M., 1978, Creutzfeldt-Jakob disease: Patterns of worldwide occurrence and the significance of familial and sporadic clustering, *Ann. Neurol.* **5**:177.

McCormick, W. F., Rodnitzky, R. L., Schochet, S. S., Jr., and McKee, A. P., 1969, Varicella-zoster encephalomyelitis: A morphologic and virologic study, *Arch. Neurol.* **21**:559.

McFarland, H. F., Griffin, D. E., and Johnson, R. T., 1972, Specificity of the inflammatory response in viral encephalitis. I. Adoptive immunization of immunosuppressed mice infected with Sindbis virus, *J. Exp. Med.* **136**:216.

McFarlin, D. E., Raff, M. C., Simpson, E., and Nehlsen, S. H., 1971, Scrapie in immunologically deficient mice, *Nature (London)* **233**:336.

Mims, C. A., 1964, Aspects of the pathogenesis of virus diseases, *Bacteriol. Rev.* **28**:30.

Mulder, D. W., Rosenbaum, R. A., and Layton, D. D., 1972, Late progression of poliomyelitis or forme fruste amyotrophic lateral sclerosis, *Mayo Clin. Proc.* **47**:756.

Murphy, F. A., 1977, Rabies pathogenesis: Brief review, *Arch. Virol.* **54**:279.

Naeye, R. L., and Blanc, W., 1965, Pathogenesis of congenital rubella, *J. Am. Med. Assoc.* **194**:1277.

Narayan, O., Griffin, D. E., and Chase, J., 1977, Antigenic shift of visna virus in persistently infected sheep, *Science* **197**:376.

Narayan, O., Griffin, D. E., and Clements, J. E., 1978, Virus mutation during "slow infection." Temporal development and characterization of mutants of visna virus recovered from sheep, *J. Gen. Virol.* **41**:343.

Norrby, E., 1978, Viral antibodies in multiple sclerosis, *Progr. Med. Virol.* **24**:1.

Ogawa, M., Okuba, H., Tsuji, Y., Yasni, N., and Someda, K., 1973, Chronic progressive encephalitis occurring 13 years after Russian-spring-summer encephalitis, *J. Neurol. Sci.* **19**:363.

Oldstone, M. B. A., Holmstoen, J., and Welsh, R. M., Jr., 1977, Alterations of acetylcholine enzymes in neuroblastoma cells persistently infected with lymphocytic choriomeningitis virus, *J. Cell. Physiol.* **91**:459.

Osburn, B. I., Johnson, R. T., Silverstein, A. M., Prendergast, R. A., Jochim, M. M., and Levy, S. E., 1971a, Experimental viral-induced congenital encephalopathies. II. The pathogenesis of bluetongue vaccine virus infection in fetal lambs, *Lab. Invest.* **25**:206.

Osburn, B. I., Silverstein, A. M., Prendergast, R. A., Johnson, R. T., and Parshall, C. J., 1971b, Experimental viral-induced congenital encephalopathies. I. Pathology of hydranencephaly and porencephaly caused by bluetongue vaccine virus, *Lab. Invest.* **25**:197.

Padgett, B. L., and Walker, D. L., 1976, New human papovaviruses, *Prog. Med. Virol.* **22**:1.

Peters, A., Palay, S. L., and Webster, H. deF., 1976, *The Fine Structure of the Nervous System: The Neurons and Supporting Cells*, Saunders, Philadelphia.

Petursson, G., Nathanson, N., Georgsson, G., Panitch, H., and Palsson, P. A., 1976, Pathogenesis of visna. I. Sequential virologic, serologic, and pathologic studies, *Lab. Invest.* **35**:402.

Prineas, J. W., 1979, Multiple sclerosis: Presence of lymphatic capillaries and lymphoid tissue in the brain and spinal cord, *Science* **203**:1123.

Prusiner, S. B., Hadlow, W. J., Eklund, C. M., and Race, R. E., 1977, Sedimentation properties of the scrapie agent, *Proc. Natl. Acad. Sci. USA* **74**:4656.

Rabinowitz, S. G., Dal Canto, M., and Johnson, T. C., 1976, Comparison of central nervous system disease produced by wild-type and temperature-sensitive mutants of vesicular stomatitis virus, *Infect. Immun.* **13**:1242.

Rawls, W. E., 1968, Congenital rubella: The significance of virus persistence, *Progr. Med. Virol* **10**:238.

Rawls, W. E., 1974, Viral persistence in congenital rubella, *Progr. Med. Virol.* **18**:273.

Rawls, W. E., and Melnick, J. L., 1966, Rubella virus carrier cultures derived from congenitally infected infants, *J. Exp. Med.* **123**:795.

Robb, J. A., 1977, Virus–cell interactions: A classification for virus-caused human disease, *Progr. Med. Virol.* **23**.51.

Roos, R., Gajdusek, D. C., and Gibbs, C. J., Jr., 1973, The clinical characteristics of transmissible Creutzfeldt-Jakob disease, *Brain* **96**:1.

Stevens, J. G., 1978, Latent characteristics of selected herpesviruses, *Adv. Cancer Res.* **26**:227.

Swarz, J. R., Brooks, B. R., and Johnson, R. T., 1978, Murine retrovirus induced spongiform encephalopathy: An ultrastructural study, *J. Neuropathol. Exp. Neurol.* **37**:696.

Tamm, I., 1975, Cell injury with viruses, *Am. J. Pathol.* **81**:163.

Tomlinson, B. E., and Irving, D., 1977, The number of limb motor neurons in the human lumbosacral cord throughout life, *J. Neurol. Sci.* **34**:213.

Vandvik, B., and Norrby, E., 1973, Oligoclonal IgG antibody response in the central nervous system to different measles virus antigens in subacute sclerosing panencephalitis, *Proc. Natl. Acad. Sci. USA* **70**:1060.

Vandvik, B., Norrby, E., Steen-Johnson, J., and Stensvold, K., 1978a, Mumps meningitis: Prolonged pleocytosis and occurrence of mumps virus-specific oligoclonal IgG in the cerebrospinal fluid, *Eur. Neurol.* **17**:13.

Vandvik B., Weil, M. L., Grandien, M., and Norrby, E., 1978*b*, Progressive rubella virus panencephalitis: Synthesis of oligoclonal virus-specific IgG antibodies and homogeneous free light chains in the central nervous system, *Acta Neurol. Scand.* **57**:53.

Vilček, J., 1964, Production of interferon by newborn and adult mice infected with Sindbis virus, *Virology* **22**:651.

Webster, A. D. B., Tripp, J. H., Hayward, A. R., Dayan, A. D., Doshi, R., Macintyre, E. H., and Tyrrell, D. A. J., 1978, Echovirus encephalitis and myositis in primary immunoglobulin deficiency, *Arch. Dis. Child.* **53**:33.

Wechsler, S. L. and Fields, B. N., 1978, Differences between the intracellular polypeptides of measles and subacute sclerosing panencephalitis virus, *Nature (London)* **272**:458.

Weinmann, E., Majer, M., and Hilfenhaus, J., 1979, Intramuscular and/or intralumbar post exposure treatment of rabies virus-infected cynomolgus monkeys with human interferon, *Infect. Immun.* **24**:24.

Westergaard, E., 1977, The blood brain barrier to horseradish peroxidase under normal and experimental conditions, *Acta Neuropathol.* **39**:181.

Wilfert, C. M., Buckley, R. H., Mohanakumar, T., Griffith, J. F., Katz, S. L., Whisnant, J. K., Eggleston, P. A., Moore, M., Treadwell, E., Oxman, M. N., and Rosen, F. S., 1977, Persistent and fatal central nervous system echovirus infections in patients with agammaglobulinemia, *New Engl. J. Med.* **296**:1485.

Willoughby, E. W., Price, R. W., Padgett, B. L., Walker, D. L., and DuPont, B., 1979, *In vitro* cell mediated immune responses to mitogens and JC virus in progressive multifocal leukoencephalopathy, *Neurology* **29**:554.

Wisniewski, H. M., Bruce, M. E., and Fraser, H., 1975, Infectious etiology of neuritic (senile) plaques in mice, *Science* **190**:1108.

Wolinsky, J., 1978, Progressive rubella panencephalitis, in: *Handbook of Clinical Neurology*, Vol. 34 (P. J. Vinken and G. W. Bruyn, eds.), pp. 331–341, North-Holland, Amsterdam.

Wolinsky, J. S., Baringer, J. R., Margolis, G., and Kilham, L., 1974, Ultrastructure of mumps virus replication in newborn hamster central nervous system, *Lab. Invest.* **31**:403.

Wolinsky, J. S., Klassen, T., and Baringer, J. R., 1976, Persistence of neuroadapted mumps virus in brains of newborn hamsters after intraperitoneal inoculation, *J. Infect. Dis.* **133**:260.

Wolinsky, J. S., Swoveland, P., Johnson, K. P., and Baringer, J. R., 1977, Subacute measles encephalitis complicating Hodgkin's disease in an adult, *Ann. Neurol.* **1**:452.

Wolinsky, J. S., Dau, P. C., Buimovici-Klein, E., Mednick, J., Berg, B. O., Lang, P. B., and Cooper, L. Z., 1979, Progressive rubella panencephalitis: Immunovirological studies and results of isoprinosine therapy, *Clin. Exp. Immunol.* **35**:397.

Woods, W. A., Johnson, R. T., Hostetler, P. D., Lepow, M. L., and Robbins, F. C., 1966, Immunofluroescent studies on rubella-infected tissue cultures and human tissues, *J. Immunol.* **96**:253.

Yamanouchi, K., Sato, T. A., Kobune, F., and Shishido, A., 1979, Antibody responses in the cerebrospinal fluid of cynomolgus monkeys after intracerebral inoculation with paramyxoviruses, *Infect. Immun.* **23**:185.

CHAPTER 7

Host Plant Responses to Virus Infection

R. E. F. Matthews

Department of Cell Biology
University of Auckland
Auckland, New Zealand

1. INTRODUCTION

The study of host responses to infection was of central importance in the development of plant virology up until the mid 1930s when the first viruses were isolated and characterized. Since 1945 development of the subject has centered on the application of molecular biological techniques to the study of virus structure and of their replication *in vitro* and *in vivo*. However, in recent years there has been a renewed interest in the study of host responses, partly because of the economic losses caused by virus diseases and partly because the wide variety of phenomena involved have substantial intrinsic biological interest.

In natural plant communities undisturbed by man it is probable that most plant–virus interactions have evolved so that the host response is minimal—that is, a symptomless or almost symptomless infection develops. However, in agricultural and horticultural plant communities both cultivated and week species often respond with some form of macroscopically observable disease. It is such host responses to infection that are most frequently studied by plant virologists. The response of plants to virus infection is extremely varied. The macroscopic symptoms characteristic of a particular disease will arise because of the effect of virus infection on particular cells or classes of cells.

These cellular responses are in turn dependent on the organelle changes which arise because of biochemical and molecular biological events that occur during the establishment and replication of the virus.

Ultimately, virologists would like to be able to explain in detail how a single virus containing a piece (or pieces) of nucleic acid sufficient to code for a few proteins is able to infect and cause the specific set of host responses which we call disease. This is a challenging task when we remember that the host plant grows continually and that it is organized into a variety of interacting tissues and organs with specific structures and functions.

We are far from attaining the above objective for any host–virus combination. Nevertheless, the knowledge about plant virus replication provided by molecular biological studies and the advances in our understanding of normal plant biochemistry, physiology, and development have allowed some progress to be made in defining possible mechanisms for the responses made by plants to infection. In addition, the widespread use of electron microscopic techniques is bridging the gap between biochemical knowledge on the one hand and descriptions of disease based on light microscope and macroscopic observations on the other. One of the most important developments has been the realization that viral gene products other than those found in the virus particle itself may play an important part in defining the hosts response to infection.

Some boundaries must be placed on the material to be discussed in a single chapter. A systematic discussion of the details of virus establishment and replication, virus-induced structures concerned with virus replication, effects on the physiology and biochemistry of the host cell, and effects of environmental factors such as light, temperature, and water supply on a plant's response to infection is beyond the scope of this chapter. Nevertheless, aspects of these topics are discussed where they may help to explain the organelle, cellular, or plant responses to infection.

2. KINDS OF HOST RESPONSE

When a virus particle successfully invades a leaf cell following mechanical inoculation, it multiplies in that cell and moves to neighboring cells where it also replicates. These initially infected cells may give rise to a macroscopically visible local lesion which, for example, may consist of a patch of dead cells or of cells that have lost some chlorophyll. Subsequently, the virus may move systemically through the plant, usually in the phloem. The kinds of symptoms which develop following systemic infection are very diverse. The major kinds of disease symptoms that occur in response to virus infection are summarized in Table 1. These various symptoms often appear in combination in particular diseases. Furthermore, the pattern of disease development for a particular host–virus combination often involves the sequential development of different kinds of symptoms.

TABLE 1

Important Host Plant Responses to Systemic Virus Infection

Plant part	Symptom	Comments
Whole plant	1. Reduction in size	Probably the commonest response
	2. Wilting	May lead to death of the plant
	3. Generalized necrosis	Leads to rapid death
Leaves	1. Vein clearing	Translucent tissue near veins
	2. Light and dark green areas giving a mosaic pattern	A very common response
	3. Blistering and distortion of lamina	Often associated with mosaic
	4. Vein banding	Darker green tissue near veins
	5. Yellowing of veins	—
	6. Generalized yellowing	—
	7. Etched ringspot and line patterns	Due to death of superficial layers of cells
	8. Reduction of lamina	In extreme examples only midrib and veins may develop
	9. Enations	Abnormal leaflike growths from veins and midrib
	10. Epinasty and leaf abcission	—
Flowers	1. Variegation or "breaking" of petal pigmentation	Often associated with mosaic in leaves
	2. Malformation	
	3. Necrosis	
Fruits	1. Mottling patterns	
	2. Ring and line patterns	
	3. Reduced size	
	4. Malformation	
	5. Necrosis	
Stems, roots, leaf veins, and petioles	Tumorlike growths	Characteristic of plant members of the Reoviridae

3.   INFLUENCE OF HOST GENOTYPE

The genotype of the host plant has a profound effect on the outcome of infection with a particular virus. There are several situations to be considered: (1) immunity, where the plant does not become infected under any circumstances; (2) resistance to infection; (3) hypersensitivity, where the host reacts by localized death of cells at the site of infection without further spread of virus; (4) tolerance, where the virus multiplies and spreads widely through the plant but the disease produced is very mild or negligible; and (5) the general influence of host genome on the kind of disease that develops.

3.1.   Immunity

A plant species or variety is said to be immune to a virus when it is totally unable to support the replication of any strain of the virus.

If we consider the possibility of exposing all plant species to all viruses, immunity may be the most common condition. However, among members of a closely related group of plants, some members of which are susceptible to a given virus, true immunity is rather rare. The potato seedling USDA 41956 has been thought to be immune to potato virus X. However, a virus which can infect this seedling and which is considered to be a strain of virus X has been found recently in Peru (Salaczar, personal communication). A few other examples of immunity have been reported, among them being the immunity of the mushroom *Agaricus bitorquis* (Quel) Sacc. to several viruses (van Zaayen, 1976) and the immunity of some soybean varieties to beet western yellows virus (Duffus and Milbrath, 1977). However, the tests applied were not sufficiently stringent to distinguish between true immunity and a high degree of resistance. These examples demonstrate the difficulties which are inherent in proving that a particular plant genotype is indeed immune.

3.2.   Resistance and Hypersensitivity

From a practical point of view, a hypersensitive reaction gives effective "field resistance" to a disease. In some instances it may be difficult to distinguish between true resistance and a hypersensitive reaction in which too few cells are killed to produce a visible lesion. Within a group of closely related plants, some of which are susceptible to a given virus, genetically controlled resistance to infection is much more common than immunity. Genetic studies with the three solanaceous species, tobacco, tomato, and pepper, will illustrate the kinds of effect that host genes may have on plant response to infection.

3.2.1. Tobacco

Some varieties of tobacco respond to infection with tobacco mosaic virus (TMV) by producing necrotic local lesions but no systemic spread, in contrast to the usual chlorotic local lesions followed by a mosaic disease. The difference in reaction between the two host varieties may be controlled by a single dominant gene pair—the necrotic reaction being dominant. The most studied example is the dominant gene N, which is found in *Nicotiana glutinosa* (Holmes, 1938). This gene has been incorporated into *N. tabacum* cv. Samsun NN (Holmes, 1938), *N. tabacum* cv. Burley NN (Valleau, 1952), and *N. tabacum* cv. Xanthi nc (Takahashi, 1956). In very young seedling plants that contain the N gene (either NN or Nn) systemic necrosis developed, whereas in older plants only localized necrotic lesions developed. Systemic mosaic disease appeared in all nn plants (Holmes, 1938). An unexplained systemic infection by TMV of some *Nicotiana* species carrying the N gene has recently been reported (Dijkstra *et al.*, 1977).

Another gene for local necrosis (N^s) has been described by Weber (1951). With this gene the heterozygote always developed systemic necrosis (Fig. 1).

Valleau and Johnson (1943) described a gene N' from *N. sylvestris*. The presence of this gene causes a necrotic local lesion response to the U_2 strain of TMV and systemic mosaic disease with U_1 (type strain). The gene EN is the same allele as N' (Melchers *et al.*, 1966). This gene also shows a clear dose effect. At temperatures of 23–26°C much more virus was produced in local lesions of EN/en plants than in EN/EN (Jockusch, 1966) (see also Section 8.1.2). A variety of tobacco known as T.I.245 tends to escape infection when lightly inoculated with TMV. This line is also partially resistant to infection with a number of other viruses (Fulton, 1953; Holmes, 1960). Holmes (1960) concluded that two genes are involved in the T.I.245 reaction. The tolerance of the Ambalema variety of tobacco to TMV is controlled by two recessive genes, r_{m1} and r_{m2}. Two dominant genes, G_1 and G_2, suppress the chlorotic halo that normally appears around N-type lesions (i.e., *N. glutinosa*-type localization of TMV). Holmes (1960) combined genes

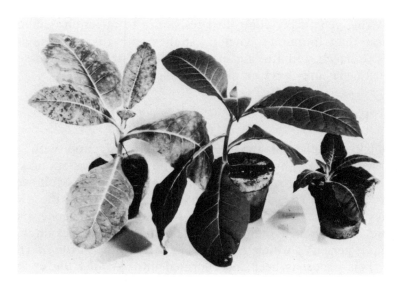

Fig. 1. Effect of host plant genotype on host response. Reaction of two varieties of tobacco to a strain of TMV from tomato. Left: Var. White Burley showing typical systemic mosaic. Center: Var. Warne's, which responds with necrotic local lesions and no systemic spread of virus (this variety probably carries the N^s gene of Weber, 1951). Right: An F_1 hybrid (Warnes ♀ × White Burley ♂) showing necrotic local lesions and severe systemic necrosis and stunting. From Matthews (1970).

for hypersensitivity, tolerance, and resistance and obtained lines of tobacco highly resistant to TMV. The new lines produced fewer, smaller, and later-developing necrotic local lesions. Holmes (1961) tested the resistance of two lines that had inherited the resistance of T.I.245 to TMV for resistance to six other viruses. Both lines were resistant to all six viruses. Since the lines were selected from a segregating population only on the basis of their resistance to TMV, it seems likely that the observed resistance to all the viruses was due to the same genetic mechanism.

3.2.2. Tomato

Tomato spotted wilt virus in tomato offers a contrast to the situation with the N gene and TMV in tobacco. Various sources of genetically controlled resistance of tomatoes to spotted wilt virus have been found. Each of these resistance factors is effective against only some strains of the virus. In Australia, where a wide range of virus strains occurs, three independently inherited recessive genes and two dominant alleles were found to control resistance to five groups of virus strains (Finlay, 1953). Certain cultivars of tomato are resistant to curly top virus, but the basis for the resistance is complex (Moser and Cannon, 1972). Resistance is in part due to lack of vector preference and in part to a more frequent failure of virus to establish itself within the plant following insect feeding on resistance varieties (Thomas and Martin, 1971, 1972). Two factors for resistance to TMV have been found in the wild *Lycopersicon* species of tomato. These are *Tm-2* and *Tm-2²*, which is probably an allele of *Tm-2*. Both are dominant for a hypersensitive response to the common strain of TMV (Pelham, 1972), but viral strain, background host genotype, and environmental conditions, especially temperature, influence the response (Cirulli and Alexander, 1969; Alexander, 1971; Pelham, 1972).

3.2.3. Pepper

Most garden peppers react to tobacco etch virus with a mosaic disease. Tabasco peppers (*Capsicum frutescens*) react with a wilting disease. The wilting reaction is controlled by a single dominant gene not present in nonwilting peppers (Greenleaf, 1959). The cultivar LP1 carried a simple dominant gene for resistance to tobacco etch virus and a recessive gene for resistance to cucumber mosaic virus (Barrios *et al.*, 1971). A gene for resistance to pepper veinal mottle virus in *C. annucum* was also recessive (Soh *et al.*, 1977). Simmonds and Harrison (1959) found that two unlinked loci, V_1 and V_2, were involved in the reactions of pepper to potato virus Y. The double recessive plants $v_1v_1v_2v_2$ were difficult to infect. When they did become infected they showed only mild mosaic symptoms and grew quite well. In the $V_1V_1v_2v_2$ state, plants were still resistant to infection, but in infected plants some abscission of leaves occurred and the plants were stunted. Introductions of the other dominant ($v_1v_1V_2V_2$) were easily infected. They developed veinal necrosis, lost their leaves, and died. Several other genes for resistance of *Capsicum* to potato virus Y are known. These may be effective under summer conditions but break down under winter conditions in the field (Shifriss and Cohen, 1971). It is possible that some genes conferring resistance to potato virus Y may also give resistance to tobacco etch virus (Smith, 1970).

3.2.4. Conclusions

The following points concerning the effects of host genes on plant response to infection emerge from the studies discussed above: (1) both dominant and recessive Mendelian genes may have effects; (2) there may or may not be a gene dose effect; (3) genes at different loci may have similar effects; (4) the genetic background of the host may affect the activity of a resistance gene; (5) genes may have their effect with all strains of a virus or with only some; (6) some genes influence the response to more than one virus; and (7) plant age and environmental conditions may interact strongly with host genotype to produce the final response.

Two further points deserve mention. While most genes known to affect host responses are inherited in a Mendelian manner, cytoplasmically transferred factors may sometimes be involved (Nagaich *et al.*, 1968), and route of infection may affect the host response. Systemic necrosis may develop following introduction of a virus by grafting into a highly resistant host that does not allow systemic spread of the same virus following mechanical inoculation (e.g., potato viruses X and Y in certain potato genotypes; Delhey, 1974, 1975).

3.3. Mechanisms of Resistance

The hypersensitive reaction is probably widespread as a basis for resistance. Experiments relating to the nature of the hypersensitive response to TMV in *Nicotiana* are discussed in Section 8.1. Various effects other than the hypersensitive response may result from the activity of resistance genes. For example, experiments on the concentration and distribution of maize dwarf mosaic virus in corn leaves suggested that host resistance involved a reduced ability of the virus to move through the host rather than reduced infection or replication of the virus locally (James and Tobin, 1972).

In cucumbers resistant to cucumber mosaic virus, resistance is associated with a much lower concentration of virus in inoculated leaves. Injection of leaves with actinomycin D within 48 hr of inoculation led to a substantial increase in virus multiplication, suggesting that the resistance mechanism may depend on transcription from cellular DNA as a first step in process giving a substance responsible for the resistance (Nachman *et al.*, 1971).

Simons and Moss (1963) suggested that the resistance of the Italian E1 variety of pepper to potato virus Y is due to the presence of a virus inhibitor. However, the presence of an inhibitor in leaf extracts does not necessarily mean that this inhibitor is active in the intact plant. No evidence for an inhibitor specific for virus Y was found in other sources of pepper resistant to the virus (Cook, 1963). Different varieties and classes of pepper differ in their resistance to various strains of the virus (Simons, 1966). Hooker and Kim (1962) could find no difference in the amounts of an inhibitor of potato virus X infection in potato varieties that were either tolerant of, hypersensitive to, or immune to potato virus X.

In a survey of over 1000 lines of cowpea for resistance to cowpea mosaic virus 65 lines were defined as operationally immune because no symptoms or virus replication could be detected following inoculation of intact plants (see also Section 9.3). The only known common feature in these various examples is a reduction in (or absence of) virus replication.

3.4. Tolerance

The classic example of genetically controlled tolerance is the Ambalema tobacco variety. TMV infects and multiplies through the plant, but in the field infected plants remain almost normal in appearance. This tolerance is due to a pair of independently segregating recessive genes r_{m1} and r_{m2}, and perhaps other genes as well which have minor effects.

Other examples are known where either a single gene or many genes control tolerance. For example, tolerance of a set of barley genotypes to barley yellow dwarf virus was controlled by a single major gene, probably with different alleles giving differing degrees of tolerance (Catherall et al., 1970). On the other hand, tolerance in Italian rye grass to both barley yellow dwarf virus (Wilkins and Catherall, 1977) and rye mosaic virus (Wilkins, 1974) appears to be polygenically inherited.

In tomatoes the gene Tm-1 is dominant or incompletely dominant for preventing symptom development following TMV infection. It was recessive or intermediate for limiting multiplication of the common strain (Pelham, 1972).

Tomatoes with the Tm-1/Tm-1 genotype are resistant to a particular type of TMV. In the heterozyous condition Tm-1 causes tolerance. When a resistant genotype was grafted onto a susceptible healthy stock, the scion became tolerant rather than resistant (Arroyo and Selman, 1977) (see also Section 9.3). Reciprocal grafting experiments between Lycopersicon species that are sugar beet curly top resistant or susceptible to sugar beet curly top virus showed that, when the root stock was of a resistant genotype, chlorophyll content in the diseased upper parts was substantially increased while other symptom features were little affected (Gardner and Cannon, 1972). Some unidentified factor diffusing from the roots was responsible for this effect. Thus the biochemical or structural basis for tolerance is not yet understood.

3.5. Kind of Symptoms

The symptoms which develop in plants which are neither immune, resistant, nor tolerant are influenced in many ways by the host genotype. For example, the difference in the mosaic disease induced by strains of turnip yellow mosaic virus (TYMV) in *Brassica pekinensis* and *B. rapa* is under the control of a nuclear gene (Matthews, 1973). The host genome influences the color pattern that develops in petals of *Matthiola incarna* (R.Br.) infected with turnip mosaic virus (Kruckelmann and Seyffert, 1970). The time taken for symptoms to develop following inoculation may be influenced by the host variety, e.g., peanut mottle virus in various soybean cultivars (Demski and Kuhn, 1975). Such differences in incubation period may be an important factor influencing the effects of viruses in the field, for example, beet curly top virus in sugar beet (Duffus and Skoyen, 1977).

4. INFLUENCE OF THE VIRAL GENOME

Studies with naturally occurring strains of viruses, with chemically induced virus mutants, and on viruses with multipartite genomes demonstrate the profound effect that even very small changes in the viral genome can have on the response of a particular plant variety to infection.

Thus naturally occurring mutants of the stock culture of turnip yellow mosaic virus (TYMV) occurring in the same individual host plant have very different effects on the cytology and biochemistry of chloroplasts (Sections 6.3 and 9.1). Figure 2 shows the responses of Chinese cabbage chloroplasts to two closely related strains of TYMV.

Sometimes a particular host species will favor a particular kind of virus strain when inoculated with a mixture of virus variants occurring naturally in another host species. For example, *Cyphomandra betacea* allows "ringspot" strains of potato virus X to multiply preferentially when inoculated with this virus from potatoes (Matthews, 1949).

Treatment of TMV with nitrous acid, a mutagen leading commonly to the base changes $C \rightarrow U$ or $A \rightarrow G$ in the RNA, can give rise to mutants which give local necrotic lesions of limited extent in a

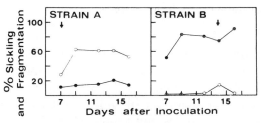

Fig. 2. An effect of the viral genome on an organelle response. Effect of strain of TYMV on proportion of Chinese cabbage leaf cells developing fragmented or sickled chloroplasts (illustrated in Fig. 6C,D). Protoplasts were made from leaves at various times after inoculation with strain A or B of TYMV (see Fig. 6A,B). They were cultured under continuous light for 24 hr before the observations were made. In inoculated plants strain A produced many necrotic lesions. Strain B produced mainly chlorotic lesions, with a few necrotic lesions developing later. Arrows indicate time of first appearance of necrotic lesions. ●, Protoplasts having sickling; ○, protoplast showing fragmentation. From Fraser and Matthews (1979).

particular host variety which normally produces chlorotic local lesions with systemic virus replication and mosaic disease. Thus mutations which may involve only a single base change in about 6500 nucleotides (Wittman and Wittman-Liebold, 1966) may produce marked changes in host response.

With multiparticle viruses it has been possible to carry out genetic reassortment experiments which allow the virus gene controlling a particular symptom in a certain host to be located on one of the viral RNA pieces (Van Vloten-Doting and Jaspars, 1977; Bruening, 1977). Perhaps the most striking effects of the viral genome have been described by Fulton for various strains of tobacco streak virus in species of *Nicotiana*. Certain variants of the virus induce profound dwarfing of the host plant, while others give rise to regularly toothed leaves in host species in which the leaves are normally entire (Fulton, 1972, 1975).

Accumulated changes in the viral genome may lead to major differences in host responses to naturally occurring strains within a group of viruses. For example, among the tymoviruses, which presumably have a common evolutionary origin, some members have no known common host.

5. POSSIBLE MECHANISMS OF DISEASE INDUCTION

Three ways in which a virus might initiate the train of events that leads to a particular host response to infection may be considered.

5.1. Sequestration of Raw Materials

The diversion of supplies of raw materials into virus production may make the host cells deficient in some metabolite or metabolites. This mechanism is very probably a factor when the host plant is under nutritional stress. For example, in mildly nitrogen-deficient Chinese cabbage plants, the local lesions produced by TYMV have a purple halo. The purple coloration is characteristic of nitrogen starvation (Diener and Jenifer, 1964). On the other hand, in well-nourished Chinese cabbage plants fully infected with TYMV, about 20% of the phosphorus in a leaf may be contained in viral RNA (Matthews *et al.*, 1963), but such plants show no symptoms of phosphorus deficiency. Another kind of specific nutritional stress can be induced by environmental conditions. For example, at least part of the effect of adverse temperature on plant growth may be due to deficiencies in specific metabolites (Ketellapper, 1963). Virus infection may well aggravate such deficiencies.

If symptoms are due to sequestration of metabolites by the virus, we would expect severe symptoms to be associated with production of large amounts of virus. In fact, an increase in severity of symptoms is sometimes associated with increased virus production. Thus, with bean pod mottle virus in soybean, Gillaspie and Bancroft (1965) observed flushes of severe symptoms followed by a recovery period of 1.5 and 4.5 weeks after inoculation. Assays of leaf extracts showed that the highest concentration of virus occurred at the first symptom flush. Concentration then fell, but rose again during the second symptom flush. Other examples of such an association are known, e.g., alfalfa mosaic virus in tobacco (Kuhn and Bancroft, 1961) and potato spindle tuber viroid in potato (Singh, 1977). However, there is no general correlation between amount of virus produced and severity of disease (e.g., Porto and Hagedorn, 1974; Palomar and Brakke, 1976). Similarly, there is no necessary correlation between the severity of macroscopic disease and various physiological and biochemical changes brought about by infection (e.g., Pring and Timian, 1969; Ziemiecki and Wood, 1975), although some correlations of this sort have been found (e.g., Huth, 1973).

In the absence of specific preexisting nutritional stress, it is unlikely that the actual sequestration of amino acids and nucleotides into virus particles has any direct connection with the induction of symptoms. The following consideration support this view. (1) Viruses are made up of the same amino acids and nucleotides in roughly the same proportions as are found in the cell's proteins and nucleic acids. Even with viruses such as TYMV, which reach a relatively high concentration in the diseased tissue ($\simeq$ 2.0 mg/g fresh weight), the amount of virus formed may be quite small relative to the reduction caused by infection in other macromolecules. For example, in Chinese cabbage plants infected with TYMV, the reduction in normal proteins and ribosomes was more than 20 times as great as the amount of virus produced (Crosbie and Matthews, 1974*b*). (2) Closely related strains of the same virus may multiply in a particular host to give the same final concentration of virus and yet have markedly different effects on host cell constituents and cause very different diseases (e.g., strains of TYMV). (3) The type strain of TMV multiplying in White Burley tobacco produces chlorotic lesions at 35°C but none at 20°C. About one-tenth as much virus is made at 35°C as at 20°C (Kassanis and Bastow, 1971). (4) A single gene change in the tobacco plant may result in a change from the typical mosaic disease produced by TMV to the hypersensitive reaction (e.g., Melchers *et al.*, 1966) (Section 3.2). F_1 hybrids between the two host genetic types may respond to TMV with a lethal systemic necrotic disease with greatly reduced virus production. (5) The fact that specific viral genes are involved in symptom induction (Section 4) makes a general nonspecific sequestration mechanism rather unlikely.

In the above discussion the amount of virus produced as measured in tissue extracts has been considered. However, the rate of virus replication in individual cells could be an important factor in influencing the course of events. Very high demand for key amino acids or other materials over a very short period perhaps of a few hours might lead to irreversible changes with major long-term effects on the cell and subsequently on tissues and organs. There is no unequivocal experimental evidence for this type of effect measured on individual cells, and such evidence might be difficult to obtain.

5.2. Direct Effects of the Virus

Structural proteins in the virus particles may play a direct and specific role in the disease process (as opposed to the nonspecific sequestration of materials discussed above). For example, a separable structural protein (the penton) of the mammalian adenovirus has been shown to cause cells to round up in culture. No such effects have been demonstrated for the proteins found in plant virus particles, although it has been suggested that a defective TMV viral coat protein may induce destruction of cell organelles (Jockusch and Jockusch 1968). Other studies with nitrous acid mutants show that TMV coat protein need not be involved in symptom induction.

Viriods consist only of RNA and yet they cause typical viruslike symptoms. It has been suggested that viroid RNA causes disease directly by acting, for example, as a repressor of some host function by combining specifically at some site in the cell (Diener and Hadidi, 1977). However, it has not been demonstrated that viroids code for no polypeptides. In principle, small segments of the genomes of normal viruses might be replicated to act directly as repressors or derepressors of host function, but there is no evidence for this.

We know that a single base change is sufficient to produce a mutant virus that produces changed symptoms. It is most improbable that such a change in one out of, say, 6500 bases in a viral RNA could bring about a change in the ability of the RNA (or even a segment of it) to bind to some specific host structure.

5.3.   Effects of Nonstructural Viral Polypeptides

The genetic reassortment experiments made possible by the existence of multiparticle viruses have demonstrated that the genetic material controlling certain symptoms is located on particular pieces of the viral genome (Section 4). None of the gene products responsible for initiating such symptoms has yet been isolated and characterized. These proteins may be very difficult to isolate and study for several reasons: (1) they may be present in very low concentration because a very few molecules per cell of a virus-specific protein might be able to block or derepress some host-cell function; (2) they may be present in the infected cells for a short period relative to that required for the completion of virus synthesis; (3) the virus-specified polypeptide may form only part of the active molecule in the cell; (4) the virus-specified polypeptide may be biologically active *in situ*, for example, in the membrane of some particular organelle. In spite of these potential difficulties, a study of the biological activities of the nonstructural viral polypeptides should prove to be most fruitful in furthering our understanding of host-plant–virus interactions.

6. ORGANELLE RESPONSES

6.1. Nuclei

Crystalline, platelike inclusions develop in nuclei of tobacco cells infected with severe etch virus (Kassanis, 1939). The plates are birefringent and are a very regular feature of severe etch infection. Intranuclear inclusions have been described for some other potyviruses. Most potyviruses also induce characteristic inclusions in the cytoplasm. The proteins of the nuclear and cytoplasmic inclusions of tobacco etch virus have been shown to be different by immunological tests (Shepard *et al.*, 1974; Knuhtsen *et al.*, 1974), and both differ from the virus coat protein. The nuclear inclusion proteins induced by tobacco etch virus in different hosts were immunologically indistinguishable suggesting that the protein is coded for by the viral genome (Knuhtsen *et al.*, 1974). Supporting this view is the fact that one strain of another potyvirus (bean yellow mosaic) produces large crystals, while another produces small ones in the same host (Mueller and Koenig, 1965). In *Gomphrena* cells infected with another potyvirus (beet mosaic), large, round, proteinaceous inclusion bodies have been observed to form in the nucleolus and migrate into the body of the nucleus, where several may accumulate (Martelli and Russo, 1969).

Shikata and Maramorosch (1966) found that, in pea leaves and pods infected with pea enation mosaic virus, particles accumulate first in the nucleus. During the course of the disease, the nucleolus disintegrates. Masses of virus particles accumulate in the nucleus and also in the cytoplasm. Virus particles of several other small isometric viruses accumulate in the nucleus (as well as in the cytoplasm). They may exist as scattered particles or in crystalline arrays (e.g., southern bean mosaic virus: Weintraub and Ragetli, 1970; tomato bushy stunt virus: Russo and Martelli, 1972). Masses of viral protein or empty viral protein shells have been observed in nuclei of cells infected with several tymoviruses (Hatta and Matthews, 1976).

Bean golden mosaic virus (a ss DNA virus) infects only phloem cells, and in these is confined to the nucleus. Nuclei of infected cells develop grossly enlarged nucleoli, which come to occupy up to 75% of the nuclear volume. The enlarged nucleoli develop distinct granular regions containing mainly ribonucleoprotein and rings of fibrillar material made up mainly of deoxyribonucleoprotein (Kim *et al.*, 1978).

Cores of some rhabdoviruses accumulate in the perinuclear space.

MacLeod *et al.* (1966) found that potato yellow dwarf virus particles accumulate as aggregates within the nucleus or in cytoplasmic invaginations into the nucleus. These inclusions may contain cytoplasmic organelles such as mitochondria or may appear to consist almost entirely of virus. Similar masses have been seen with other rhabdoviruses.

6.2. Mitochondria

The long rods of isolates of tobacco rattle virus are associated with the mitochondria in infected cells (Harrison and Roberts, 1968; Kitajima and Costa, 1969). The ends of the rods are closely appressed to the mitochondrial membrane but do not penetrate it. A defective strain of tobacco rattle virus (CAM/DF) which produces no virus rods causes the mitochondria to develop peripheral membraneous sacs and membrane-bound vesicles, and to become clumped into large masses that persist in the cell and which eventually become amorphous (Harrison *et al.*, 1970). The bodies formed of aggregated mitochondria are rich in RNA, and in cells infected with the normal strain they contain aggregates of virus rods.

The mitochondria in cells of various hosts infected with cucumber green mottle mosaic virus develop small vesicles bounded by a membrane and lying within the perimitochondrial space and in the cristae (Hatta *et al.*, 1971; Hatta and Ushiyama, 1973; Sugimura and Ushiyama, 1975). Aggregated mitochondria have been observed in *Datura* cells infected by a potyvirus (Kitajima and Lovisolo, 1972), but there was no indication that these aggregates were involved in virus synthesis. The development of abnormal membrane systems within mitochondria has been described for several virus infections (e.g., Kim and Fulton, 1972; Robleda, 1973). They resemble degenerative effects.

6.3. Chloroplasts

TYMV-infected Chinese cabbage leaf cells have been the most extensively studied system with respect to the responses of chloroplasts to infection. During the phase of active TYMV replication, the Hill reaction and cyclic and noncyclic phosphorylation were all increased (Goffeau and Bové, 1965). There was also a substantial diversion of the early products of carbon fixation away from sugars and into organic acids and amino acids (Bedbrook and Matthews, 1972). During the phase of virus replication the overall rate of carbon fixation was not affected, but, as replication neared completion, the efficiency of carbon fixation decreased; this was associated with reduction in amounts of various chloroplast components (see Section 8.3.2a).

Magyarosy *et al.* (1973) found a shift from the production of sugars to amino acids and organic acids in squash plants systemically infected with squash mosaic virus. A reduction in carbon fixation has been the most commonly reported effect on photosynthesis in leaves showing other mosaic or yellows diseases. The reduction usually becomes detectable some days after infection and is usually associated with a reduction in the amounts of photosynthetic pigments and ribulose 1'-5'-biphosphate carboxylase.

Tymoviruses such as TYMV induce the formation of numerous small flask-shaped vesicles near the periphery of the chloroplasts. They are the first detectable cytological change induced by the virus. These vesicles appear to be formed by the invagination of both chloroplast membranes. Virus infection induces changes in the distribution and size of particles within the membranes (Hatta *et al.*, 1973; Hatta and Matthews, 1976). The vesicles are the sites of viral RNA synthesis. There may be some direct relationship between the biochemical changes noted above and the formation and functioning of these vesicles, but so far there is no convincing evidence for this hypothesis.

TYMV infection can cause many other cytological changes in the chloroplasts, most of which appear to constitute a structural and biochemical degeneration of the organelles. The exact response of the chloroplasts of any particular mesophyll cell depends on the developmental stage at which it was infected, the strain of virus infecting, the time after infection, and the environmental conditions (Chalcroft and Matthews, 1966, 1967*a,b*; Ushiyama and Matthews, 1970; Hatta and Matthews, 1974).

In leaves inoculated with TYMV the chloroplasts become rounded and clumped together; most strains of the virus produce rather similar effects. There is little effect on grana or stroma lamellae, but the chloroplasts become cupshaped, with the opening of the cup generally facing the cell wall. Starch grains accumulate. "White" strains of the virus cause degeneration of the grana in inoculated leaves. Expanded leaves located above the inoculated leaf may become fully infected without the appearance of mosaic symptoms. In such leaves the effects of infection on chloroplasts are similar to those seen in isolated leaves.

In leaves that were small at the time of infection and that develop the typical mosaic, a variety of different pathological states in the chloroplasts can readily be distinguished by light microscopy in fresh leaf sections. Islands of tissue in the mosaic that show various shades of green, yellow, and white have been found to contain different strains of the virus which affect the chloroplasts in recognizably distinct ways. In contrast, the dark green islands of tissue that contain very little virus possess chloroplasts that appear normal.

The most important changes in the chloroplasts are (1) Color—ranging from almost normal green to colorless. (2) Clumping—in the mildest form of clumping, individual chloroplasts may be arranged in rows in contact with each other. In more severely affected tissue, chloroplasts are grouped into an irregular clump in which the outlines of the chloroplasts are barely discernible. In very severely affected tissue containing white strains of the virus, the clump of chloroplasts is a spherical, amorphous mass. (3) Presence of large vesicles—large vesicles tend to appear more frequently in leaves that have been infected for some time, but with certain strains these vesicles appear much sooner. They are variable in size up to several microns in diameter and usually have no electron-dense contents. (4) Fragmentation of chloroplasts—some strains of the virus cause fragmentation of the clumped chloroplasts. Fragmentation is a fairly synchronous process in any cell, thus differing from the situation in isolated protoplasts (see Section 9.3). Further rounds of fragmentation may give rise to very small pieces of chloroplast. The fragments are membrane bound and contain lamellae. (5) Grana—the numbers of grana per chloroplast and average granal stack size may be reduced. In pale green strains these effects either are absent or are of minimal extent. They are most marked in white strains. There are increasing effects on the grana as infection proceeds, and a fairly close correspondence exists between the reduction in the number of grana and the chlorophyll content of the chloroplast. (6) Osmiophilic globules, about 100 nm diameter, are seen occasionally in normal mature chloroplasts. Virus infection had no effect on these except in the white strain in old local lesions when many large osmiophilic globules occur. They are also seen in other infections (e.g., Milkus, 1975). (7) Arrays of phytoferritin molecules may be more frequent in chloroplasts of TYMV-infected cells (Chalcroft and Matthews, 1966) and also in those infected by some other viruses (Craig and Williamson, 1969; Shukla and Hiruki, 1975).

Different strains of TYMV produce particular combinations of abnormalities in the chloroplasts. Within the virus-infected leaf tissue, blocks of tissue of one type are composed of cells which show the same abnormalities.

In contrast to the small peripheral vesicles which appear to be induced by all tymoviruses in the chloroplasts of all infected cells, none of the changes noted above is an essential consequence of tymovirus infection, nor can they be regarded as diagnostic for the group. For example, no clumping of the chloroplasts occurs in cucumbers infected with okra mosaic virus. On the other hand, clumping of chloroplasts is induced by turnip mosaic virus in *Chenopodium* (Kitajima and Costa, 1973).

Several viruses outside the tymovirus group induce small vesicles near the periphery of the chloroplasts. Most of these vesicles differ from the tymovirus type in that they do not appear to have necks connecting them to the cytoplasm nor do they contain stranded material (e.g, Carroll, 1970; Betto *et al.*, 1972; Mohamed, 1973; Murant *et al.*, 1975). McMullen *et al.* (1978) have described a varied assortment of cytological abnormalities induced in chloroplasts of barley leaf cells infected with barley stripe mosaic virus. These abnormalities include the occurrence of small peripheral vesicles having wide opening to the cytoplasm, but most of the changes appeared to be degenerative responses in cells destined to undergo necrosis. Degenerative changes in the chloroplasts are a common feature of some other virus infections, for example, cucumber mosaic virus in tobacco leaf (Ehara and Misawa, 1975) and beet western yellow virus in lettuce (Tomlinson and Webb, 1978).

In many infections, the size and number of starch grains seen in leaf cells are abnormal. Generally speaking, in mosaic diseases there is less starch than normal, but in some diseases (e.g., sugar beet curly top, potato leaf roll) excessive amounts of starch may accumulate. Similarly, in local lesions induced by TMV in cucumber cotyledons, chloroplasts become greatly enlarged and filled with starch grains (Cohen and Loebenstein, 1975). These effects are probably due to metabolic changes rather than mechanical obstruction (see Matthews, 1970).

6.4. Cell Walls

The plant cell wall tends to be regarded mainly as a physical barrier and supporting structure. In fact, the cell wall is a distinct biochemical and physiological compartment containing a substantial proportion of the total activity of certain enzymes in the leaf, particularly peroxidase activity (85%) (Yung and Northcote, 1975). Three kinds of cytological abnormality have been observed in or near the walls of virus-diseased cells:

1. Abnormal thickening, due to the deposition of callose may occur in cells near the edge of virus-induced lesions (e.g., Tu and Hiruki, 1971; Hiruki and Tu, 1972). Chemical changes in the walls may be complex and difficult to study (Faulkner and Kimmins, 1975).
2. Cell wall protrusions involving the plasmodesmata have been reported for dahlia mosaic virus (Kitajima and Lauritis, 1969) and for several unrelated viruses. The protrusions from the plasodesmata into the cell have one or more canals. They may be quite short or of considerable length. They appear to be due to deposition of new wall material induced by the virus, and they may be lined inside and out with plasma membrane (e.g., Murant *et al.*, 1973; Bassi *et al.*, 1974; Allison and Shalla, 1974). The function of these protuberances has not been established.
3. Depositions of electron-dense material between the cell wall and the plasma membrane. These deposits may extend over substantial areas of the cell wall (as with oat necrotic mottle virus, Gill, 1974) or may be limited in extent and occur in association with plasmodesmata (as with barley stripe mosaic virus, McMullen *et al.*, 1977). They have been termed "paramural bodies." The major cytopathic effect of citrus exocortis viroid is the induction near the cell surface of numerous small membrane-bound bodies with an electron density similar to that of the plasma membrane (Semancik and Vanderwoude, 1976). They are found in all cell types.

7. CELLULAR RESPONSES

7.1. Necrosis

Necrosis (cell death) may be the major response of the plant to virus infection. In some diseases necrosis may be confined to particular organs and tissues and may remain very localized. It may be the first visible effect or may occur as the last stage in a sequence. For example, necrosis of epidermal cells or of midrib parenchyma may be caused by lettuce mosaic virus in lettuce (Coakley *et al.*, 1973). Necrosis caused by tobacco necrosis virus (TNV) is usually confined to localized areas of the roots (e.g., Lange, 1975). Late infection of virus-free tomato plants with TMV may give rise to internal necrosis in the immature fruits (e.g.,

Taylor *et al.*, 1969). Patches of necrosis on the seed are characteristic of broad bean stain virus in *Vicia faba* (Cockbain *et al.*, 1976).

In potato leaf roll disease the phloem develops normally but is killed by the infection. Necrosis may spread in phloem throughout the plant but is limited to this tissue. In *Pelargonium* infected with tomato ringspot virus histological effects seen by light microscopy were confined to reproductive tissues (Murdock *et al.*, 1976). Pollen grain abortion and abnormal and aborted ovules were common. The symptoms could be confused with genetic male sterility.

Drastic cytological changes occur in cells as they approach death. These changes have been studied by both light and electron microscopy, but such studies do not tell us how virus infection actually kills the cell. For example, Hayashi and Matsui (1965) examined the fine structure of cells at the periphery of expanding necrotic local lesions produced by TMV in *N. glutinosa*. In chloroplasts in altered cells, the stroma disappeared first. Then the grana and lamellae became amorphous, and the chloroplast disintegrated. In the nucleus, the ground substance disappeared first. Materials in the cytoplasm aggregated and the interface between cytoplasm and vacuole became obscure. At the edge of the lesion, cells in all stages of degeneration were intermingled.

7.2. Hypoplasia

Leaves with mosaic symptoms frequently show hypoplasia (deficient growth or development) in the yellow areas. The lamina is thinner than in the dark green areas, and the mesophyll cells are less differentiated with fewer chloroplasts and fewer or no intercellular spaces. The general appearance of the yellowed tissue in a nature leaf is like that of a leaf at an early stage of development.

In stem-pitting disease of apples, pitting is shown on the surface of the wood when the bark is lifted. The pitting is due to the failure of some cambial initial cells to differentiate cells normally, and a wedge of phloem tissue is formed that becomes embedded in newly formed xylem tissue (Hilborn *et al.*, 1965). The affected phloem becomes necrotic, and after a time the tree may die. The major anatomical effect of apple stem grooving virus in apple stems is the disappearance of the cambium in the region of the groove. Normal phloem and xylem elements are replaced by a largely undifferentiated parenchyma (Pleše *et al.*, 1975). Reduced size of pollen grains (e.g., Nyéki and Vértesy, 1974) and reduced growth of pollen tubes from virus-infected pollen also may be regarded as a hypoplastic effect.

7.3. Hyperplasia

Vein-clearing symptoms are due, with some viruses at least, to enlargement of cells near the veins (Esau, 1956). The intercellular spaces are obliterated and, since there is little chlorophyll present, the tissue may become abnormally translucent.

The vascular tissues appear to be particularly prone to virus-induced hyperplasia (excessive growth or development). In the diseased shoots found in swollen shoot disease of cocoa, abnormal amounts of xylem tissue are produced, but the cells appear structurally normal (Posnette, 1947). In plants infected by sugar beet curly top virus, a large number of abnormal sieve elements develop, sometimes associated with companion cells. The arrangement of the cells is disorderly, and they subsequently die (Esau, 1956). Oat blue dwarf virus causes abnormalities of the development of phloem in oats involving hyperplasia and limited hypertrophy of the phloem procambium (Zeyen and Banttari, 1972).

In crimson clover infected by wound tumor virus, there is abnormal development of phloem cambium cells. Phloem parenchyma forms meristematic tumor cells in the phloem of leaf, stem, and root (Lee and Black, 1955). The galls on sugar cane leaves arise from virus-induced cell proliferation. This gives rise in the mature leaf to a region in the vein where the vascular bundle is grossly enlarged (Fig. 4). Two main types of abnormal cell are present: lignified gall xylem cells and nonlignified gall phloem (Hatta and Francki, 1976).

7.4. Cell Division in Differentiated Cells

The development of a wound periderm in response to virus-induced necrosis is a typical wound-healing response (see Section 8.1.2f).

7.5. Reduced Responsiveness to Stimuli

Various experiments have shown that chronic infection of Chinese cabbage by TYMV lowers the responsiveness of the stomata to changes in light intensity. Thus Bedbrook (1972) used the cobalt chloride paper method (Stahl, 1894) to estimate relative transpiration rates and to give a measure of stomatal opening. In intact Chinese cabbage plants he compared dark green islands in leaves showing mosaic patterns with various island of tissue fully invaded by the virus. In darkness or low light intensity, stomata in darker green and pale green islands were closed, while those in islands of more severely affected lamina were open. In plants that had been held in full daylight, the dark and pale green islands were transpiring rapidly. Transpiration from severely affected islands was much less. The lowered response to light was most marked with strains of virus causing the greatest reduction in chlorophyll.

7.6. Responses of Cultured Plant Cells

The effects of virus infection on plant cells in continuous culture have not been extensively studied. Sacristan and Melchers (1969) found no effect of TMV on regeneration of plants from tobacco callus cultures or on chromosome numbers. Viruslike particles were observed in the nuclei of a cultured line of *Strepanthus* cells that had lost the ability to differentiate (Sjolund and Shih, 1970). However, it was not shown that the virus was responsible for the effect.

Strains of potato virus X of varying symptom severity in tobacco plants had no significant effect on the ease with which whole tobacco plants could be regenerated from single protoplasts (Shepard, 1975). However, when leaves were doubly infected with potato viruses X and Y, there was a pronounced selective advantage for regeneration of protoplasts that were not doubly infected.

7.7. Nodulation in Legumes

Nodulation of various legume species is adversely affected by virus infection. For example, nodulation of soybean plants by *Rhizobium* was reduced by infection with soybean mosaic virus, bean pod mottle virus, or both viruses. Greatest reduction (about 80%) occurred when plants were inoculated with virus at an early stage of growth (Tu *et al.*, 1970). The first phase in the infection of soybean root cells by *Rhizobia* (i.e., development of an infection thread and release of rhizobia into the cytoplasm) appears not to be affected by infection of the plant with soybean mosaic virus (Tu, 1973). In the second stage of infection a membrane envelope forms around the bacteria cell to form a bacteroid. Structural differences such as decreased vesiculation of this membrane envelope were observed in virus-infected roots (Tu, 1977*a*).

8. PLANT RESPONSES

8.1. Limitation of Infection Near the Site of Infection

Local lesions may be chlorotic or necrotic, they may be very limited in size or may continue to spread radially, and virus may or may not leave them and invade the plant systemically. There is no consistent correlation between any of these phenomena.

8.1.1. Nonnecrotic Local Lesions

Almost nothing is known about the mechanism of the limitation of virus movement in local lesions where necrosis does not occur. The process is controlled in part at least by the viral genome. Closely related strains of virus may differ markedly in the extent to which local infection is limited. No necrosis followed infection of cucumber cotyledons by TMV, but the virus was limited to local infections which could be revealed by staining for starch grains since cells containing virus in the center of the lesion accumulated starch. In the zone of cells surrounding the lesion some contained virus but otherwise were cytologically normal. Others contained virus and abnormal chloroplasts. Normal plasmodesmata connected infected and noninfected cells (Cohen and Loebenstein, 1975). Thus localization in this host must be a biochemical rather than a structural phenomenon.

8.1.2. Necrotic Lesions

The mechanism by which virus spread may be localized near necrotic local lesions has received a great deal of study, but we still have no coherent picture of the sequence of events involved. Most work has been carried out with TMV in tobacco var. Samsun NN or *N. glutinosa*, and TMV or TNV in *Phaseolus*. An early view was that the zone of necrotic cells might extend radially faster than the virus so that the virus then had no viable cells into which it could move. As will become apparent below, this idea is no longer valid.

8.1.2a. Genetics of the Reaction

The reaction is under the control of both the host and viral genes (see Sections 3.2.1 and 4).

8.1.2b.   Requirement for Intact Tissue

Necrotic local lesions will develop on pieces of excised leaf, but the tissue must be otherwise intact. Shimomura (1971) used TMV to inoculate the lower surface of *Nicotiana* leaves from which the lower epidermis had been removed. Control tissue developed necrotic lesions but the stripped tissue did not, although about half as much TMV was produced.

Callus cultures from the various *Nicotiana* sources carrying the NN gene gave reddish-brown necrotic local lesions when they were infected with TMV *in vitro*. This response occurred only if the tissue culture medium was supplemented with additional growth factors (Beachy and Murakishi, 1971). In a similarly supplemented medium, chains of Samsun NN cells in suspension culture responded to TMV infection with a loss of cell integrity which was not evident in cells derived from Samsun (Russell and Halliwell, 1974). For experiments with protoplasts see Section 9.3.

8.1.2c.   Localized Acquired Resistance

Ross (1961*a*) showed that a high degree of resistance to TMV developed in a 1–2 mm zone surrounding TMV local lesions in Samsun NN tobacco. The zone increased in size and resistance for about 6 days after inoculation. Greatest resistance developed in plants grown at 20–24°C. Resistance was not found in plants grown at 30°C, and no necrotic lesions formed at this temperature. Leaves infected with potato virus X did not develop zones resistant to TMV. The zones around TMV lesions were resistant to inoculation with tobacco necrosis virus and several other viruses, demonstrating a lack of specificity in the resistance.

8.1.2d.   Protein Synthesis in the Resistant Zone

In a narrow band (about 10 cell diameters) around TMV necrotic lesions in Samsun NN, mesophyll cells showed clear cytological evidence of active protein synthesis (Israel and Ross, 1967). These included more ribosomes and membrane-bound organelles and an extensive continuous endoplasmic reticulum with bound ribosomes.

Development of acquired resistance is inhibited completely by treatment of the tissue with actinomycin D before the challenge inoculation (Loebenstein *et al.*, 1968). The size of the local lesions resulting from the primary inoculation in several hypersensitive reactions was increased by prior actinomycin D treatment (Loebenstein *et al.*, 1969). These results support the idea that both the limitation of lesion size and the localized acquired resistance may involve an induced host DNA-dependent RNA synthesis. The possibility that the acquired resistance involves the synthesis of new host proteins is strengthened by the fact that chloramphenicol treatment and ultraviolet irradiation can also cause a substantial increase in lesion size and virus replication (Sela *et al.*, 1969; Loebenstein *et al.*, 1970).

Electrophoretic analyses of extracts of Samsun NN leaves with necrotic local lesions revealed four proteins not detectable in healthy tissue (van Loon and van Kammen, 1970). No such bands were found in infected Samsun tobacco. In infected *N. glutinosa* one "new" band and an increase in two other components was detected. Gianinazzi *et al.* (1970) demonstrated the presence of four similar new leaf protein components (which they called b_1–b_4) in the living tissue surrounding necrotic lesions in *N. tabacum* c.v. Xanthi n.c.

The expression of the N gene is temperature sensitive. At 30°C it is no longer expressed, and varieties like Samsun NN develop typical mosaic disease. Proteins from the two infected genotypes at 30°C were indistinguishable (van Loon, 1975a). Studies with various host genotypes and TMV strains showed that the differences in the soluble proteins are associated with a particular symptom type—localized necrosis or mosaic—and are not confined to the NN genotype.

In resistant leaves the b_1 protein may come to represent 1% of the soluble leaf protein (Antoniw and Pierpont, 1978). The four proteins appear in high concentration only in the tissue very close to the lesions (Rohloff and Lerch, 1977). Gianinazzi *et al.* (1977b) considered that b_2 and b_3 from Xanthi n.c. tobacco were oligomers of a 16,000 molecular-weight monomer (b_1), b_4 being a monomer of 29,500 molecular weight. However, more recent work has shown that b_1, b_2, and b_3 are charge isomers of similar molecular weight and amino acid composition (Antoniw *et al.*, 1979).

These proteins are not detected in healthy tissue, but they are induced by stimuli other than virus infection—for example, polyacrylic acid (Gianinazzi and Kassanis, 1974; Kassanis and White, 1978) and ethephon (a compound releasing ethylene) (van Loon, 1977). These treatments also induced resistance to infection by TMV. Development of resistance and the appearance of the proteins are suppressed by actinomycin D (Kassanis and White, 1974), lending support to the idea that they might be involved in the resistance phenomenon. In summary, some viruses, by causing localized necrosis, induce a nonspecific host response to such necrosis, which includes the *de novo* synthesis of two new polypeptides. These polypeptides may play some as yet undefined role in the resistance phenomenon.

8.1.2e. Metabolic Changes Near the Lesions

While some p-quinones are essential normal cell constituents, o-quinones are highly reactive, unstable compounds that can combine with proteins and inactivate them (Pierpont, 1970; Walker, 1975). It has been suggested that cell death in necrotic local lesions may be due to the production of such o-quinones. In the localized necrotic reaction, enzymes involved in the synthesis of phenolic compounds (e.g., phenylalanine ammonia lyase, cinnamic acid-4-hydroxylase, and catechol-O-methyltransferase are markedly stimulated (reviewed by Duchesne et al., 1977), and there is an increase in phenolic compounds. Furthermore, there is a stimulation of peroxidase and polyphenol oxidase activity reported by many workers (reviewed by Solymosy, 1970; Weststeijn, 1976).

In the few millimeters of tissue around each lesion there is a gradient of phenylalanine ammonia lyase activity (Fritig et al., 1973) and of peroxidase (Weststeijn, 1976). The increase in the first of these activities has been shown to be due to the synthesis of new enzyme (Duchesne et al., 1977). The accumulation of phenolic materials in the interveinal areas around the lesion sites is readily demonstrated because of their bright blue fluorescene under ultraviolet light.

It seems quite likely that the formation of o-quinones is a factor leading to cell death and that dying cells may stimulate the enzyme activities noted above. However, a role for these enzymes and products in the localization of virus infection remains to be established. Various lines of evidence make it unlikely that they are directly responsible for a cell's resistance to infection. Weststeijn (1976) has suggested that virus localization and the necrotic reaction are both brought about by an increased permeability of cell membranes. Such an increase has been detected at an early stage in the hypersensitive response (Weststeijn, 1978).

In cowpea leaves infected with cowpea mosaic virus, the enzymes concerned with phenol metabolism increased after necrotic lesions began to appear. In marked contrast, lipoxygenase activity increased and decreased again before lesion appearance (Kato and Misawa, 1976a). Biochemical studies indicate that lipid peroxidation takes place at an early stage following inoculation (Kato and Misawa, 1976c). Furthermore, loss of electrolytes indicating increased permeability of cell membranes begins well before lesions appear.

When TMV or TNV infect tobacco varieties that develop necrotic local lesions, there is an increase in the release of ethylene from the leaves during the period of lesion formation (Balázs et al., 1969; Nakagaki et al., 1970; Gáborjanyi et al., 1971). Systemic infection without necrosis did not give rise to such an increase. It should be remembered that a decreased release of ethylene from infected leaves may mean an increase in the internal concentration of this hormone. The relationships between ethylene release, the necrotic process, and other factors are not established. However, the fact that ethephon introduced into leaves with a needle can mimic all the specific changes associated with the response of Samsun NN and TMV is strong evidence that ethylene is involved in the initiation of this hypersensitive response (van Loon, 1977).

8.1.2f. Wound-Healing Responses

Plant tissue frequently reacts to wounds caused by mechanical injury, insects, and various pathogens by a series of wound healing responses. The most important of these are the development of a wound periderm and cell wall changes, including lignification, suberization, and the deposition of callose. Virus-induced necrosis may lead to such wound responses. For example, periderm formed in young bean leaves inoculated with the VM strain of TMV which gives very small lesions, but did not form in old leaves or in leaves inoculated with the U_1 strain which gives large lesions (Wu, 1973).

Various workers have noted a deposition of callose in cells around necrotic local lesions, leading to thickening of cell walls and probably to blocking of plasmodesmata (e.g., Hiruki and Tu, 1972; Wu, 1973). Stobbs et al. (1977) found that callose deposition in live cells extended beyond the margin of detectable virus, while remaining within the zone of fluorescent metabolite accumulation in Pinto bean leaves infected with TMV. Kimmins and Brown (1973) found an accumulation of cell wall glycoproteins following inoculation of hypersensitive hosts with TMV or TNV. An identical response occurred in leaves that had been sham inoculated.

Other observations suggest that cell wall modifications may not be a factor limiting spread. Appiano et al. (1977) considered that the conspicuous cell wall lignification seen in lesions caused by tomato bushy stunt virus in Gomphrena leaves was not a barrier to spread of virus, because lignification did not follow the whole cell perimeter and because virus could be detected beyond the cells with modified walls. In a further detailed study Pennazio *et al.* (1978) could detect no cell structure active in limiting spread of virus. Shimomura and Dijkstra (1975) found callose deposition to occur in walls of cells around necrotic local lesions in host–virus combinations where systemic infection took place.

When [^{35}S]methionine, ^{32}P, or ^{45}Ca was supplied through the petioles to *N. glutinosa* or Samsun EN leaves with developing TMV lesions, these substances accumulated in a sharply defined zone of cells around the lesion. The zone included the cells with increased callose deposition (Schuster and Flemming, 1976). A similar zone developed around necrosis induced by physical means, both in hypersensitive varieties and in Samsun tobacco. Since this latter variety does not contain the NN gene responsible the hypersensitive reaction, callose deposition and the diffusion barrier are unlikely to be the result of NN gene activity in hypersensitive hosts.

8.1.2g.   Antiviral Factors

Sela and his colleagues have isolated a material which they call an antiviral factor from virus-infected leaves of hosts containing the NN gene (Antignus *et al.*, 1975, 1977; Mozes *et al.*, 1978). However, the substance (or substances) has not yet been sufficiently characterized to permit assessment of its significance.

An antiviral factor of a different kind has been identified in cowpea leaves infected with cowpea mosaic virus (Kato and Misawa, 1976*b*). Traumatic acid, a known wound hormone, was isolated from infected but not from healthy leaves. Its appearance may be due to the increased lipoxygenase activity noted above. The acid inhibited lesion production in cowpea but did not inhibit TMV replication in tobacco.

Besides inhibitory compounds, factors stimulating virus infection may also be induced during virus replication—for example, the nonspecific stimulating factor (protein) induced in *N. glutinosa* by TMV infection (Khurana and Hidaka, 1977). The existence of such factors will obviously complicate the study of antiviral factors.

8.1.2h.   Changes in the Vascular Tissue

The discussion above has been concerned with structural and biochemical changes in mesophyll cells surrounding a localized infection. Long-distance systemic movement of virus from such lesions normally involves the vascular tissue. Favali *et al.* (1978) have shown that, in the zone surrounding lesions induced by TMV in *N. glutinosa*, phloem and xylem elements became occluded by callose or plugs of electron-dense material. It is not yet certain whether such occlusion plays a role in preventing movement of virus out of the lesion zone.

8.2.   Systemic Acquired Resistance

Our knowledge about systemic acquired resistance has come mainly from the work of Ross and his colleagues (Ross, 1961*a,b*, 1966; Loebenstein and Ross, 1963; Loebenstein *et al.*, 1966) on TMV in the tobacco variety Samsun NN and on tobacco necrosis virus in the pinto bean. In tests with tobacco, lower leaves are inoculated with TMV and then some days later the same leaves or upper leaves may be challenged by a second inoculation with TMV (Fig. 3). Acquired resistance is measured by the reduction in diameter of the lesions (and with some viruses, reduction in number). With bean, one primary leaf is inoculated and the opposite primary leaf challenged with an inoculation some days later.

Lesions were about one-fifth to one-third the size found in control leaves, but lesion number was not reduced with TMV in Samsun NN tobacco. Resistance was detectable in 2–3 days, rose to a maximum in about 7 days, and persisted for about 20 days. Leaves that developed

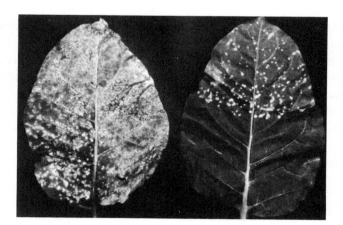

Fig. 3.   Resistance acquired at a distance from the site of inoculation. Right: Samsun NN tobacco leaf inoculated first on the apical half with TMV and 7 days later given a challenge inoculation over its whole surface with TMV. Left: Control leaf given only the second inoculation. From Ross (1961*b*).

resistance were free of virus before the challenge inoculation. No conditions have been found which would give complete resistance. In plants held at 30°C, no resistance developed. Mechanical or chemical injury that killed cells did not lead to resistance, nor did infection with viruses that do not cause necrotic local lesions. On the other hand many other nonspecific agents applied to leaves will induce the phenomenon (Solymosy, 1970; Gupta et al., 1974). In such experiments it is not possible to be sure that the same phenomenon is being studied since many treatments affect lesion size.

The resistance induced by TMV was not specific for TMV but was effective for tobacco necrosis virus and several other viruses. A similar lack of specificity in the resistance acquired following the development of necrotic local lesions was found with various other host–virus combinations giving the hypersensitive response. However, virus-specific factors may regulate the extent of the resistance (van Loon and Dijkstra, 1976).

Ross (1966) pointed out that effects on lesion number tend to be more variable and to develop later. He considered that a fall in lesion number merely means that, in highly resistant leaves, lesions do not become large enough to be countable. The action at a distance involved in systemic acquired resistance presumably involves the translocation of some substance or substances. Ross (1966) has presented good evidence that transport of a resistance-inducing material is involved. For example, when the midrib of an upper tobacco leaf was cut, resistance did not develop in the portion of the lamina distal to the cut. Similarly, killing sections of petiole of inoculated leaves with boiling water while allowing the leaf to remain turgid prevented development of resistance in other leaves. Other experiments showed that in large tobacco plants the material moved equally well both up and down the stems.

The nature of the material that migrates is unknown, as is the actual mechanism of resistance in the resistant uninfected leaves. This mechanism may or may not be the same as that in the zone of tissue around necrotic lesions. New protein bands can be detected by gel electrophoresis in extracts from leaves that have developed systemic acquired resistance, and these have the same electrophoretic mobilities as some of the proteins that appear in tissue near local lesions (van Loon, 1975b; Rohloff and Lerch, 1977).

A marked increase in phenylalanine ammonia lygase about the time necrotic lesions could first be detected appeared in leaves showing acquired resistance (Simons and Ross, 1971; Vegetti et al., 1975). Conflicting results were obtained by Fritig et al. (1973). Increased peroxidase activity in these leaves does not appear to be directly concerned

with their acquired resistance (van Loon, 1976). Finally, Balázs *et al.*
(1977) found that cytokinin content of resistant Xanthi NN tobacco
leaves was increased. A reduction in size and number of necrotic local
lesions in the systemically "resistant" leaves may not be associated with
a reduction in the actual amount of TMV produced (Balázs *et al.*,
1977). Our ignorance of the factors that either initiate or limit systemic
necrosis is emphasized by the fact that, in some infections where the
virus invades the whole organ without causing symptoms, limited
patches of necrotic tissue may later develop (e.g., Hanchey *et al.*, 1975).

8.3. Stunting

There appear to be two probable general mechanisms by which
virus infection could cause stunting of growth: a change in the activity
of growth hormones and a reduction in the availability of the products
of carbon fixation.

8.3.1. Changes in Growth Hormones

There is little doubt that a virus-induced change in hormone
concentration is one of the ways in which virus infection causes stunting. It should be remembered that plant hormones have been defined
chemically and biologically in controlled growth tests on excised tissues
or organs. In the intact plant, however, each of the groups of hormones
induces many physiological effects. Their functions overlap to some
extent and their interactions are complex. For a given process their
effects may be similar, synergistic, or antagonistic. In the intact plant,
members of all or most of the groups are involved in any particular
developmental process. Their mode of action is not yet understood.
There is indirect evidence that specific receptor sites are involved, but
none of these has been fully characterized. There are many possible
ways in which virus infection could influence plant growth by increasing
or decreasing the synthesis, translocation, or effectiveness of these
various hormones in different organs and at different stages of growth.
In view of our ignorance of the biochemistry and molecular biology of
hormone action in the healthy plant, it is not surprising that our understanding of the interactions between viruses and hormones is extremely
sketchy. As a result of earlier work, it was widely believed that infection resulted in reduced concentrations of auxinlike substances (e.g.,
Diener, 1963) but the procedures and materials used make such studies

impossible to interpret. Some examples from more recent work are considered here.

The growth inhibition and increased respiration of cowpea hypocotyls induced by infection with cowpea mosaic virus may be caused by an interference with indole acetic acid (IAA) metabolism, mediated somehow by changes in ethylene and IAA oxidase activity (Lockhart and Semancik 1970a,b). These results merely provided correlations between various activities so that no cause and effect relationships could be established.

Application of giberellic acid can partially annul the growth-stunting effect of tobacco etch virus infection in tobacco (Chessin, 1957) and of wound tumor virus in clover (Maramorosch, 1957), but other symptoms, and active virus, were still present. Stein (1962) found that when tobacco plants infected with severe etch virus were treated with giberellic acid plant height and leaf growth were greatly stimulated. Treated infected plants were about 2.5 times taller than untreated infected plants but only about 0.8 times as tall as treated healthy plants.

The stunting of barley leaves caused by barley yellow dwarf virus infection was due to a reduction in cell number (i.e., reduced mitotic activity) rather than any effect on cell size (Russell and Kimmins, 1971). There was a reduction in endogenous giberellins but not of auxin. Spraying infected plants with giberellin (A_3) allowed infected plants to grow taller than uninfected unsprayed plants but not as tall as uninfected, hormone-treated plants. The reversal of dwarfing was due solely to elongation. Thus the exogenous hormone was not annulling the virus-induced reduction in mitotic activity which must have occurred in the basal cell division zone of the leaves at an earlier stage in the life of the leaf. Fifty-two giberellins are now known, and several are usually present in a single plant so that interpretation of their effects is even more difficult than with IAA.

Ethylene production was enhanced in cucumber cotyledons infected with cucumber mosaic virus. The increase began just before hypocotyl elongation rate was slowed (Marco et al., 1976). Reducing the ethylene content enhanced elongation of infected seedlings but not as much as it did healthy seedlings, suggesting some other factors were involved. This was borne out by further work showing that suppression of hypocotyl elongation was also accompanied by a reduction in giberellinlike substances and an increase in abscisic acid (Aharoni et al., 1977). This work illustrates well the complex effects of infection on hormone balance and the difficulty involved in establishing cause-and-effect relationships.

8.3.2. Reduction in the Availability of Fixed Carbon

Apart from any effects on hormone balance, plants will become stunted (on a dry weight basis, at least) if the availability of carbon fixed in photosynthesis is limiting. A reduction in available fixed carbon could be brought about in several ways.

8.3.2a. Direct Effects on the Photosynthetic Apparatus

The most obvious and perhaps the most common way by which infection reduces plant size is through direct effects on the photosynthetic apparatus. For example, infection of Chinese cabbage leaves with TYMV reduced the three major chloroplast components, chlorophyll a, ribulose biphosphate carboxylase, and 68 S ribosomes, to about the same extent on a per plant basis (Crosbie and Matthews, 1974b). These changes took place after most virus replication was completed, and reduction in the first two began before the ribosomes were affected.

The initial events that lead to reduced carbon fixation in the chloroplasts are not known for any host–virus combination. Hormones may play a role in the initiation of chlorophyll degradation. In leaves of *Tetragona expansa* inoculated with bean yellow mosaic virus, chlorotic local lesions develop. Shortly after their appearance there is a substantial increase in ethylene release from the leaves (Gáborjanyi *et al.*, 1971). In cucumber cotyledons infected with cucumber mosaic virus, Marco and Levy (unpublished) have shown that ethylene is produced before local lesion appearance. They were able to delay the appearance of chlorotic local lesions by removing the ethylene by hypobaric ventilation.

8.3.2b. Starch Accumulation in Chloroplasts

The accumulation of starch in chloroplasts, commonly seen in virus infections, must deprive the growing parts of the plant of some newly fixed carbon. This accumulation may be due to reduced permeability of the chloroplast membrane or to changes in enzyme activities within the chloroplast.

cAMP has been detected in white clover plants, the concentration being higher in leaves of healthy clover than in those infected with clover yellow mosaic virus (Tu, 1977b). Tu supplied clover cuttings with cAMP and showed that this treatment caused the starch grains to disappear from both healthy and diseased leaves. The role of cAMP in starch metabolism is not known, but Tu suggested that disappearance of the starch grains might be due to an increase in β-amylase activity. Plants contain substantial phosphodiesterase activity so that at least some of the cAMP supplied to the clover cuttings was probably degraded to adenosine, A 5'p, and A 3'p. These compounds should be tested for their effects on starch accumulation.

8.3.2c. Stomatal Opening

Lowered photosynthesis in yellows-infected sugar beet could be accounted for in part by a virus-induced reduction in stomatal opening (Hall and Loomis, 1972). The reduced responsiveness of stomata to changes in light intensity might be a factor limiting carbon fixation in TYMV-infected leaves during the earlier part of the day (see also Section 7.5).

8.3.2d. Translocation of Fixed Carbon

Any effect of virus infection, such as necrosis, that reduces the efficiency of phloem tissues must limit translocation of fixed carbon from mature leaves to growing tissues. However, reduced permeability of leaf cells to the migration of sugars into the phloem may be more commonly the limiting factor.

8.3.2e. Leaf Posture

Leaf posture may affect the overall efficiency of photosynthesis in the field. For example, a wheat variety with an erect habit fixed more CO_2 than one with a lax posture (Austin *et al.*, 1976). Virus infection can affect growth habit, but no studies have been made of this factor in relation to carbon fixation per plant.

8.3.3. Growth Analysis

Analysis of the stunting process during the development of a mosaic disease is an extremely complex problem which has not been adequately investigated even in experimental herbaceous hosts. Crosbie and Matthews (1974a,b) investigated the overall effects of infection of Chinese cabbage plants with a severe white strain of TYMV.

Healthy plant growth was approximately logarithmic over the period we studied, as was the amount of chlorophyll per plant. Virus infection caused a virtual cessation of chlorophyll A production for several weeks. Growth of the diseased plant was almost linear over this period, and it can be assumed that this was because chlorophyll content increased very little for several weeks. The diseased Chinese cabbage plant responded to the reduction in chlorophyll in two ways. First, a higher proportion of the material available for growth was used to make leaf lamina rather than midrib, petiole, stem, or roots. Second, the proportion of dark green island tissue (see Section 8.6.7) increased in later formed leaves so that chlorophyll in these islands came to form a significant proportion of the total. As the disease progressed, plant growth became critically dependent on the presence of tissue containing normal amounts of chlorophyll. Most of such tissue was located in a group of about three fully expanded leaves located just above the inoculated leaves, and which usually escape infection by TYMV for several weeks. If these leaves were removed at 3 weeks after inoculation, subsequent net increase in fresh weight was halted for at least 4 weeks. A further consequence of removing these leaves was that the proportion of the lamina that consisted of dark green islands subsequently increased to 40% compared with 17% for plants retaining the lower green leaves.

This last result shows that the mechanism which leads to the formation of islands of potential dark green tissue in the short apex must be a dynamic one responding to events taking place elsewhere in the plant.

The "white" strain of TYMV used in the above experiments causes an apparently much more severe disease than mild "pale green" strains of the virus. However, closer analysis showed there was little difference in total fresh weight of aerial parts or of roots between plants infected with the two kinds of strain. The gross differences were mainly due to different distribution of total chlorophyll within the plant, and a more extreme alteration in growth form with the severe strain (i.e., reduction in stem, petiole, and midrib). In another study on growth, Takahashi (1972) examined systematically the effect of TMV infection of leaf size and shape and on internode length, but he did not relate the effects to chlorophyll loss.

8.4. Epinasty and Leaf Abscission

The experiments of Ross and Williamson (1951) indicated that the epinastic response and leaf abscission in *Physalis floridiana* infected with potato virus Y was associated with the evolution of a physiologically active gas which was probably ethylene.

Beginning about 48 hr after inoculation of cucumber cotyledons with cucumber mosaic virus, there was a decrease in ethylene emanation compared with controls (Levy and Marco, 1976). Over the same period there was an increase in the resistance of infected leaves to gaseous diffusion and an increase in the internal concentration of ethylene. Infection gave rise to a marked epinastic response in the cotyledons. The following evidence strongly suggests that the epinasty was due to the increased ethylene concentration: (1) Ethylene reached a peak concentration before the epinastic response began. (2) Treatment of healthy cucumbers with ethylene caused epinasty. (3) Epinasty could be prevented in infected cotyledons by hypobaric ventilation, which facilitates removal of the internal ethylene.

This is the best evidence showing that a hormone is directly involved in the production of symptoms induced by virus infection. How virus infection stimulates ethylene production and how the hormone has its effects are not known. Phospholipase D reversibly inhibits ethylene production in healthy tissue, suggesting that some membrane function is involved (Odawara *et al.*, 1977). Ethylene release caused changes in the distribution of peroxidase activity within cells in the abscission zone, suggesting that ethylene may cause changes in membrane permeability (Webster *et al.*, 1976). Peroxidase is active during abscission, but its role in the process is not clear.

8.5. Abnormal Growth

8.5.1. Virus-Induced Tumors

All the plant viruses belonging to the Reoviridae except rice dwarf virus induce galls or tumors in their plant hosts (but not in the insect vectors in which they also multiply) (Fig. 4).

There is a clear organ or tissue specificity for the different viruses. For example, tumors caused by wound tumor viruses predominate on roots and, to a lesser extent, on stems and petioles (Lee and Black 1955). Fiji disease virus causes neoplastic growths on veins of stems and leaves. Thus we can be reasonably certain that some function of the viral genome induces tumor formation, but we are quite ignorant as to how this is brought about. Wounding plays an important role as an inducer or promoter of tumors caused by wound tumor virus. Hormones released on wounding may play some part in this process.

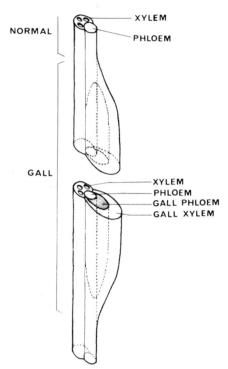

Fig. 4. An abnormal growth response. Diagrammatic representation of the vascular anatomy of a galled vascular bundle in a sugar cane leaf infected with Fijivirus. Only the distribution of phloem and xylem tissues is shown. A section of the bundle through the galled area has been removed to expose the tissues in transverse section. From Hatta and Francki (1976).

Microscopic tumor initials which normally do not develop into macroscopic tumors occur in the stem apices of sweet clover infected with wound tumor virus. Application of IAA stimulates the growth of these tumors to macroscopic size (Black, 1972).

8.5.2. Distortion or Reduction of Tissues

In leaves showing mosaic disease, the dark green islands of tissue frequently show blistering or distortion. This is due to the reduced cell size in the surrounding tissues and the reduced size of the leaf as a whole. The cells in the dark green island are much less affected and may not have room to expand in the plane of the lamina. The lamina then becomes convex or concave to accommodate this expansion. In some diseases the lamina is greatly reduced in area. In extreme examples only the midrib and lateral veins are formed.

8.6. Mosaic Disease and Leaf Development

Solberg and Bald (1962) noted that there was a relationship between the physiological maturity of *Nicotiana glauca* leaves and the pattern of symptoms induced by TMV. Others have suggested that mosaic patterns are laid down in the short apex (Chalcroft and Matthews, 1966; Reid and Matthews, 1966). These workers assumed that, in a plant infected with a mixture of virus strains, the first virus particle to establish itself in a dividing cell preempts that cell and all or almost all its progeny, giving rise in the mature leaf to a macroscopic or microscopic island of tissue occupied by the initial strain. Since that time detailed evidence has accumulated to support this view.

8.6.1. Cell Lineages in Normal Leaf Ontogeny

8.6.1a. Dicotyledons

As pointed out by Stewart and Dermen (1975) and outlined below, the position of green and white cells in the leaf of a homoplastidic periclinal chimera provides a visible record of the orientation and sequence of cell divisions during the ontogeny of that leaf—information that would be impossible to obtain from histological observation of the orientation of cell plates during cell division.

Much of our understanding of the ontogeny of the dicotyledon leaf has come from the study of such chimeras (e.g., Stewart and Dermen, 1970, 1975; Stewart and Burk, 1970).

In the apical dome there are three independent layers of cells that give rise to all primary growth. The outermost layer, LI, and the next layer, LII, consist of one cell layer. Beneath this, LIII consists of a less-well-defined layer more than one cell thick. All primary growth arises from division in one to three apical cells (usually three) in each of these three layers (Stewart and Dermen, 1970). The development of an individual leaf begins with a lateral protrusion on the apical dome called a leaf buttress. Next, the leaf axis is formed as the buttress elongates. Then lamina development begins. In the mature lamina the final distribution of cells that originated in LI, LII, and LIII depends successively on the pattern of cell divisions in the buttress, the axis, and the lamina. The basic general pattern in the mature leaf is as follows: LI gives rise to the epidermis. LII gives rise to all the internal layers of cells around a variable proportion of the leaf margins and to two single layers of cells immediately below the epidermis over a wide area. LIII give rise to midrib tissues and to the internal layers of the leaf in irregular areas near the midrib.

The pattern of contribution from the three layers may vary widely in successive leaves. This is best seen in a periclinal chimera with a G-W-G constitution (i.e., LI apical initials are green, LII are mutant (white), and LIII are green). The following are the major variables: (1) The relative extents of divisions of LII and LIII cells at all three stages of leaf development. At one extreme LIII may occupy most of the lamina; at the other, it may contribute small irregular islands of tissue near the midrib at the base of the leaf. Temperatures at which the plants are grown may affect the relative contributions of the three apical layers. (2) At a relatively late stage, periclinal divisions may occur in LI (green), giving rise to a G cell in the hypodermal palisade layer. Subsequent anticlinal divisions of the G cell gives rise to a small island of green cells surrounded by white cells derived from LII. (3) There may be rather frequent periclinal intercalary divisions in either LII or LIII cells. With a G-W-G chimera these give rise by further anticlinal divisions to isolated island of dark green (GGG) or pale tissue (GWW). (4) There may be differences in the number of layers involved in vertical extension of the lamina. The minimal number of layers for a typical dicotyledon leaf like tobacco would be five (two from LI, two from LII, and one from LIII). In fact, seven are found in tobacco.

8.6.1b. Monocotyledons

Cell lineages have not been studied in the same detail in monocotyledons. However, it is well established that, once the developing leaf primorium reaches a certain size, new cells contributing to elongation arise from a basal intercalary meristem (e.g., Stevenson, 1973; Kirchanski, 1975). In chimeras containing a plastid mutation, this form of development gives rise to longitudinal stripes of mutant and normal tissue—a situation commonly found in ornamental monocotyledons. As one proceeds acropetally along a monocotyledon leaf, the cells become older.

8.6.2. Role of Virus Strains and Dark Green Tissue in Mosaic Disease

In some infections such as TMV in tobacco, the disease in individual plants appears to be produced largely by a single strain of the virus. However, it has been known for many years that occasional bright yellow islands of tissue in the mosaic contain different strains of the virus. Such strains probably arise by mutation and during leaf development come to exclude the original mild strain from a block of tissue. In Chinese cabbage plants infected with TYMV there may be many islands of tissue of slightly different color from which different strains of the virus can be isolated (Chalcroft and Matthews, 1967a,b).

Dark green islands of tissue that superficially appear normal occur in these two diseases and in many other mosaics. They are a prominent component of the mosaics and may be important in the growth of the diseased plant. Dark green tissue is discussed further in Section 8.6.7.

8.6.3.   Evidence That Mosaic Development Depends on Leaf Ontogeny

8.6.3a.   Leaf Age at Time of Infection

By inoculating plants at various stages of growth it has been demonstrated for TYMV (Chalcroft and Matthews, 1966) and TMV (Atkinson and Matthews, 1970; Takahashi, 1971; Suwa and Takahashi, 1975) that the type of mosaic pattern developing in a leaf at a particular position on the plant depends not on its position but on its stage of development when infected by the virus. There is a critical leaf size at the time of infection above which mosaic disease does not develop. This critical size is about 1.5 cm (length) for tobacco leaves infected with TMV (Atkinson and Matthews, 1970; Gianinazzi et al., 1977a).

8.6.3b.   Gradients in Size of Islands

Although the size of macroscopic islands in a mosaic are very variable, there tends to be a definite gradient up the plant. Leaves that were younger when systemically infected tend to have a mosaic made up of larger islands of tissue. Even within one leaf there may be a relationship between both the number and size of islands and the age of different parts of the lamina as determined by frequency of cell division.

8.6.3c.   Presence of Virus, and the Mosaic Pattern in Very Young Leaves

Many viruses can invade the apical dome. The mosaic pattern is already laid in very small TYMV infected Chinese cabbage leaves that have not yet developed significant amounts of chlorophyll (Matthews, 1973).

8.6.3d. Patterns in the Macroscopic Mosaic

Patterns in a macroscopic mosaic are often so jumbled that an ontogenetic origin for them cannot be deduced. Occasionally, patterns that are clearly derived from the apical initials have been observed. For example, Chinese cabbage leaves (or several successive leaves) have been observed to be divided about the midrib into two islands of tissue—one half dark green and the other containing a uniform virus infection (Matthews, 1973). These observations show that individual apical initials must have been infected either with virus or with the agent that induces dark green tissue.

8.6.3e. The Microscopic Mosaic

The existence of microscopic mosaics provides the strongest evidence that mosaic patterns depend on leaf ontogeny. In Chinese cabbage leaves infected with TYMV the microscopic mosaic develops only on leaves that were less than about 1–2 mm long at the time of infection. In such leaves, areas in the mosaic pattern that macroscopically appear to be a uniform color may on microscopic examination be found to consist of mixed tissue in which different horizontal layers of the mesophyll have different chloroplast types. A wide variety of mixed tissues can be found. Perhaps the most common type is one in which the upper one or two layers of palisade cells are of one type, dark green or pale green, the rest of the mesophyll being yellow green or white. Alternatively, the lower one or two cell layers of spongy mesophyll may be dark green, the rest of the mesophyll being abnormal tissue. In some areas, both palisade and the lower layers of the spongy tissue may consist of dark green tissue while the central zone of cells in the lamina is white or yellow green (Fig. 5A). This situation may be reversed, with the central layer being dark green and the upper and lower layers consisting of diseased cells (Fig. 5B).

As seen in fresh leaf sections, these areas of horizontal layering may extend for several millimeters or they may be quite small, grading down to islands of a few cells or even one cell of a different type. The junction between islands of dark green cells and abnormal cells in the microscopic mosaic is often very sharp.

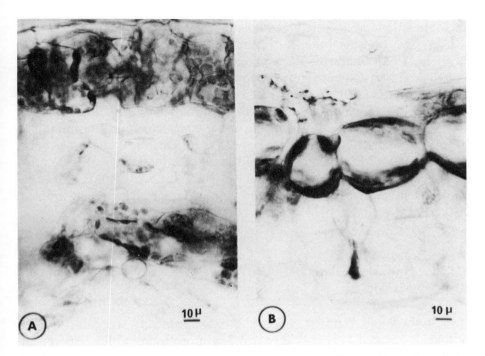

Fig. 5.   Relationship between leaf ontogeny and mosaic disease. Examples of the microscopic mosaic in Chinese cabbage leaves infected with TYMV. A: Upper and lower cell layers consist of dark green cells. (presumably contributed by LII) The central zone is infected by a severe white strain. This layer was presumably contributed by LI. B: The reverse of A. From Chalcroft and Matthews (1967*b*).

Such arrangements are not confined to dark green vs. virus-infected layers. The microscopic mosaic also includes cell layers infected by different strains of the virus with distinctive effects on chloroplasts. These arrangements can all be interpreted in terms of the ontogenic processes described for healthy leaves from observations on chimeras.

In many leaves showing mosaic, there are areas of leaf which consist of one tissue type interspersed with small islands of another type. Many of these islands may be visible to the naked eye. The background color of this stipple tissue is frequently white or yellowish white, with numerous dark green or pale green small islands. The dark green islands appear on the upper surface of the leaf and are not usually apparent when viewed from the underside. Cytologically, stipple areas in the microscopic mosaic usually consist of an island of tissue that is white, nearwhite, or a shade of yellow, but in which there are numerous small islands of palisade cells which are either dark green or pale green.

In some stipple areas, the green islands are raised above the rest of the leaf surface. In others, the leaf surface is flat.

The small island of dark green cells in otherwise diseased mesophyll could arise by occasional periclinal division of a "dark green" LI cell with subsequent migration of one daughter cell into the palisade layer, followed by limited subsequent anticlinal division. If this explanation is correct, we would expect the upper epidermis to be normal (dark green) in the area of a patch of stipple tissue. This expectation has been confirmed (Matthews, 1973). In epidermal cells infected by TYMV, the small chloroplasts have peripheral vesicles, but these were absent in chloroplasts of epidermal cells overlying an area of dark green stippled tissue.

8.6.3f. How Many Initially Infected Cells Give Rise to an Island in the Mosaic?

Stewart and Dermen (1975) showed that at any stage during leaf ontogeny one cell may divide only a few more times while a sister cell may give rise to a substantial area of tissue. The simplest assumption is that in cells still undergoing division the first virus particle to establish itself in a cell preempts that cell and its progeny. The progeny give rise in the mature leaf to a macroscopic or microscopic island of tissue occupied by that particular strain of virus. Alternatively, the cell is converted to a dark green state and gives rise to a dark green island in the mature leaf.

In some circumstances cell-to-cell spread and infection by the virus in the short apex must be possible, for example, early after infection of the apex. Following such spread some islands of tissue in the mature mosaic will arise from the progeny of a group of neighboring cells in the apex rather than as a clone from a single cell.

Islands of dark green tissue which extend through all the histological layers of a leaf must have arisen by cell-to-cell spread of an agent during leaf ontogeny (Atkinson and Matthews, 1970). Experiments using a tobacco variety in which the mesophyll cells and epidermal cells were genetically distinguishable confirm the idea that some diffusible substance may be involved in the establishment of such dark green islands (Carlson and Murakishi, 1978). On the other hand the small dark green islands described in Section 8.6.3e almost certainly arise as clones from single cells.

8.6.4. Additional Variables in Mosaic Disease

The extreme variability in direction and frequency in cell division during leaf ontogeny, with the consequent variation in contribution from the three cell layers in the apical meristem, was summarized in Section 8.6.1. Several additional variables are introduced by virus infection. First, a virus particle infecting a cell in the initial invasion of a leaf primordium may replicate in that cell and then spread to neighboring cells before other virus particles establish there. The extent of such spread will affect the size of and the cell layers involved in the island of tissue. Second, viruses may invade the apical meristem to different extents. Different viruses and virus strains may vary in the extent of such invasion, which may also be influenced by environmental conditions. Third, a virus replicating in a developing leaf may mutate at any stage during leaf ontogeny. Fourth, an important variable might be the differing extent to which strains of the virus affected the rate of cell division. A cell infected by a mutant that doubled the time between successive divisions compared with the parent strain would produce only about 6% as many progeny as the cell infected with the parent strain after ten divisions of this latter cell. There are very few data on the differential effects of strains on cell division rate. However, such differences or lack of them could be a potent factor determining the gross appearance of a mosaic. For example, many mutants of TYMV may have little differential effect on the rate of cell division so that many strains survive to give islands in the mosaic. It is possible that most TMV mutants affecting chlorophyll content may, in addition, reduce cell division rate and thus become lost in a mass of tissue infected with the parent strain. There is good evidence that suppressed strains exist. For example, Shepard (1975) regenerated plants from protoplasts isolated from a tobacco plant showing a mild diffuse mottle due to potato virus X. About 10% of the regenerated plants were infected with strains giving a different symptom type.

8.6.5. Genetic Control of Mosaics

In spite of the fact that the most striking effects of TYMV infection in *Brassica* spp. are on the chloroplasts, the response of these organelles to infection is under some degree of nuclear control. Certain varieties of *B. rapa* respond to all the strains isolated from *B. pekinensis* with a mild diffuse mottle. In reciprocal crosses between *B.*

rapa and *B. chinensis* all the progeny gave a *B. chinensis* type of response to the strains (Matthews, 1973).

8.6.6. Mosiac Disease in Monocotyledons

The macroscopic islands of tissue in mosaic diseases in monocotyledons almost always consist of stripes, streaks, or elongated blocks of tissue lying parallel to the axis of the leaf rather than in an irregular pattern. This arrangement is almost certainly due to the fact that these leaves elongate by means of a basal meristem, producing files of cells. Undoubtedly there are other variations that are not yet understood.

8.6.7. The Nature of Dark Green Tissue

Dark green islands in the mosaic pattern are cytologically and biochemically normal as far as has been tested. They contain low or zero amounts of infectious virus and no detectable viral protein or viral dsRNA (Reid and Matthews, 1966; Chalcroft and Matthews, 1967*a,b*; Fulton, 1951; Atkinson and Matthews, 1970; Verhoyen, 1962; Honda and Matsui, 1974; Loebenstein *et al.*, 1977; Chamberlain *et al.*, 1977).

Various lines of evidence show that dark green islands are resistant to superinfection with the same virus or closely related viruses (Fulton 1951; Atkinson and Matthews, 1970; Reid and Matthews, 1966; Chalcroft and Matthews, 1967*b*; Matthews, 1973; Loebenstein *et al.*, 1977).

Various factors can influence the proportion of leaf tissue that develops as green islands in a mosaic. These include leaf age, strain of virus, season of the year, and removal of the lower leaves on the plant (Crosbie and Matthews, 1974*b*). The dark green islands of tissue may not persist in an essentially virus-free state for the life of the leaf. "Breakdown" leading to virus replication usually takes place after a period of weeks or after a sudden elevation in temperature (Atkinson and Matthews, 1970; Matthews, 1973; Loebenstein, *et al.*, 1977).

There is no convincing evidence for any of the various theories that have been put forward to explain the nature of dark green islands. They certainly do not consist merely of tissue that has escaped infection, as was suggested by Goldstein (1926). There is no evidence for the presence of very mild strains of virus in dark green islands nor is there any good evidence for the presence of virus-specific inhibitors. It is possible that the cells in dark green islands are occupied by defective strains, but such strains would have to produce little or no intact virus or viral antigen and would have to replicate without detectable cytological effects. These cannot be ruled out at present but, on the other hand, there is no positive evidence for their presence.

The phenomenon of lysogeny has been known among bacterial viruses for a long time. Noting that dark green islands of tissue appeared in the TYMV-induced mosaic only in leaves that were still undergoing cell division at the time of infection, Reid and Matthews (1966) speculated that some process like lysogeny might be taking place to give dark green tissue its resistance to infection. This suggestion is somewhat more credible now that integration into the host genome, in DNA form, of the genomes of RNA tumor viruses is an established phenomenon (Vogt, 1977). There is no experimental evidence to indicate such integration with RNA plant viruses, but the possibility cannot be ruled out. The frequent presence of very small contaminating blocks of infected cells in dark green islands makes it difficult to investigate this problem by conventional molecular biological techniques.

8.7. Responses of the Host Plant Genome

There is another kind of experimental observation indicating that an RNA virus can interact with the host genome to produce a persistent effect. A genetic abnormality is induced in *Zea mays* by infection with barley stripe mosaic virus, a virus which is transmitted through the pollen (Sprague *et al.*, 1963; Sprague and McKinney, 1966, 1971). If pollen from a virus-infected parent having the genetic constitution A_1A_1, *PrPr*, *SuSu* was crossed with a homozygous recessive line (a_1a_1, *prpr*, *susu*,) that was resistant to the virus, a low frequency of the progeny lines gave significant distortion from the expected ratios for one or more of the genetic markers (A_1-a_1, presence of absence of aleurone color; *Pr-pr*, purple or red aleurone color; *Su-su*, starchy or sugary seed). This aberrant ratio (AR) effect was observed only when the original parent supplying the pollen was infected and showed virus symptoms on the upper leaves. The AR effect was inherited in a stable manner in infected lines, with a low frequency of reversion to normal ratios. Wheat streak mosaic virus and lily fleck corn virus also induced the AR effect. More is known about the genetics of *Zea mays* than any other angiosperm, and this may account for the discovery of the AR effect in this species. Further work may show that similar phenomena occur in other virus-infected plants.

9. USE OF PROTOPLASTS TO STUDY HOST RESPONSES

Protoplasts infected *in vitro* have been used mainly to study the molecular biological aspects of plant virus replication. In principle, they should also be of considerable value in the study of host plant responses to infection. A few experiments have been reported with this objective in view. However, various limitations are becoming apparent: (1) Some ultrastructural features seen in TMV-infected tobacco leaf cells were not observed during TMV replication in protoplasts (Otsuki *et al.*, 1972*b*). (2) Crystalline inclusion bodies in TMV-infected leaf cells were degraded in protoplasts made from such leaves (Föglein *et al.*, 1976). (3) The development of cytological changes in Chinese cabbage protoplasts infected with TYMV *in vitro* is less synchronous than is generally believed (Sugimura and Matthews, unpublished). Some other discrepancies between observations in the intact plant and in protoplasts are noted in the following sections.

9.1. Structural Changes in Organelles

TYMV infection in Chinese cabbage provides particularly favorable material for the study of virus-induced structural changes in chloroplasts. This is because virus-induced clumping of chloroplasts and some other changes such as the formation of large vesicles (sickling) and fragmentation (Fig. 6A,B) can be monitored in large numbers of cells by light microscopy. Protoplasts isolated from leaves inoculated with TYMV can be used to study the effects of various factors on these virus-induced structural changes.

In the sickling process a large clear vesicle appears in chloroplasts of an infected protoplast, the chlorophyll-bearing structures being confined to a cup-shaped fraction of the chloroplast volume that is seen as a crescent in section. The vesicle is bounded by a membrane which appears to arise from stroma lamellae (Fraser and Matthews, 1979). Red and blue light are equally effective inducers of sickling, which does not occur in the dark (Matthews and Sarkar, 1976). At 6–8 days after inoculation of leaves, very few protoplasts show sickling when freshly isolated, although the light intensity received by the leaves is more than adequate to induce sickling in isolated protoplasts. Thus some factor partially represses the sickling process in intact leaves.

We have recently developed a method permitting the repeated examination by light microscopy of the same individual protoplasts (Fraser and Matthews, 1979). Examination of many cells from leaves

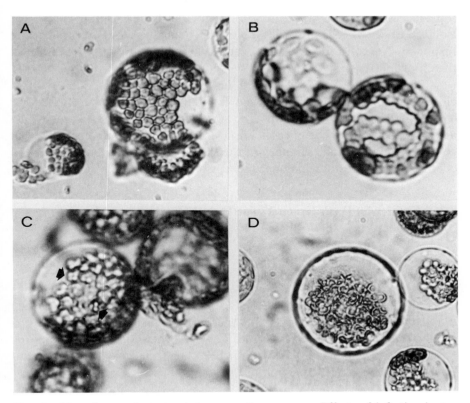

Fig. 6.   Use of protoplasts to study organelle responses. Effects of infection by two strains of TYMV on chloroplasts in Chinese cabbage mesophyll protoplasts. A: Angular clumped chloroplasts (strain A of Fig. 1). B: Rounded and clumped chloroplasts in larger cell (strain B of Fig. 1). Smaller cell is healthy. C: Fragmenting chloroplasts arising from type A on exposure to light (arrows indicate fragmentation). D: Sickled chloroplasts arising from type B cells on exposure to light. From Fraser and Matthews (1979).

inoculated with different strains of the virus has shown the following: (1) Light-induced structural changes are of two quite distinct types—sickling and fragmentation (Fig. 6A,B). (2) The two processes are mutually exclusive. In individual protoplasts only one type of change is observed. (3) Sickled chloroplasts occur in cells with rounded clumped chloroplasts (Fig. 6D). Fragmentation develops in cells with chloroplasts that are clumped in an angular manner (Fig. 6C). (4) The processes are highly asynchronous in individual protoplasts. (5) Both processes require active electron transport since they are inhibited by 10^{-6} M 3-(3,4,-dichlorophenyl)-1,1-dimethylurea (DCMU). (6) The proportion of protoplasts showing the two kinds of change depends on the strain (or isolate) or virus. Strains with chlorotic local lesions gave a sickling response. Necrotic local lesions were associated with fragmentation in the chloroplasts (Fig. 2).

The isolates of TYMV used in these experiments are certainly closely related, both being derived from the stock culture of TYMV. The experiments show that specific series of cytological changes which are not essential for virus replication are under the control of the viral genome. Small genetic changes in the virus may bring about substantial changes in the cytological consequences of infection.

9.2. Studies on Dark Green Tissue from Virus-Induced Mosaics

9.2.1. Cells Free of Virus

The existence in dark green tissue of cells that are free of infectious virus has been confirmed by the isolation of protoplasts from dark green islands and the regeneration from these protoplasts of intact plants, a proportion of which were virus free. This has been done for potato virus X in tobacco (Shepard, 1975) and TMV in tobacco (Murakishi and Carlson, 1976).

9.2.2. Resistance to Infection

Apparently virus-free plants regenerated from protoplasts from dark green tissue have been tested for resistance to inoculation with the original virus. All the virus-free plants regenerated from dark green islands of tobacco infected with TMV were able to be reinfected (Murakishi and Carlson, 1976), but they showed an apparent transitory resistance to infection in the first few leaves produced by the plantlets. Of 200 plants regenerated from apparently dark green islands in tobacco infected with potato virus X, only ten were free of infection and all were readily reinfected (Shepard, 1975). The published photograph suggests that not all the tissue used in this experiment came from true dark green island tissue.

9.2.3. Renewed Virus Synthesis in Protoplasts

Föglein *et al.* (1975) showed that when protoplasts are prepared from tobacco leaf tissue fully infected with TMV, there is a renewal of viral RNA synthesis. They also found a renewal of TMV-RNA synthesis and an increase in infectivity over 24 hr incubation in protoplasts prepared from dark green island tissue. However, even when freshly isolated, about 30% of these protoplasts were infected as judged by fluorescent antibody staining, and no increase in this number was seen during incubation. Therefore, the observed increase in infectivity and TMV RNA synthesis probably took place in the cells that were already infected. Incubation of protoplasts isolated from green islands in tobacco leaves infected with cucumber mosaic virus led to no increase in the infectivity of extracts made from them (Loebenstein *et al.*, 1977).

9.3. Nature of the Hypersensitive Response

Inoculation of isolated protoplasts may be a useful technique for distinguishing between true immunity and an extreme hypersensitive reaction where only microscopic necroses develop. For example, protoplasts from 64 lines of cowpeas that were apparently immune to cowpea mosaic virus supported virus replication when infected *in vitro* (Beier *et al.*, 1977).

Several genes that induce a hypersensitive necrotic reaction in intact plants or excised leaf pieces fail to do so when isolated protoplasts are infected. This has been found for the *NN* gene in tobacco (Otsuki *et al.*, 1972a) and for *Tm-2* and *Tm-2²* in tomato (Motoyoshi and Oshima 1975, 1977). Protoplasts from plants carrying these genes in the homozygous condition allowed replication of TMV without death of the cells. It has been suggested that this effect might be due to the epidermis being involved in the necrotic response (Motoyoshi and Oshima, 1975) or that cell to cell connections are necessary for the hypersensitive phenotype to be expressed (Motoyoshi and Oshima, 1977). Another and possibly more likely explanation could be that the presence of the cell wall is necessary for expression of the *N* gene. Peroxidase enzymes appear to be involved in the necrotic response (Section 8.1.2e). These enzymes may be located mainly in the cell wall compartment (Section 6.4). Thus removal of the wall may cause a gap in the chain of biochemical events leading to cell death.

10. REFERENCES

Aharoni, N., Marco, S., and Levy, D., 1977, Involvement of gibberellins and abscisic acid in the suppression of hypocotyl elongation in CMV-infected cucumbers, *Physiol. Plant Pathol.* **11**:189.

Alexander, L. J., 1971, Host-pathogen dynamics of tobacco mosaic virus on tomato, *Phytopathology* **61**:611.

Allison, A. V., and Shalla, T. A., 1974, The ultrastructure of local lesions induced by potato virus X: A sequence of cytological changes, *Phytopathology* **64**:784.

Antignus, Y., Sela, I., and Harpaz, I., 1975, A phosphorus containing fraction associated with antiviral activity in *Nicotiana* spp. carrying the gene for localization of TMV infection, *Physiol. Plant Pathol.* **6**:159.

Antignus, Y., Sela, I., and Harpaz, I., 1977, Further studies on the biology of an antiviral factor (AVF) from virus-infected plants and its association with the N gene of *Nicotiana* species, *J. Gen. Virol.* **35**:107.

Antoniw, J. F., and Pierpont, W. S., 1978, Purification of a tobacco leaf protein associated with resistance to virus infection, *Biochem. Soc. Tr.* **6**:248.

Antoniw, J. F., Ritter, C. E., Pierpont, W. S., and van Loon, L. C., 1980, Separation and comparison of three pathogenesis-related proteins from two cultivars of virus-infected tobacco plants, *J. Gen. Virol.* **47**:79–87.

Appiano, A., Pennazio, S., D'Agostino, G., and Redolfi, P., 1977, Fine structure of necrotic local lesions induced by tomato bushy stunt virus in *Gomphrena globosa* leaves, *Physiol. Plant Pathol.* **11**:327.

Arroyo, A., and Selman, I. W., 1977, The effects of rootstock and scion on tobacco mosaic virus infection in susceptible, tolerant and immune cultivars of tomato, *Ann. Appl. Biol.* **85**:249.

Atkinson, P. H., and Matthews, R. E. F., 1970, On the origin of dark green tissue in tobacco leaves infected with tobacco mosaic virus, *Virology* **40**:344.

Austin, R. B., Ford, M. A., Edrich, J. A., and Hooper, B. E., 1976, Some effects of leaf posture on photosynthesis and yield in wheat, *Ann. Appl. Biol.* **83**:425.

Balázs, E., Gáborjányi, R., Tóth, Á., and Király, Z., 1969, Ethylene production in Xanthi tobacco after systemic and local virus infections, *Acta Phytopathol. Acad. Sci. Hung.* **4**:355.

Balázs, E., Sziráki, I., and Király, Z., 1977, The role of cytokinins in the systemic acquired resistance of tobacco hypersensitive to tobacco mosaic virus, *Physiol. Plant Pathol.* **11**:29.

Barrios, E. P., Mosokar, H. I., and Black, L. L., 1971, Inheritance of resistance to tobacco etch and cucumber mosaic viruses in *Capsicum frutesceus*, *Phytopathology* **61**:1318.

Bassi, M., Favali, M. A., and Conti, G. G., 1974, Cell wall protrusions induced by cauliflower mosaic virus in Chinese cabbage leaves: A cytochemical and autoradiographic study, *Virology* **60**:353.

Beachy, R. N., and Murakishi, H. H., 1971, Local lesion formation in tobacco tissue culture, *Phytopathology* **61**:877.

Bedbrook J. R., 1972, The effects of TYMV infection on photosynthetic carbon metabolism, MSc Thesis, University of Auckland, Auckland, New Zealand.

Bedbrook J. R., and Matthews, R. E. F., 1972, Changes in the proportions of early products of photosynthetic carbon fixation induced by TYMV infection, *Virology* **48**:255.

Beier, H., Siler, D. J., Russell, M. L., and Bruening, G., 1977, Survey of susceptibility to cowpea mosaic virus among protoplasts and intact plants from *Vigna sinensis* lines, *Phytopathology* **67**:917.

Betto, E., Bassi, M., Favali, M. A., and Conti, G. G., 1972, An electron microscopic and autoradiographic study of tobacco leaves infected with the U5 strain of tobacco mosaic virus, *Phytopathol. Z.* **75**:193.

Black, L. M. 1972, Plant tumors of viral origin, *Prog. Exp. Tumor Res.* **15**:110.

Bruening, G., 1977, Plant covirus systems: Two-component systems, *Comp. Virol.* **11**:55.

Carlson, P. S., and Murakishi, H. H., 1978, Evidence on the clonal versus non-clonal origin of dark green islands in virus-infected tobacco leaves, *Plant Sci. Lett.* **13**:377.

Carroll, T. W., 1970, Relation of barley stripe mosaic virus to plastids, *Virology* **42**:1015.

Catherall, P. L., Jones, A. T., and Hayes, J. D., 1970, Inheritance and effectiveness of genes in barley that condition tolerance to barley yellow dwarf virus, *Ann. Appl. Biol.* **65**:153.

Chalcroft, J. P., and Matthews, R. E. F., 1966, Cytological changes induced by turnip yellow mosaic virus infections, *Virology* **28**:555.

Chalcroft, J. P., and Matthews, R. E. F., 1967a, Virus strains and leaf ontogeny as factors in the production of leaf mosaic patterns by turnip yellow mosaic virus, *Virology* **33**:167.

Chalcroft, J. P., and Matthews, R. E. F., 1967b, Role of virus strains and leaf ontogeny in the production of mosaic patterns by turnip yellow mosaic virus, *Virology* **33**:659.

Chamberlain, J. A., Catherall, P. L., and Jellings, A. J., 1977, Symptoms and electron microscopy of ryegrass mosaic virus in different grass species, *J. Gen. Virol.* **36**:297.

Chessin, M., 1957, Growth substances and stunting in virus infected plants, in: *Proceedings of the Third Conference on Potato Virus Diseases*, p. 80, Lisse-Wageningen, Netherlands.

Cirulli, M., and Alexander, L. J., 1969, Influence of temperature and strain of tobacco mosaic virus on resistance in a tomato breeding line derived from *Lycopersicon peruvianum*, *Phytopathology* **59**:1287.

Coakley, S. M., Campbell, R. N., and Kimble, K. A., 1973, Internal rib necrosis and rusty brown discoloration of Climax lettuce induced by lettuce mosaic virus, *Phytopathology* **63**:1191.

Cockbain, A. J., Bowen, R., and Vorra-Urai, S., 1976, Seed transmission of broad bean stain virus and Echtes Ackerbohnenmosaik-Virus in field beans (*Vicia faba*), *Ann. Appl. Biol.* **84**:321.

Cohen, J., and Loebenstein, G., 1975, An electron microscope study of starch lesions in cucumber cotyledons infected with tobacco mosaic virus, *Phytopathology* **65**:32.

Cook, A. A., 1963, Genetics of response in pepper to three strains of potato virus Y, *Phytopathology* **53**:720.

Craig, A. S., and Williamson, K. I., 1969, Phytoferritin and virus infection, *Virology* **39**:616.

Crosbie, E. S., and Matthews, R. E. F., 1974a, Effects of TYMV infection on leaf pigments in *Brassica pekinensis* Rupr, *Physiol. Plant Pathol.* **4**:379.

Crosbie, E. S., and Matthews, R. E. F., 1974b, Effects of TYMV infection on growth of *Brassica pekinensis* Rupr, *Physiol. Plant Pathol.* **4**:389.

Delhey, R., 1974, Zur Natur der extremen Virusresistenz bei der Kartoffel. I. Das X-virus, *Phytopathol. Z.* **80**:97.

Delhey, R., 1975, Zur Natur der extremen Virusresistenz bei der Kartoffel. II. Das Y-Virus, *Phytopathol. Z.* **82**:163.

Demski, J. W., and Kuhn, C. W., 1975, Resistant and susceptible reaction of soybeans to peanut mottle virus, *Phytopathology* **65**:95.

Diener, T. O., 1963, Physiology of virus-infected plants, *Am. Rev. Phytopathol.* **1**:197.

Diener, T. O., and Hadidi, A., 1977, Viroids, *Comp. Virol.* **11**:285.

Diener, T. O., and Jenifer, F. G., 1964, A dependable local lesion assay for turnip yellow mosaic virus, *Phytopathology* **54**:1258.

Dijkstra, J., Bruin, G. C. A., Burgers, A. C., van Loon, L. C., Ritter, C., van de Sanden, P. A. C. M., and Wieringa-Brants, D. H., 1977, Systemic infection of some N-gene-carrying *Nicotiana* cultivars after inoculation with tobacco mosaic virus, *Neth. J. Plant Pathol.* **83**:41.

Duchesne, M., Fritig, B., and Hirth, L., 1977, Phenylalanine ammonia-lyase in tobacco mosaic virus-infected hypersensitive tobacco. Density-labelling evidence of *de novo* synthesis, *Biochim. Biophys. Acta* **485**:465.

Duffus, J. E., and Milbrath, G. M., 1977, Susceptibility and immunity in soybean to beet western yellow virus, *Phytopathology* **67**:269.

Duffus, J. E., and Skoyen, O., 1977, Relationship of age of plants and resistance to a severe isolate of the beet curly top virus, *Phytopathology* **67**:151.

Ehara, Y., and Misawa, T., 1975, Occurrence of abnormal chloroplasts in tobacco leaves infected systemically with the ordinary strain of cucumber mosaic virus, *Phytopathol. Z.* **84**:233.

Esau, K., 1956, An anatomist's view of virus diseases, *Am. J. Bot.* **43**:739.

Faulkner, G., and Kimmins, W. C., 1975, Staining reactions of the tissue bordering lesions induced by wounding tobacco mosaic virus, and tobacco necrosis virus in bean, *Phytopathology* **65**:1396.

Favali, M. A., Conti, G. G., and Bassi, M., 1978, Modifications of the vascular bundle ultrastructure in the "resistant zone" around necrotic lesions induced by tobacco mosaic virus, *Physiol. Plant Pathol.* **13**:247.

Finley, K. W., 1953, Inheritance of spotted wilt resistance in the tomato. II. Give genes controlling spotted wilt resistance in four tomato types, *Aust. J. Biol. Sci.* **6**:153.

Föglein, F. J., Kalpagam, C., Bates, D. C., Premecz, G., Nyitrai, A., and Farkas, G. L., 1975, Viral RNA synthesis is renewed in protoplasts isolated from TMV-infected Xanthi tobacco leaves in an advanced stage of virus infection, *Virology* **67**:74–79.

Föglein, F. J., Nyitrai, A., Gulyás, A., Premecz, G., Oláh, T., and Farkas, G. L., 1976, Crystalline inclusion bodies are degraded in protoplasts isolated from TMV-infected tobacco leaves, *Phytopathol. Z.* **86**:266.

Fraser, L., and Matthews, R. E. F., 1979, Strain-specific pathways of cytological change in individual chinese cabbage protoplasts infected with turnip yellow mosaic virus, *J. Gen. Virol.* (in press).

Fritig, B., Gosse, J., Legrand, M., and Hirth, L., 1973, Changes in phenylalanine ammonia-lyase during the hypersensitive reaction of tobacco to TMV, *Virology* **55**:371.

Fulton, R. W., 1951, Superinfection by strains of tobacco mosaic virus, *Phytopathology* **41**:579.

Fulton, R. W., 1953, Resistance in tobacco to cucumber mosaic virus infection, *Phytopathology* **43**:472.

Fulton, R. W., 1972, Inheritance and recombination of strain-specific characters in tobacco streak virus, *Virology* **50**:810.

Fulton, R. W., 1975, The role of top particles in recombination of some characters of tobacco streak virus, *Virology* **67**:188.

Gáborjanyi, R., Balázs, E., and Király, Z., 1971, Ethylene production, tissue senescent and local virus infections, *Acta Phytopathol. Acad. Sci. Hung.* **6**:51.

Gardner, D. E., and Cannon, O. S., 1972, Unusual symptomatology of curly top in sus-
    ceptible-resistant grafted tomato plants, *Phytopathology* **62**:187.
Gianinazzi, S., and Kassanis, B., 1974, Virus resistance induced in plants by polyacrylic
    acid, *J. Gen. Virol.* **23**:1.
Gianinazzi, S., Martin, C., and Vallée, J. C., 1970, Hypersensibilitié aux virus,
    temperature et protéines solubles chez le *Nicotiana* Xanthi N. C. Apparition de
    nouvelles macrolécules lors de la répression de la synthese virale, *C. R. Acad. Sci.
    Ser. D* **270**:2383.
Gianinazzi, S., Deshayes, A., Martin, C., and Vernoy, R., 1977a, Differential reactions
    to tobacco mosaic virus infection in Samsun 'NN' tobacco plants. I. Necrosis,
    mosaic symptoms and symptomless leaves following the ontogenic gradient, *Phy-
    topathol. Z.* **88**:347.
Gianinazzi, S., Pratt, H. M., Shewry, P. R., and Miflin, B. J., 1977b, Partial purifica-
    tion and preliminary characterization of soluble leaf proteins specific to virus
    infected tobacco plants, *J. Gen. Virol.* **34**:345.
Gill, C. C., 1974, Inclusions and wall deposits in cells of plants infected with oat ne-
    crotic mottle virus, *Can. J. Bot.* **52**:621.
Gillaspie, A. G., and Bancroft, J. B., 1965, The rate of accumulation, specific
    infectivity and electrophoretic characteristics of bean pod mottle virus in bean and
    soybean, *Phytopathology* **55**:906.
Goffeau, A., and Bové, J. M., 1965, Virus infection and photosynthesis. I. Increased
    photophosphorylation by chloroplasts from Chinese cabbage infected with turnip
    yellow mosaic virus, *Virology* **27**:243.
Goldstein, B., 1926, A cytological study of the leaves and growing points of healthy and
    mosaic-diseased plants, *Bull. Torrey Bot. Club* **53**:499.
Greenleaf, W. H., 1959, Breeding tobacco-etch virus-resistance Tabasco-type peppers,
    Phytopathology **49**:317.
Gupta, B. M., Chandra, K., Vermas, H. N., and Verma, G. S., 1974, Induction of
    antiviral resistance in *Nicotiana glutinosa* plants by treatment with *Trichothecium*
    polysaccharide and its reversal by actinomycin D, *J. Gen. Virol.* **24**:211.
Hall, A. E., and Loomis, R. S., 1972, An explanation for the difference in
    photosynthetic capabilities of healthy and beet yellows virus-infected sugar beets
    (*Beta vulgaris* L), *Plant Physiol.* **50**:576.
Hanchey, P., Livingston, C. H., and Reeves, F. B., 1975, Cytology of flower necrosis in
    Cattleyas infected by Cymbidium mosaic virus, *Physiol. Plant Pathol.* **6**:227.
Harrison, B. D., and Roberts, I. M., 1968, Association of tobacco rattle virus with
    mitochondria, *J. Gen. Virol.* **3**:121.
Harrison, B. D., Stefanac, Z., and Roberts, I. M., 1970, Role of mitochondria in the
    formation of X-bodies in the cells of *Nicotiana clevelandii* infected by tobacco rat-
    tle viruses, *J. Gen. Virol.* **6**:127.
Hatta, T., and Francki, R. I. B., 1976, Anatomy of virus-induced galls on leaves of
    sugarcane infected with Fiji disease virus and the cellular distribution of virus
    particles, *Physiol. Plant Pathol.* **9**:321.
Hatta, T., and Matthews, R. E. F., 1974, The sequence of early cytological changes in
    Chinese cabbage leaf cells following systemic infection with turnip yellow mosaic
    virus, *Virology* **59**:383.
Hatta, T., and Matthews, R. E. F., 1976, Sites of coat protein accumulation in turnip
    yellow mosaic virus-infected cells, *Virology* **73**:1.

Hatta, T., and Ushiyama, R., 1973, Mitochondrial vesiculation associated with cucumber green mottle mosaic virus-infected plants, *J. Gen. Virol.* **21**:9.

Hatta, T., Nakamoto, T., Takagi, Y., and Ushiyama, R., 1971, Cytological abnormalities of mitochondria induced by infection with cucumber green mottle mosaic virus, *Virology* **45**:292.

Hatta, T., Bullivant, S., and Matthews, R. E. F., 1973, Fine structure of vesicles induced in chloroplasts of Chinese cabbage leaves by infection with turnip yellow mosaic virus, *J. Gen. Virol.* **20**:37.

Hayashi, T., and Matsui, C., 1965, Fine structure in the lesion periphery produced by tobacco mosaic virus, *Phytopathology* **55**:387.

Hilborn, M. T., Hyland, F., and McCrum, R. C., 1965, Pathological anatomy of apple trees affected by the stem-pitting virus, *Phytopathology* **55**:34.

Hiruki, C., and Tu, J. C., 1972, Light and electron microscopy of potato virus M lesions and marginal tissue in red kidney bean, *Phytopathology* **62**:77.

Holmes, F. O., 1938, Inheritance of resistance to tobacco-mosaic disease in tobacco, *Phytopathology* **28**:553.

Holmes, F. O., 1960, Inheritance in tobacco of an improved resistance to infection by tobacco mosaic virus, *Virology* **12**:59.

Holmes, F. O., 1961, Concomitant inheritance of resistance to several viral diseases in tobacco, *Virology* **13**:409.

Honda, Y., and Matsui, C., 1974, Electron microscopy of cucumber mosaic virus-infected tobacco leaves showing mosaic symptoms, *Phytopathology* **64**:534.

Hooker, W. J., and Kim, W. S., 1962, Inhibitors of potato virus X in potato leaves with different types of virus resistance, *Phytopathology* **52**:688.

Huth, W., 1973, Das Verhalten einiger Enzyme des Kohlenhydratstoffwechsels in Kartoffel-X-virus-kranken Tabakpflanzen, *Phytopathol. Z.* **77**:117.

Israel, H. W., and Ross, A. F., 1967, The fine structure of local lesions induced by tobacco mosaic virus in tobacco, *Virology* **33**:272.

James, R. K., and Tobin, S. A., 1972, Factors affecting purification of maize dwarf mosaic virus from corn, *Phytopathology* **62**:812.

Jockusch, H., 1966, The role of host genes temperature and polyphenoloxidase in the necrotization of TMV infected tobacco tissue, *Phytopathol. Z.* **55**:185.

Jockusch, H., and Jockusch, B., 1968, Early cell death caused by TMV mutants with defective coat proteins, *Mol. Gen. Genet.* **102**:204.

Kassants, B., 1939, Intranuclear inclusions in virus-infected plants, *Ann. Appl. Biol.* **26**:705.

Kassanis, B., and Bastow, C., 1971, The relative concentration of infective intact virus and RNA of four strains of tobacco mosaic virus as influenced by temperature, *J. Gen. Virol.* **11**:157.

Kassanis, B., and White, R. F., 1974, Inhibition of acquired resistance to tobacco mosaic virus by actinomycin D, *J. Gen. Virol.* **25**:323.

Kassanis, B., and White, R. F., 1978, Effect of polyacrylic acid and b proteins on TMV multiplication in tobacco protoplasts, *Phytopathol. Z.* **91**:269

Kato, S., and Misawa, T., 1976a, Hypersensitive reaction of cowpea leaves to cucumber mosaic virus, *Tohoku J. Agric. Res.* **26**:49.

Kato, S., and Misawa, T., 1976b, Isolation and identification of a substance interfering with local lesion formation produced in cowpea leaves locally infected with cucumber mosaic virus, *Ann. Phytopathol. Soc. Jpn.* **42**:450.

Kato, S., and Misawa, T., 1976c, Lipid peroxidation during the appearance of hypersensitive reaction in cowpea leaves infected with cucumber mosaic virus. *Ann. Phytopathol. Soc. Jpn.* **42**:472.

Ketellapper, H. J., 1963, Temperature induced chemical defects in higher plants, *Plant Physiol.* **38**:175.

Khurana, S. M. P., and Hidaka, Z., 1977, Virus-infection stimulating factor(s) induced by tobacco mosaic virus infection in *Nicotiana glutinosa* plants, *Phytopathol. Z.* **88**:140.

Kim, K. S., and Fulton, J. P., 1972, Fine structure of plant cells infected with bean pod mottle virus, *Virology* **49**:112.

Kim, K. S., Shock, T. L., and Goodman, R. M., 1978, Infection of *Phaseolus vulgaris* by bean golden mosaic virus: Ultrastructural aspects, *Virology* **89**:22.

Kimmins, W. C., and Brown, R. G., 1973, Hypersensitive resistance. The role of cell wall glycoproteins in virus localization, *Can. J. Bot.* **51**:1923.

Kirchanski, S. J., 1975, The ultrastructural development of the dimorphic plastids of *Zea mays* L, *Am. J. Bot.* **62**:695.

Kitajima, E. W., and Costa, A. S., 1969, Association of pepper ringspot virus (Brazilian tobacco rattle virus) with mitochondria, *J. Gen. Virol.* **4**:177.

Kitajima, E. W., and Costa, A. S., 1973, Aggregates of chloroplasts in local lesions induced in *Chenopodium quinoa* Wild, by turnip mosaic virus, *J. Gen. Virol.* **20**:413.

Kitajima, E. W., and Lauritis, J. A., 1969, Plant virions in plasmodesmata, *Virology* **37**:68.

Kitajima, E. W., and Lovisolo, O., 1972, Mitochondrial aggregates in *Datura* leaf cells infected with henbane mosaic virus, *J. Gen. Virol.* **16**:265.

Knuhtsen, H. H. E., Hiebert, E., and Purcifull, D. E., 1974, Partial purification and some properties of tobacco etch virus-induced intranuclear inclusions, *Virology* **61**:200.

Kruckelmann, H. W., and Seyffert, W., 1970, Wechselwirkung zwischen einem turnip mosaic virus und dem Genom des Wirtes, *Theor. Appl. Genet.* **40**:121.

Kuhn, C. W., and Bancroft, J. B., 1961, Concentration and specific infectivity changes of alfalfa mosaic virus during systemic infection, *Virology* **15**:281.

Lange, L., 1975, Infection of *Daucus carota* by tobacco necrosis virus, *Phytopathol. Z.* **83**:136.

Lee, C. L., and Black, L. M., 1955, Anatomical studies of *Trifolium incarnatum* infected by wound tumor virus, *Am. J. Bot.* **42**:160.

Levy, D., and Marco, S., 1976, Involvement of ethylene in epinasty of CMV-infected cucumber cotyledons which exhibit increased resistance to gaseous diffusion, *Physiol. Plant Pathol.* **9**:121.

Lockhart, B. E. L., and Semancik, J. S., 1970a, Growth inhibition peroxidase and 3-indoleacetic acid oxidase activity, and ethylene production in cowpea mosaic virus-infected cowpea seedlings, *Phytopathology* **60**:553.

Lockhart, B. E. L., and Semancik, J. S., 1970b, Respiration and nucleic acid metabolism changes in cowpea mosaic virus-infected etiolated cowpea seedlings, *Phytopathology* **60**:1852.

Loebenstein, G., and Ross, A. F., 1963, An extractable agent induced in uninfected tissues by localized virus infections, that interferes with infection by tobacco mosaic virus, *Virology* **20**:507.

Loebenstein, G., Rabina, S., and van Praagh, T., 1966, Induced interference phenomena in virus infections, in: *Viruses of Plants* (A. B. R. Beemstern and J. Dijkstra, eds.), p. 151, North-Holland, Amsterdam.

Loebenstein, G., Rabina, S., and van Praagh, T., 1968, Sensitivity of induced localized acquired resistance to actinomycin D, *Virology* **34**:264.

Loebenstein, G., Sela, B., and van Praagh, T., 1969, Increase of tobacco mosaic local lesion size and virus multiplication in hypersensitive hosts in the presence of actinomycin D, *Virology* **37**:42.

Loebenstein, G., Chazan, R., and Eisenberg, M., 1970, Partial suppression of the localizing mechanism to tobacco mosaic virus by u.v. irradiation, *Virology* **41**:373.

Loebenstein, G., Cohen, J., Shabtai, S., Coutts, R. H. A., and Wood, K. R., 1977, Distribution of cucumber mosaic virus in systemically infected tobacco leaves, *Virology* **81**:117.

MacLeod, R., Black, L. M., and Moyer, F. H., 1966, The fine structure and intracellular localization of potato yellow dwarf virus, *Virology* **29**:540.

McMullen, C. R., Gardner, W. S., and Myers, G. A., 1977, Ultrastructure of cell-wall thickenings and paramural bodies induced by barley stripe mosaic virus, *Phytopathology* **67**:462.

McMullen, C. R., Gardner, W. S., and Myers, G. A., 1978, Aberrant plastids in barley leaf tissue infected with barley stripe mosaic virus, *Phytopathology* **68**:317.

Magyarosy, A. C., Buchanan, B. B., and Schürmann, P., 1973, Effect of a systemic virus infection on chloroplast function and structure, *Virology* **55**:426.

Maramorosch, K., 1957, Reversal of virus-caused stunting in plants by Giberellic acid, *Science* **126**:651.

Marco, S., Levy, D., and Aharoni, N., 1976, Involvement of ethylene in the suppression of hypocotyl elongation in CMV-infected cucumbers, *Physiol. Plant Pathol.* **8**:1.

Martelli, G. P., and Russo, M., 1969, Nuclear changes in mesophyll cells of *Gomphrena globosa* L associated with infection by beet mosaic virus, *Virology* **38**:297.

Matthews, R. E. F., 1949, Reactions of *Cyphomandra betacea* to strains of potato virus X, *Parasitology* **39**:241.

Matthews, R. E. F., 1970, *Plant Virology*, 778 pp., Academic Press, New York.

Matthews, R. E. F., 1973, Induction of disease by viruses with special reference to turnip yellow mosaic virus, *Annu. Rev. Phytopathol.* **11**:147.

Matthews, R. E. F., and Sarkar, S., 1976, A light-induced structural change in chloroplasts of Chinese cabbage cells infected with turnip yellow mosaic virus, *J. Gen. Virol.* **33**:435.

Matthews, R. E. F., Bolton, E. T., and Thompson, H. R., 1963, Kinetics of labeling of turnip yellow mosaic virus with P^{32} and S^{35}, *Virology* **19**:179.

Melchers, G., Jockusch, H., and Sengbusch, P. V., 1966, A tobacco-mutant with a dominant allele for hypersensitivity against some TMV strains, *Phytopathol. Z.* **55**:86.

Milkus, B. N., 1975, The influence of the grapevine infectious chlorosis virus on chloroplast ultrastructure, *Acta Phytopathol. Acad. Sci. Hung.* **10**:179.

Mohamed, N. A., 1973, Some effects of systemic infection by tomato spotted wilt virus on chloroplasts of *Nicotiana tabacum* leaves, *Physiol. Plant Pathol.* **3**:509.

Moser, P. E., and Cannon, O. S., 1972, An analysis of plant breeding procedures for obtaining curly top resistance in tomato, *Phytopathology* **62**:564.

Motoyoshi, F., and Oshima, N., 1975, Infection with tobacco mosaic virus of leaf mesophyll protoplasts from susceptible and resistant lines of tomato, *J. Gen. Virol.* **29**:81.

Motoyoshi, F., and Oshima, N., 1977, Expression of genetically controlled resistance to tobacco mosaic virus infection in isolated tomato leaf mesophyll protoplasts, *J. Gen. Virol.* **34**:499.

Mozes, R., Antignus, Y., Sela, I. and Harpaz, I., 1978, The chemical nature of an antiviral factor (AVF) from virus-infected plants, *J. Gen. Virol.* **38**:241.

Mueller, W. C., and Koenig, R., 1965, Nuclear inclusions produced by bean yellow mosaic virus as indicators of cross protection, *Phytopathology* **65**:242.

Murakishi, H. H., and Carlson, P. S., 1976, Regeneration of virus-free plants from dark green islands of tobacco mosaic virus infected tobacco leaves, *Phytopathology* **66**:931.

Murant, A. F., Mayo, M. A., Harrison, B. D., and Goold, R. A., 1973, Evidence for two functional RNA species and a "satellite" RNA in tomato black ring virus, *J. Gen. Virol.* **19**:275.

Murant, A. F., Roberts, I. M., and Hutcheson, A. M., 1975, Effects of parsnip yellow fleck virus on plant cells, *J. Gen. Virol.* **26**:277.

Murdock, D. J., Nelson, P. E., and Smith, S. H., 1976, Histopathological examination of *Pelargonium* infected with tomato ringspot virus, *Phytopathology* **66**:844.

Nachman, I., Loebenstein, G., van Praagh, T., and Zelcer, A., 1971, Increased multiplication of cucumber mosaic virus in a resistant cucumber cultivar caused by actinomycin D, *Physiol. Plant Pathol.* **1**:67.

Nagaich, B. B., Upadhya, M. D., Prakash, O., and Singh, S. J., 1968, Cytoplasmically determined expression of symptoms of potato virus X crosses between species of Capsicum, *Nature (London)* **220**:1341.

Nakagaki, Y., Hirai, T., and Stahmann, M. A., 1970, Ethylene production by detached leaves infected with tobacco mosaic virus, *Virology* **40**:1.

Nyéki, J., and Vértesy, J., 1974, Effect of different ringspot viruses on the physiological and morphological properties of montmorency sour cherry pollen. II, *Acta Phytopathol. Acad. Sci. Hung.* **9**:23.

Odawara, S., Watanabe, A., and Imaseki, H., 1977, Involvement of cellular membrane in regulation of ethylene production, *Plant Cell Physiol.* **18**:569.

Otsuki, Y., Shimomura, T., and Takebe, I., 1972a, Tobacco mosaic virus multiplication and expression of the N gene in necrotic responding tobacco varieties, *Virology* **50**:45.

Otsuki, Y., Takebe, I., Honda, Y., and Matsui, C., 1972b, Ultrastructure of infection of tobacco mesophyll protoplasts by tobacco mosaic virus, *Virology* **49**:188.

Palomar, M. K., and Brakke, M. K., 1976, Concentration and infectivity of barley stripe mosaic virus in barley, *Phytopathology* **66**:1422.

Pelham, J., 1972, Strain-genotype interaction of tobacco mosaic virus in tomato, *Ann. Appl. Biol.* **71**:219.

Pennazio, S., D'Agostino, G., Appiano, A., and Redolfi, P., 1978, Ultrastructure and histochemistry of the resistant tissue surrounding lesions of tomato bushy stunt virus in *Gomphrena globosa* leaves, *Physiol. Plant Pathol.* **13**:165.

Pierpont, W. S., 1970, Formation and behavior of o-quinones in some processes of agricultural importance, *Rep. Rothamsted Exp. Sta. 1970*, p. 199.

Pleše, N., Hoxha, E., and Miličič, D., 1975, Pathological anatomy of trees affected with apple stem grooving virus, *Phytopathol. Z.* **82**:315.

Porto, M. D. M., and Hagedorn, D. J., 1974, Susceptibility of *Phaseolus lathyroides* to soybean mosaic virus, *Plant Dis. Rep.* **58**:322.

Posnette, A. F., 1947, Virus diseases of cacao in West Africa. I. Cacao viruses 1A, 1B, 1C, and 1D, *Ann. Appl. Biol.* **34**:388.

Pring, D. R., and Timian, R. G., 1969, Physiological effects of barley stripe mosaic virus infection, *Phytopathology* **59**:1381.

Reid, M. S., and Matthews, R. E. F., 1966, On the origin of the mosaic induced by turnip yellow mosaic virus, *Virology* **28**:563.

Robleda, S. C., 1973, Ultrastructure of cells infected with carnation mottle virus, *Phytopathol. Z.* **78**:134.

Rohloff, H., and Lerch, B., 1977, Soluble leaf proteins in virus infected plants and acquired resistance. I. Investigations on *Nicotiana tabacum* cvs 'Xanthi-NC' and Samsun, *Phytopathol. Z.* **89**:306.

Ross, A. F., 1961a, Localized acquired resistance to plant virus infection in hypersensitive hosts, *Virology* **14**:329.

Ross, A. F., 1961b, Systemic acquired resistance induced by localised virus infections in plants, *Virology* **14**:340.

Ross, A. F., 1966, Systemic effects of local lesion formation in viruses of plants (A. B. R. Beemster and J. Dijkstra, eds.), p. 127, North Holland, Amsterdam.

Ross, A. F., and Williamson, C. E., 1951, Physiologically active emanations from virus infected plants, *Phytopathology* **41**:431.

Russell, S. L., and Kimmins, W. C., 1971, Growth regulators and the effect of barley yellow dwarf virus on Barley (*Hordeum vulgare* L), *Ann. Bot.* **35**:1037.

Russell, T. E., and Halliwell, R. S., 1974, Response of cultured cells of systemic and local lesion tobacco hosts to microinjection with TMV,

Russo, M., and Martelli, G. P., 1972, Ultrastructural observations on tomato bushy stunt virus in plant cells, *Virology* **49**:122.

Sacristan, M. D., and Melchers, G., 1969, The caryological analysis of plants regenerated from tumorous and other callus cells of tobacco, *Mol. Gen. Genet.* **105**:317.

Schuster, G., and Flemming, M., 1976, Studies on the formation of diffusion barriers in hypersensitive hosts of tobacco mosaic virus and the role of necrotisation in the formation of diffusion barriers as well as the localization of virus infection, *Phytopathol. Z.* **87**:345.

Sela, B., Loebenstein, G., and van Praagh, T., 1969, Increase of tobacco mosaic virus multiplication and lesion size in hypersensitive hosts in the presence of chloramophenicol, *Virology* **39**:260.

Semancik, J. S., and Vanderwoude, W. J., 1976, Exocortis Viroid: Cytopathic effects at the plasma membrane in association with pathogenic RNA, *Virology* **69**:719.

Shepard, J. F., 1975, Regeneration of plants from protoplasts of potato virus X-infected tobacco leaves, *Virology* **66**:492.

Shepard, J. F., Gaard, G., and Purcifull, D. E., 1974, A study of tobacco etch virus-induced inclusions using indirect immunoferritin procedures, *Phytopathology* **64**:418.

Shifriss, C., and Cohen, S., 1971, Environmental modification of heritable resistance to potato virus Y in peppers (*Capsicum annuum*), *Plant Dis. Rep.* **55**:604.

Shikata, E., and Maramorosch, K., 1966, Electron microscopy of pea enation mosaic virus in plant cell nuclei, *Virology* **30**:439.

Shimomura, T., 1971, Necrosis and localization of infection in local lesion hosts, *Phytopathol. Z.* **70**:185.

Shimomura, T., and Dijkstra, J., 1975, The occurrence of callose during the process of local lesion formation, *Neth. J. Plant Pathol.* **81**:107.

Shukla, P., and Hiruki, C., 1975, Ultrastructural changes in leaf cells of *Chenopodium quinoa* infected with potato virus S, *Physiol. Plant Pathol.* **7**:189.

Simmonds, N. W., and Harrison, E., 1959, The genetics of reaction to pepper vein-banding virus, *Genetics* **44**:1281.

Simons, J. N., 1966, Resistance of *Capsicum annuum* "Italian El" to infection with potato virus Y, *Phytopathology* **56**:1370.

Simons, J. N., and Moss, L. M., 1963, The mechanism of resistance to potato virus Y infection in *Capsicum annuum* var Italian El, *Phytopathology* **53**:684.

Simons, T. J., and Ross, A. F., 1971, Changes in phenol metabolism associated with induced systemic resistance to tobacco mosaic virus in Samsun NN tobacco, *Phytopathology* **61**:1261.

Singh, R. P., 1977, Infectivity of potato spindle tuber viroid in potato plant parts, *Phytopathology* **67**:15.

Sjolund, R. D., and Shih, C. Y., 1970, Virus-like particles in nuclei of cultured plant cells which have lost the ability to differentiate, *Proc. Natl. Acad. Sci. USA* **66**:25.

Smith, P. G., 1970, Tobacco etch strains on peppers, *Plant Dis. Rep.* **54**:786.

Soh, A. C., Yap, T. C., and Graham, K. M., 1977, Inheritance of resistance to pepper veinal mottle virus in chilli, *Phytopathology* **67**:115.

Solberg, R. A., and Bald, J. G., 1962, Virus invasion and multiplication during leaf histogenesis, *Virology* **17**:359.

Solymosy, F., 1970, Biochemical aspects of hypersensitivity to virus infection in plants, *Acta Phytopathol. Acad. Sci. Hung.* **5**:55.

Sprague, G. F, and McKinney, H. H., 1966, Aberrant ratio; an anomaly in maize associated with virus infection, *Genetics* **54**:1287.

Sprague, G. F., and McKinney, H. H., 1971, Further evidence on the genetic behavior of AR in maize, *Genetics* **67**:533.

Sprague, G. F., and McKinney, H. H., and Greeley, L. W., 1963, Virus as a mutagenic agent in maize, *Science* **141**:1052.

Stahl, E., 1894, Einige Versuche üher Transpiration und Assimilation, *Bot. Ztg.* **52**:117.

Stein, D. B., 1962, The developmental morphology of *Nicotiana tabacum* "White Burley" as influenced by virus infection and gibberellic acid, *Am. J. Bot.* **49**:437.

Stevenson, D. W., 1973, Phyllode theory in relation to leaf ontogeny in *Sansevieria trifasciata, Am. J. Bot.* **60**:387.

Stewart, R. N., and Burk, L. G., 1970, Independence of tissues derived from apical layers in ontogeny of the tobacco leaf and ovary, *Am. J. Bot.* **57**:1010.

Stewart, R. N., and Dermen, H., 1970, Determination of number and mitotic activity of shoot apical initial cells by analysis of mericlinal chimeras, *Am. J. Bot.* **57**:816.

Stewart, R. N., and Dermen, H., 1975, Flexibility in ontogeny as shown by the contribution of shoot apical layers to leaves of periclinal chimeras, *Am. J. Bot.* **62**:935.

Stobbs, L. W., Manocha, M. S., and Dias, H. F., 1977, Histological changes associated with virus localization in TMV-infected pinto beans, *Physiol. Plant Pathol.* **11**:87.

Sugimura, Y., and Ushiyama, R., 1975, Cucumber green mottle mosaic virus infection and its bearing on cytological alterations in tobacco mesophyll protoplasts, *J. Gen. Virol.* **29**:93.

Suwa, M., and Takahashi, T., 1975, Studies on viral pathogenesis in plant hosts. VII. Symptoms and external morphology of "Samsun" tobacco plants following systemic infection with tobacco mosaic virus, *Phytopathol. Z.* **83**:348.

Takahashi, T., 1971, Studies on viral pathogenesis in host plants. I. Relation between host leaf age and the formation of systemic symptoms induced by tobacco mosaic virus, *Phytopathol. Z.* **71**:275.

Takahashi, T., 1972, Studies on viral pathogenesis on plant hosts. II. Changes in developmental morphology of tobacco plants infected systemically with tobacco mosaic virus, *Phytopathol. Z.* **74**:37.

Takahashi, W. N., 1956, Increasing the sensitivity of the local-lesion method of virus assay, *Phytopathology* **46**:654.

Taylor, G. A., Lewis, G. D., and Rubatzky, V. E., 1969, The influence of time of tobacco mosaic inoculation and stage of fruit maturity upon the incidence of tomato internal browning, *Phytopathology* **59**:732.

Thomas, P. E., and Martin, M. W., 1971, Apparent resistance to establishment of infection by curly top virus in tomato breeding lines, *Phytopathology* **61**:550.

Thomas, P. E., and Martin, M. W., 1972, Characterization of a factor of resistance in curly top virus-resistant tomatoes, *Phytopathology* **62**:954.

Tomlinson, J. A., and Webb, M. J. W., 1978, Ultrastructural changes in chloroplasts of lettuce infected with beet western yellow virus, *Physiol. Plant Pathol.* **12**:13.

Tu, J. C., 1973, Electron microscopy of soybean root nodules infected with soybean mosaic virus, *Phytopathology* **63**:1011.

Tu, J. C., 1977a, Effects of soybean mosaic virus infection on ultrastructure of bacteriodal cells in soybean root nodules, *Phytopathology* **67**:199.

Tu, J. C., 1977b, Cyclic AMP in clover and its possible role in clover yellow mosaic virus-infected tissue, *Physiol. Plant Pathol.* **10**:117.

Tu, J. C., and Hiruki, C., 1971, Electron microscopy of cell well thickening in local lesions of potato virus M infected red kidney bean, *Phytopathology* **61**:862.

Tu, J. C., Ford, R. E., and Quiniones, S. S., 1970. Effect of soybean mosaic virus and/or bean pod mottle virus infection on soybean nodulation, *Phytopathology* **60**:518.

Ushiyama, R., and Matthews, R. E. F., 1970, The significance of chloroplast abnormalities associated with infection by turnip yellow mosaic virus, *Virology* **42**:293.

Valleau, W. D., 1952, Breeding tobacco for disease resistance, *Econ. Bot.* **6**:69.

Valleau, W. D., and Johnson, E. M., 1943, An outbreak of *Plantago* virus in Burley tobacco, *Phytopathology* **33**:210.

van Loon, L. C., 1975a, Polyacrylamide disc electrophoresis of the soluble leaf proteins from *Nicotiana tabacum* var "Samsun" and "Samsun" NN. III. Influence of temperature and virus strain on changes induced by tobacco mosaic virus, *Physiol. Plant Pathol.* **6**:289.

van Loon, L. C., 1975b, Polyacrylamide disc electrophoresis of the soluble leaf proteins from *Nicotiana tabacum* var "Samsun" and "Samsun" NN. IV. Similarity of qualitative changes of specific proteins after infection with different viruses and their relationship to acquired resistance, *Virology* **67**:566.

van Loon, L. C., 1976, Systemic acquired resistance, peroxidase activity and lesion size in tobacco reacting hypersensitivity to tobacco mosaic virus, *Physiol. Plant Pathol.* **8**:231.

van Loon, L. C., 1977, Induction by 2-chloroethylphosphonic acid of viral-like lesions, associated proteins, and systemic resistance in tobacco, *Virology* **80**:417.

van Loon, L. C., and Dijkstra, J., 1976, Virus-specific expression of systemic acquired resistance in tobacco mosaic virus and tobacco necrosis virus-infected "Samsun" NN and "Samsun" tobacco, *Neth. J. Plant Pathol.* **82**:231.

van Loon, L. C., and van Kammen, A., 1970, Polyacrylamide disc electrophoresis of the soluble leaf proteins from *Nicotiana tabacum* var "Samsun" and "Samsun" NN. II. Changes in protein constitution after infection with tobacco mosaic virus, *Virology* **40**:199.

van Vloten-Doting, L., and Jaspars, E. M. J., 1977, Plant covirus systems: Three component systems, *Comp. Virol.* **11**:1.

van Zaayen, A., 1976, Immunity of strains of *Agaricus bitorquis* to mushroom virus disease, *Neth. J. Plant Pathol.* **82**:121.

Vegetti, G., Conti, G. G., and Pesci, P., 1975, Changes in phenylalamine, ammonia-lyase, peroxidase, and polyphenoloxidase during the development of local necrotic lesions in pinto bean leaves infected with alfalfa mosaic virus, *Phytopathol. Z.* **84**:153.

Verhoyen, M., 1962, Quelques Researches sur deux variantes particulières du virus de la mosaique du concombre, *Agricultura* **10**:359.

Vogt, P. K., 1977, Genetics of RNA tumor viruses, in: *Comprehensive Virology*, Vol. 9 (H. Fraenkel-Conrat and R. R. Wagner, eds.), p. 341, Plenum Press, New York and London.

Walker, J. R. L., 1975, *The Biology of Plant Phenolics: Studies in Biology No.* **54**, 57 pp., Edward Arnold, London.

Weber, P. V. V., 1951, Inheritance of a necrotic-lesion reaction to a mild strain of tobacco mosaic virus, *Phytopathology* **41**:593.

Webster, B. D., Dunlap, T. W., and Craig, M. E., 1976, Ultrastructural studies of abscission in *Phaseolus:* localization of peroxidase, *Am. J. Bot.* **63**:759.

Weintraub, M., and Ragetli, H. W. J., 1970, Electron microscopy of the bean and cowpea strains of southern bean mosaic virus within leaf cells, *J. Ultrastruc. Res.* **32**:167.

Weststeijn, E. A., 1976, Peroxidase activity in leaves of *Nicotiana tabacum* var. Xanthi NC before and after infection with tobacco mosaic virus, *Physiol. Plant Pathol.* **8**:63.

Weststeijn, E. A., 1978, Permeability changes in the hypersensitive reaction of *Nicotiana tabacum* CV Xanthi NC after infection with tobacco mosaic virus, *Physiol. Plant Pathol.* **13**:253.

Wilkins, P. W., 1974, Tolerance to ryegrass mosaic virus and its inheritance, *Ann. Appl. Biol.* **78**:187.

Wilkins, P. W., and Catherall, P. L., 1977, Variation in reaction to barley yellow dwarf virus in ryegrass and its inheritance, *Ann. Appl. Biol.* **85**:257.

Wittman, H. G., and Wittman-Liebold, B., 1966, Protein chemical studies of two RNA viruses and their mutants, *Cold Spring Harbor Symp. Quant. Biol.* **31**:163.

Wu, J. H., 1973, Wound-healing as a factor in limiting the size of lesions in *Nicotiana glutinosa* leaves infected by the very mild strain of tobacco mosaic virus (TMV-VM), *Virology* **51**:474.

Yung, K. H., and Northcote, D. H., 1975, Some enzymes present in the walls of mesophyll cells of tobacco leaves, *Biochem. J.* **151**:141.

Zeyen, R. J., and Banttari, E. E., 1972, Histology and ultrastructure of oat blue dwarf virus infected oats, *Can. J. Bot.* **50**:2511.

Ziemiecki, A., and Wood, K. R., 1975, Changes in the soluble protein constitution of cucumber cotyledons following infection with two strains of cucumber mosaic virus, *Physiol. Plant Pathol.* **7**:79.

Index

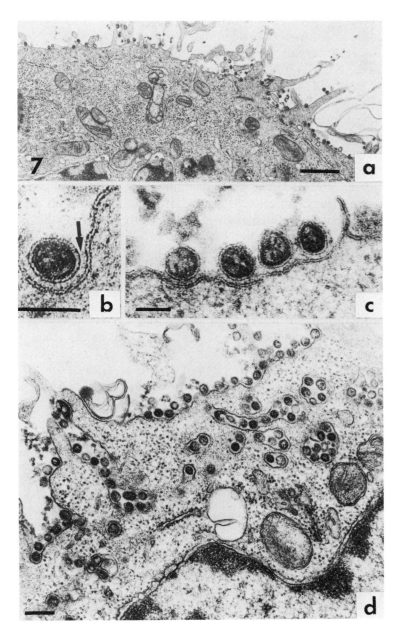

Fig. 7. Ehrlich ascites tumor cells exposed to influenza virus at MOI 200–300 at 4°C, showing (a) massive adsorption of particles and at high magnification (b,c) showing the envelope spikes interposed between virion and invaginated (?prephagocytic) segments of membrane. (d) After 10 min at 36°C, many virions, still apparently intact, are in various stages of engulfment and enclosure into cytoplasmic vacuoles. Courtesy, T. Bächi. Reprinted by permission of the publisher. Bar = 100 nm.

virus alone, or active monodisperse virus without histone. Electron microscopic analyses clearly demonstrated that aggregates of whole viral particles were internalized by phagocytosis, without evidence of interaction between virions and cell membranes other than initial attachment through envelope spikes (Dales and Pons, 1976). Moreover, virus rendered noninfectious by prior complexing with antibody, when similarly incorporated into histone aggregates with inactivated virus, regained infectivity after internalization by viropexis.

Influenza virus adsorbs rather specifically to cilia and to surfaces of respiratory epithelial cells in culture, in which viral replication occurs (Gould *et al.*, 1972). However, morphological analyses of interactions of influenza virus with ciliated epithelial cells have yielded discrepant results. In one study influenza virus appeared to attach to cilia and then to enter apparently by fusion with ciliated as well as with unciliated epithelial cells, no phagocytosis being observed (Blaskovic *et al.*, 1972). In contrast, with guinea pig tracheal epithelial cells, influenza virus was seen to adhere to cilia but not to undergo fusion with them, whereas parainfluenza type 1 (Sendai) virus in the same system penetrated by envelope-membrane fusion (Dourmashkin and Tyrrell, 1970).

The weight of evidence then points to viropexis as the mode of entry by orthomyxoviruses in which discernible fusion of viral envelope with cell membrane appears not to be involved. However, host-specific enzymatic cleavage activation of HA glycoprotein (to yield HA_2) accompanies penetration and is required for initiation of infection. Here there is a functional analogy with fusing paramyxoviruses (e.g., Sendai, NDV) in which intramembranal cleavage of F glycoprotein (to yield F_1) is prerequisite to infectivity. Accordingly, there is also striking homology between HA_2 and F_1 in N-terminal amino acid sequences, the region which in each of these molecules is apparently involved in viral penetration infection (Choppin and Scheid, 1980). Studies with electron spin resonance have indicated that there is an increase in the fluidity of the lipid bilayer of chicken erythrocytes on primary reaction of influenza virus with surface glycoprotein receptors (Lyles and Landsberger, 1976). Similar changes were not observed with human erythrocytes or with isolated plasma membranes, neither of which retain the microtubular systems found in chicken erythrocytes. A similar signal may trigger viropexis by fully susceptible cells.

5.2. Paramyxoviruses

In paramyxoviruses, hemagglutinin and neuraminidase activity both reside in one glycoprotein (HN, molecular weight 65,000). In